D1557679

COMMUNITY MEDIATION

COMMUNITY MEDIATION

A Handbook for Practitioners and Researchers

Edited by

KAREN GROVER DUFFY
State University of New York at Geneseo

JAMES W. GROSCH
Colgate University

PAUL V. OLCZAK
State University of New York at Geneseo
Family Court Psychiatric Center, Buffalo

THE GUILFORD PRESS
New York   London

© 1991 The Guilford Press
A Division of Guilford Publications, Inc.
72 Spring Street, New York, NY 10012

Printed in the United States of America

This book is printed on acid-free paper.

Last digit is print number: 9 8 7 6 5 4 3 2 1

Library of Congress Cataloging-in-Publication Data

Community mediation: a handbook for practitioners and researchers /
edited by Karen Grover Duffy, James W. Grosch, Paul V. Olczak.
     p. cm.
  Includes bibliographical references and index.
  ISBN 0-89862-561-0
  1. Social service—United States.   2. Dispute resolution (Law)—
United States.   3. Mediation—United States.   4. Neighborhood
justice centers—United States.   5. Conflict management—United
States.   I. Duffy, Karen Grover.   II. Grosch, James W.
III. Olczak, Paul V.
  [DNLM: 1. Community Psychiatry.   2. Conflict (Psychology)
3. Agonistic Behavior.   WM 30.6 C7335]
HV91.C67534   1991
306.2—dc20
DNLM/DLC
for Library of Congress   91-6640
                                                                  CIP

The cover design is an adaptation, used by permission, of the logo of The Center of Dispute Settlement, Inc.

To Paul J., who was more patient during this project than the best of mediators. And to Mom and Dad, who first taught my twin sister and me about peaceful dispute resolution.

K. G. D.

To my mother and father, with whom I experienced my first conflict in life and from whom I learned about the many constructive ways in which conflicts can be resolved.

J. W. G.

To my parents and my wife, Marie, for their many years of unconditional support, and my three *amigos*, Paul, Patrick, and Drew, who occasionally remind me of the ongoing need for alternative dispute resolution forums.

P. V. O.

And to all the peacemakers of the world.

Foreword

Living in harmony in a world full of conflict requires energies from many sources. Individuals need mechanisms to help solve everyday problems; family members need simple, practical methods to enhance communication, grow as persons, and live in harmony; and communities need resources to resolve disputes and manage conflicts. Many problems that people experience every day are labeled as "crimes," but in reality are interpersonal conflicts. In these instances, we do not have to summon the police, sue in court, or fine and incarcerate our fellow citizens. Many can be handled through communication and problem solving in mediation. The State of New York Unified Court System is answering these challenges by promoting community mediation. These are neighborhood-based nonprofit dispute resolution centers, available to every citizen across the state in all 62 counties. They serve as a resource for disputes as varied as racial conflicts in New York City, trailer court disagreements in a rural area, or intratribal disputes on Mohawk lands. The centers can be available for neighbor–neighbor conflicts such as noise problems, or for victim–offender mediation, which can involve restitution and an opportunity to express feelings and frustrations. Each center can adapt to the needs of its community and address conflicts with an emphasis on cooperation and collaboration.

With the increase in violence in our society, people are too ready to see one another as actual or potential adversaries. They need the opportunity to respect one another's perceptions and to learn from the diversity in society. Responsible citizens are coming forward in our communities to assist this process by receiving training to serve as volunteer mediators. There is a particular need to train our young people in mediation skills, in order for them to be able to solve problems and take responsibility for their own situations. Instead of dropping out and escaping reality through drugs or acting out through confrontation and violence, they can experience the success of cooperative and collaborative efforts through mediation. They grow in mind and spirit and achieve satisfaction with life through successful problem solving.

It is with this background that I am particularly happy to see the publication of *Community Mediation: A Handbook for Practitioners and Researchers*. It provides the opportunity to learn more about dispute resolution techniques and enables individuals to benefit from research in the field.

I am particularly pleased that this book was inspired by one of our New York conferences on dispute resolution. Our centers are always open to research that will improve their services. In our performance guidelines, the Unified Court System encourages the partnership between institutions of higher learning and community dispute resolution centers. One of our requirements on this relationship is to have researchers share their findings with our centers through reports, seminars at our conferences, and practical publications. This timely volume is a product of a number of people from academic disciplines and the dispute resolution trenches. It provides a balance that should satisfy a number of audiences.

If the art and science of community mediation can be cultivated and developed throughout our society, it presents the possibility that every citizen, young and old, can be exposed to peaceful methods of working with each other. It opens up avenues for the acceptance of diversity and a sharing of perceptions and experiences. On behalf of the mediation community, I thank the editors and chapter authors of *Community Mediation: A Handbook for Practitioners and Researchers* for their role in promoting resources that enhance peace and harmony throughout our communities.

Thomas F. Christian, PhD
State Director, Community Dispute
Resolution Centers Program
Unified Court System, State of New York

Preface

Nothing can bring you peace, but yourself.
—Ralph Waldo Emerson

Most people have come to think of mediation as a dialogue between two parties or sets of parties. The dialogue is facilitated by an intermediary or third party, and the goal of the dialogue is to enhance problem solving where conflict exists. If this approximates our readers' definition, then this book offers a mediation of sorts, too. Our book is intended to be the intermediary or catalyst in the furtherance of dialogue between practitioners and researchers in the field of alternative dispute resolution (ADR)—in particular, among those individuals interested in the peaceful management of conflict in our communities across the country. However, those individuals might not always agree on the best avenue for the promotion of conflict resolution.

Several years ago, all three of us were pleased to participate for the first time in New York State's Conference on Dispute Resolution, the largest conference of its kind outside of the international conference. As we attended one meeting and workshop after another, we realized that scientists and practitioners, while emotionally sympathetic to each other, were not cognitively in synchrony. When researchers (mostly academics) discussed the need for the mediation centers to obtain sophisticated computers to enhance data collection, program directors introduced the researchers to the reality that computers were far down the list of priorities. Some programs operate with part-time staffs in small, donated offices. As scientists pushed for more grant and research money, mediators pressed for money for better training and intercoms or "panic buttons" in their hearing rooms. Scientists expressed preferences for random assignment of cases to research conditions; intake workers bemoaned either the lack of cases or case overload.

Although these two groups, scientists and practitioners, cherish the same goal—the peaceful resolution of conflict—their means of studying and understanding that process often seem divergent, if not altogether at odds with each other. One simply cannot randomly assign cases to treatment conditions when sufficient cases do not exist. Although we contend that conflict can often be healthy, the divergent demands of the researchers and practitioners for the young but rapidly expanding ADR field may not always be constructive. Practitioners and scientists do have much to learn from each other, as became apparent during our conference attendance. To that end, we welcome readers—whether scientists or mediators—to our book, which we believe integrates the art and the science of community mediation.

We do not pretend that this volume supplies the definitive answers to the questions practitioners and researchers ask of each other. Rather, we see this book as fostering a useful and productive dialogue between these two groups, the two groups we feel can justly serve the ADR field in the future. Because we have learned much while assembling this book, we are sure readers will too. We certainly hope that the book is followed by similar others promoting such exchanges.

The book is divided into five parts, with chapters authored by both practitioners and researchers in each part. The first part, entitled "The Beginnings," provides background information to both practitioners and researchers on the nature of conflict, the state of the field of mediation, the process of conducting applied research, and useful methods both for assessing the need for ADR services and for promoting the services once established. From this common ground, Part II provides more detailed information about the actual process of mediation in four chapters. The first chapter delineates the stages of mediation from intake to follow-up. The other chapters examine research on each component of the process (the mediator, the parties, and their complex interactions).

In Part III of the book, readers are introduced to critical and timely issues regarding the practice of mediation. One chapter offers thoughtful commentary on resistance to mediation, while others discuss perceptions of ADR by the legal profession, credentialing and quality control, and the role of mental health professionals in mediation forums. Part IV of the book extends mediation services to other settings. The special arenas discussed include the mediation of family, school, victim–offender, consumer, and environmental disputes. Finally, in Part V, a concluding chapter summarizes findings, suggests issues for further research, and considers future directions for the field.

Welcome to *Community Mediation: A Handbook for Practitioners and Researchers*. We wish our readers joy in the reading of the book and peace in their lives.

About Our Authors

ARTHUR BEST, JD, is currently professor of law at the University of Denver College of Law. He is the author of *When Consumers Complain,* an analysis of consumer problem resolution in the United States, and of several articles on consumer law. He has served as deputy commissioner of the New York City Department of Consumer Affairs, and in the 1970s participated in research at Ralph Nader's Center for the Study of Responsive Law.

CRAIG H. BLAKELY, PhD, received his graduate training in psychology at Michigan State University. He is currently associate director of the Public Policy Resources Laboratory at Texas A&M University where his research interests include public health and the transfer and use of innovation and technology. Before being affiliated with Texas A&M, Craig was a senior policy analyst at the Stanford Research Institute.

PETER J. CARNEVALE, of the Department of Psychology and the Institute of Labor and Industrial Relations at the University of Illinois, received his PhD from the State University of New York at Buffalo. His research focuses on negotiation, mediation, and dispute resolution systems in organizations. He is also an active mediator for the Neighborhood Justice of Chicago dispute resolution center.

SUSAN CARPENTER has spent two decades designing and managing programs to resolve complex public disputes, most recently serving as the first director of the Program for Community Problem Solving in Washington, D.C. She is the coauthor of *Managing Public Disputes: A Practical Guide to Handling Conflicts and Reaching Agreements,* in addition to numerous journal articles. She holds a doctorate in future studies from the University of Massachusetts and presently is a free-lance consultant in public policy and dispute resolution in Riverside, California.

ELLEN S. COHN is an associate professor in the Department of Psychology at the University of New Hampshire. She received her BA (1974) from Clark University in psychology, and her PhD from Temple University in social psychology. She specializes in the study of legal socialization and reasoning.

DONALD E. CONLON, PhD, is an assistant professor of management in the Department of Business Administration at the University of Delaware. His research interests include third-party dispute resolution, procedural justice, and decision making. He is a member of the Academy of Management and the International Association for Conflict Management.

ALBIE M. DAVIS is director of mediation for the District Court Department of the Commonwealth of Massachusetts, Salem, Massachusetts. She has been a mediator with the Urban Community Mediators in Dorchester since 1980 and is cofounder of the National Association for Mediation in Education. She is a member of the Society for Professionals in Dispute Resolution (SPIDR) ethics committee and helped draft the current SPIDR ethics code. Previously, she directed a multicultural awareness program for the city and suburban students and teachers in the greater Boston area. She is currently writing a book on Mary Parker Follett (1868–1933), a pioneer of creative conflict resolution.

KAREN GROVER DUFFY is currently a professor of psychology at the State University of New York at Geneseo, and received her PhD from Michigan State University in personality and social psychology. Her research program includes studies on the topics of mediation, conflict, and interpersonal attraction. She has edited a book of readings on personal adjustment for Dushkin Press and assisted with the writing of a human sexuality text. She is trained as a mediator and hears primarily juvenile and family cases.

JOSEPH P. FOLGER received his PhD from the University of Wisconsin and is an associate professor in the Department of Rhetoric and Communication at Temple University. He has published in journals such as *The Harvard Negotiation Journal*, *Mediation Quarterly*, and *Communication Monographs*. He is coauthor of *Working through Conflict: A Communication Perspective*. He has also worked at the Center for Conflict Resolution, Madison, Wisconsin, and the Ann Arbor Mediation Center, Ann Arbor, Michigan.

SAMUEL G. FORLENZA is the developer and director of the Essex County Family Mediation Program, a service of the family section of the Superior Court of New Jersey, Newark, New Jersey. He has a master's degree and a professional diploma in counseling. Currently he is pursuing doctoral studies in the Department of Counseling Psychology at Seton Hall University. He is a member of the Academy of Family Mediators and the SPIDR.

JAMES W. GROSCH received his PhD from the University of New Hampshire and is currently an assistant professor of psychology at Colgate University. He has been a mediator for the past 5 years in New Hampshire and, most recently, in New York for the Center for Dispute Settlement of Livingston County. He has been actively engaged in research on mediation as well as issues related to the quality of work life.

LISA HICKS has been the program coordinator for the Wayne County office of the Center for Dispute Settlement in Lyons, New York, for the past 5 years; during this time, the program expanded from a part-time to a full-time service. Prior to this she worked for the Wayne County District Attorney's Office and was a mediator for the Center for Dispute Settlement. Having received a BS from the State University College of New York at Buffalo, she has taught special education in Buffalo.

SHARON LUNDGREN is a graduate student in social psychology at Texas A&M University. She received her undergraduate degree in psychology at Southwestern University. Her research interests are in the areas of consumer behavior, attitude change, and group behavior.

NEIL B. McGILLICUDDY is a research project director at the Research Institute on Alcoholism, Buffalo, New York. He received his PhD from the State University of New York at Buffalo in 1989. His research interests include the role of mediator power, prevention of alcohol problems among special populations, and family issues related to alcoholism. He also served as a volunteer mediator at the Dispute Settlement Center in Buffalo for 7 years.

MAE LYNN NEYHART is a graduate student in social psychology in the Department of Psychology at the University of New Hampshire. She received her BA (1985) in psychology at Moravian College. She is currently conducting research on self-presentation styles, including work on gender schemas and politeness.

KATHLEEN M. O'CONNOR is a graduate student in the Department of Psychology at the University of Illinois. She received her BS from the New York State School of Industrial and Labor Relations, Cornell University. She is currently completing a master's thesis on negotiation strategy.

PAUL V. OLCZAK is currently professor of psychology at the State University of New York at Geneseo. He received his PhD from Northern Illinois University with training in both social and clinical psychology. A licensed clinical psychologist, he has published over 30 articles on a variety of topics, including psychology and the law, interpersonal psychiatry, individual differences, and mediation. He also serves as a consulting supervising clinical psychologist to the Family Court Psychiatric Clinic in Buffalo, New York.

MELINDA OSTERMEYER has been the director of the Multi-Door Dispute Resolution Division of the Superior Court of the District of Columbia since 1989. She was previously the director of the Dispute Resolution Centers in Houston, Texas for 5 years, where she also served as staff director of the Alternative Dispute Resolution Committees of the Houston Bar Association and the state bar of Texas.

ROBERT S. PEIRCE received his BA in psychology at Hope College and his MA in social and organizational psychology at the State University of New York at Buffalo. He is currently a doctoral student at the latter institution. His research interests include mediation and other topics in conflict resolution.

DEAN G. PRUITT is a Distinguished Professor of Psychology at the State University of New York at Buffalo. He received his PhD from Yale University in 1957. He did postdoctoral work in psychology at the University of Michigan and in international relations at Northwestern University. He specializes in the psychology of social conflict and does laboratory and field research on negotiation and mediation. He is the author of *Theory and Research on the Causes of War* (with Richard C. Snyder); *Negotiation Behavior, Social Conflict: Escalation, Stalemate, and Settlement* (with Jeffrey Z. Rubin), and *The Mediation of Disputes: Empirical Studies in the Resolution of Conflict* (with Kenneth Kressel).

LINDA L. PUTNAM is a professor in the Department of Communication at Purdue University. Having received her PhD in speech and communication, she focuses in her research on communication strategies in negotiation, mediation, and organizational conflict. She was the coeditor of two special issues on dispute resolution for *Communication Research* and *Management Communication Quarterly*, and is currently editing a book, *Communication Perspectives on Negotiation*.

LARRY RAY is presently the executive director of the American Bar Association (ABA) Standing Committee on Dispute Resolution, Washington, D.C. He serves as a consultant for the Federal Departments of Justice and of Health and Human Resources on dispute resolution issues. Larry recently served as a consultant for the Ohio Governor's Commission on Peace and Conflict Management. Previously, Larry served as assistant city prosecutor in Columbus, Ohio, and directed the Night Prosecutor's Mediation Program, which was designated "an exemplary project" by the ABA and the Department of Justice. Larry received his JD from Capital University Law School and his BA from Muskingum College.

LETITIA J. ROSENTHAL received her degree in management science from the State University of New York at Geneseo, with a concentration in labor–management relations. As program coordinator for 4 years for the Center for Dispute Settlement of Livingston County, she has seen her programs in community, juvenile, and family mediation double in referrals.

LYNNE STANDISH received her BS in criminal justice from the Rochester Institute of Technology. For 6 years Lynne worked as program coordinator for the Center for Dispute Settlement in Rochester, New York. She started two county programs and was promoted to tri-county coordinator for Seneca, Yates, and Ontario Counties. She is now Expansion Coordinator for Lifeline, Inc., which is part of the Health Association of Rochester, New York.

MARILYN STERN holds a PhD in counseling from the State University of New York at Buffalo. She is currently assistant professor of counseling psychology at the State University of New York at Albany. Her research interests include the impact of stereotyping processes on the development of vulnerable children, coping with stress, and adolescent health care issues; she has conducted many seminars and workshops on these topics. She is a corecipient of a grant from the Fund for Research on Dispute Resolution to study parent–child mediation.

ELSJE H. van MUNSTER, JD, is currently the deputy executive director of the Center for Dispute Settlement, Inc. in Rochester, New York. She is vice president of the New York State Association of Community Dispute Centers and is president of the Rochester Association of Family Mediators. Her previous experience includes the practice of corporate law and some teaching at the college level.

MICHAEL VAN SLYCK holds an MA and is completing a PhD in psychology at the State University of New York at Buffalo in social conflict. Mediation-related positions include several research fellowships for the study of conflict and the directorship of research and training at the Community Dispute Resolution Centers Program for New York State. He is currently the director of the Research Institute for Dispute Resolution and principal author of a grant from the Fund for Research on Dispute Resolution.

GARY L. WELTON is an assistant professor of psychology at Tabor College, Hillsboro, Kansas. He holds a PhD (State University of New York at Buffalo) in social and organizational psychology. His research interests include mediation, social dilemmas, statistics and measurement, and religiosity. His articles have appeared in the *Journal of Conflict Resolution, Journal of Personality and Social Psychology,* and *Personality and Social Psychology Bulletin*.

STEPHEN WOOLPERT received his PhD from Stanford University and currently teaches in the Department of Government at St. Mary's College, Moraga, California. He has published several articles on criminal justice reform. As a member of his county's Juvenile Justice and Delinquency Prevention Commission, he helped establish a victim–offender reconciliation program in his community. He is an associate editor of the *Journal of Humanistic Psychology* and is currently editing an anthology of readings in political psychology.

FRANK Y. WONG, PhD, is assistant professor of psychology at Hofstra University. He received his doctorate from Texas A&M University and held an assistantship in the Public Policy Resources Laboratory. His research and teaching interests include public health, intergroup relations, sex roles, and research methods.

STEPHEN WORCHEL, PhD, is professor and department head of psychology at Texas A&M University. He received his PhD from Duke University and taught at the Universities of North Carolina and of Virginia before going to Texas. His research has recently focused on how groups develop and establish their identity. He is presently doing research in the People's Republic of China, Poland, and Israel on the influence of culture on responses to conflict, especially political conflict. He has authored many journal articles and books in social psychology.

STACIE L. WORSHAM holds a BS but is currently a graduate student enrolled in management classes at Texas A&M University. She holds an assistantship in the Public Policy Resources Laboratory and plans to obtain a master's degree in business administration.

JO M. ZUBEK received her BA in psychology from the State University of New York at Buffalo. She is a doctoral student in the university's social and organizational psychology program. Her research interests include mediation, intergroup conflict, the dual-career lifestyle, and work–family interrole conflict. She also has a background in social gerontology.

Contents

12. The Legal System Discovers New Tools: 185
Dispute Resolution Techniques
LARRY RAY

13. How to Ensure High-Quality Mediation   203
Services: The Issue of Credentialing
ALBIE M. DAVIS

14. Mediation and Psychotherapy: Parallel Processes   227
SAMUEL G. FORLENZA

COMMUNITY MEDIATION

PART I

THE BEGINNINGS

"The beginnings": What do we mean by that? This first part of the book is held together by our desire to ensure that all readers speak the same language—that is, that all readers commence this book with the same common information before proceeding to the other parts of the book. It should be recalled in reading this unit that we are serving two audiences: practitioners, including mediators, arbitrators, legal professionals, and program directors; and also researchers or scientists. We are, after all, attempting to stimulate dialogue between these two diverse although not always mutually exclusive groups.

We begin our book with a stimulating chapter on conflict by Stephen Worchel and Sharon Lundgren. Worchel and Lundgren look at what conflict is, how it escalates, and how it is often managed or mismanaged. In so doing, they remind us that conflict is both intrapersonal and interpersonal, as well as regressive and progressive. Their engaging writing style, replete with examples, illustrates many important points about conflict.

The second chapter, by Karen Duffy, contains historical and other background information for both sets of readers—practitioners and researchers. After highlighting the history of mediation, the chapter delineates how mediation centers typically function (who mediates, the demography of the parties, etc.) and debates the merits of the centers today.

Frank Wong and his colleagues introduce research strategies in applied settings in the next chapter. While researchers, of course, need to worry about problems of design, control, and analysis, practitioners will also want to understand this chapter, since they too are often asked to present and interpret data to funders, public policy makers, and others. The chapter is written at a level that will not insult the experienced researcher, yet is accessible and understandable to practitioners so that they will feel comfortable with and be able to utilize the information.

Using needs assessment, a common research technique, Joseph Folger shows us in Chapter 4 how he and his colleagues conducted an actual assessment of the need for a mediation center in a real community. As more centers become established, and as existing centers expand their services and markets, the ability to conduct such an assessment becomes more and more valuable. We offer here a template for others to follow.

1

Finally, three highly experienced program coordinators, Lisa Hicks, Letitia Rosenthal, and Lynne Standish, share in Chapter 5 how they have marketed their now well-established programs. Although insiders are convinced that mediation works, outsiders remain not only unconvinced but even unaware and sometimes skeptical about mediation. Proactive marketing is therefore essential. These last two chapters will be especially useful for program directors, but, because they challenge some of the myths and misconceptions about mediation, these chapters will also be relevant to researchers.

1

The Nature of Conflict and Conflict Resolution

STEPHEN WORCHEL and SHARON LUNDGREN
Texas A&M University

No one paid much attention to Floyd Hatfield on that day in 1873 when he drove a sow and her piglets into his pigsty near his home in Stringtown, Kentucky. It was not until a day or two later, when Randolph McCoy happened by the Hatfields' farm, that those pigs received any notice at all. For the past few years, Randolph and his brother-in-law Floyd had had a series of minor disagreements, but this was the last straw. When Randolph spotted the pigs, he immediately accused Floyd of stealing them. The argument between the two men heated up, and a crowd quickly gathered. Nothing Floyd could say would convince Randolph that those were not his pigs. The dispute finally ended up in the court of Preacher Anse Hatfield. Witness after witness paraded up to testify about the ownership of the pigs. To the surprise of few, those whose last name was Hatfield swore the pigs belonged to Floyd, while the McCoys swore with equal conviction that "those were Randolph's pigs." Possession being nine-tenths of the law, and with testimony equally divided, Floyd Hatfield retained possession of the pigs.

> There have been bigger trials, bigger courts, bigger crimes, but rarely a verdict so ponderous. In this outcome, the die was cast. Years would pass before the hatred thus engendered would fade; generations would follow in which the family names of Hatfield and McCoy could never be mentioned without thought of feuds. (Jones, 1948, p. 21)

The feud lasted 55 years with over 100 people killed. The states of Kentucky and West Virginia were drawn into the conflict as each tried to protect the rights of its native clan (the McCoys of Kentucky and the Hatfields of West Virginia). As the feud raged on, few participants remembered or cared about the events that started it; the pigs had long since gone to bacon. But the anger and hatred persisted and grew.

While the accounts of the Hatfield–McCoy feud make for fascinating

3

reading, they also provide a clear lesson on the topic of conflict. The story is so filled with examples of conflict that it is difficult to know where to begin, so we take the safe route and begin with a definition.

DEFINING CONFLICT: A ROAD WITH MANY FORKS

We all know what conflict is. We deal with it in our work, in our play, and in our relationships. Defining it should therefore be rather easy. But as the Zen proverb warns us, "it is the straight road that often has the most curves." So, too, do we find the task of defining conflict to be a formidable task. In order to understand the difficulty, let us consider the account of the Hatfield–McCoy feud.

Randolph had suspected Floyd of dirty dealing for some time. He had struggled with trying to decide whether to confront Floyd or not. Here, then, we have our first example of conflict. "Intrapersonal conflict" is "a state that obtains for an individual when he is motivated to make two or more mutually incompatible responses" (Jones & Gerard, 1967, p. 709). Examples of intrapersonal conflict are almost endless. In fact, this conflict arises every time we are faced with making a decision.

There is a wonderfully rich literature on the processes that are set into motion each time we face the ordeal of having to make a decision. Leon Festinger (1957) suggested that we are motivated to maintain consistency between our attitudes and behaviors. When a discrepancy (or "dissonance") occurs, we begin the mental work necessary to restore consistency ("consonance"). The greater the degree of cognitive dissonance we experience, the greater will be our efforts to restore consonance. Festinger argued that each time we make a decision between alternatives, we will experience dissonance. At the root of the dissonance is our desire to perceive the decision as a good decision. The positive aspects of the chosen alternative and the negative characteristics of the rejected alternative support the image of the good decision. However, the negative features of the chosen alternative and the positive features of the rejected alternative question the correctness of the decision. Herein lies the cast of characters that determine the degree of conflict associated with a decision: The more nearly equal the supporting and detracting features of the decision, the greater the conflict involved in the decision.

Festinger (1957) took this view of intrapersonal conflict one step further when he hypothesized about the consequences of making a decision. In order to reduce the conflict (dissonance) associated with a decision, we are motivated to enhance the value of the chosen alternative and to depreciate the rejected alternative *after* the decision. Therefore, following a decision, we will focus our attention on the features that support the chosen alternative and ignore those that cast doubt on it. For example, an individual may be in a quandary about whether to submit a dispute to a mediator or take it to court. Dissonance theory argues that *after* the individual decides to go through mediation, he or she will focus on the positive aspects of mediation and the negative features of a court trial. This mental work reduces the dissonance and increases the individual's conviction that he or she has made the right choice. There is extensive literature supporting the dissonance theory analysis of the decision-making process (Brehm & Cohen, 1962; Wicklund & Brehm, 1976). Our interest here, however, is not in wandering through the archives of dissonance theory. Rather, we wish to illustrate the pervasiveness of intrapersonal conflict before dealing with the major focus of this chapter: conflict between people.

The incident that led to the Hatfield–McCoy feud began as a case of interpersonal conflict and escalated into intergroup conflict. A generic definition of "interpersonal conflict" is as follows: "tension between two or more social entities (individuals, groups, or larger organizations) which arises from incompatibility of actual or desired responses" (Raven & Kruglanski, 1970, p. 70). Bringing this definition to life, we can see the existence of conflict between Floyd Hatfield and Randolph McCoy because both of them wanted the same sow. Although this definition seems straightforward enough, it fails to draw an important distinction between types of interpersonal conflict.

Going back to Floyd and Randolph, we find an example of true "competition" or "zero-sum conflict," to use the language of game theorists (Rapoport, 1974). Both men wanted the same pig, and unless King Solomon were to step in, one man would come away a winner with the pig and the other would be the loser. The gain of one is exactly the loss of the other; hence the term "zero-sum conflict." Board games such as chess and checkers also represent zero-sum conflicts. Ex-spouses dividing up their possessions as part of a divorce settlement may also view their situation as a zero-sum conflict.

While these are examples of true competition, most types of interpersonal conflict are not zero-sum. In fact, most conflicts fall under the heading of "non-zero-sum conflict" or "mixed-motive conflict." As the name implies, these conflicts have a range of solutions beyond the win–lose alternative. The adversary in these conflicts is not only the other party, but also our own motives. In the mixed-motive conflict we have parties faced with alternatives of trying to maximize their own gain versus working for the best collective solution. As readers can imagine, those nasty human frailties of distrust, greed, and fear rear their ugly heads as the parties wrestle with the conflict. In order to bring the mixed-motive conflict to life, let us consider two classic examples.

The first example is affectionately called the "Prisoner's Dilemma." The prototype situation involves a district attorney who is trying to get a conviction of murder in the first degree for two defendants. (To simplify the pronouns, let us assume that the attorney is female and the defendants are male.) The attorney knows that she does not have sufficient evidence to get the first-degree murder convictions without confessions from either or both of the defendants. She knows, however, that she can get a manslaughter conviction for both defendants with no confession. But she wants the murder conviction, so she sets up a diabolical conflict for the defendants. She first isolates the two in separate cells and approaches each man with a set of alternatives (see Figure 1.1). She tells each defendant that if neither he nor his partner confess, she will get the manslaughter conviction and each will serve 4 years. However, if the defendant confesses and turns state's evidence, and the partner does not confess, she will free the confessor and get the maximum sentence for the partner (99 years). If both men confess, she will get murder convictions for both, but with a reduced sentence (20 years). Here, then, is the conflict for each man! The best *joint* payoff occurs if neither confesses and both receive a light sentence. On the other hand, each man can see that his best *individual* option results if he confesses and his partner does not. At the same time, each man can see that if the partner confesses and he does not, he will spend his life in jail while the double-crossing partner goes free. Clearly, this conflict is a stew of mixed motives—trust and greed.

A bit closer to home for most of us is the "social dilemma," which also places desire for individual short-term gain against the good of the collective (Hardin, 1968; Samuelson & Messick, 1986). For example, one of us (Stephen Worchel), as the father of new twins, believed that plastic disposable diapers were a gift from heaven. But just as he was about to give thanks

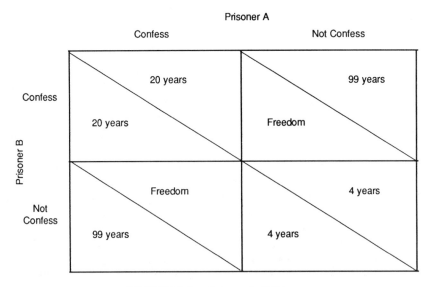

FIGURE 1.1.   Prisoner's Dilemma

for this wonderful invention, environmentalists captured the media and painted the horrifying picture of the billions of plastic diapers clogging our landfills. If everyone continued using these plastic diapers, the end result would be certain disaster for the environment. Worchel's personal convenience and best option for coping with his twins was suddenly in conflict with the fate of his fellow inhabitants of the world. After a bit of thought, he arrived at a tremendous solution: If all other suffering parents paid heed to the environment and ceased using plastic diapers, he could continue using them. Certainly the world's landfills could absorb the 20 diapers a day he was using! But then the social psychologist side of Worchel's mind took over, and the flaw in his reasoning became clear. If all of us who are parents adopt this line of thinking, we will all survive our children's infancy, only to be killed along with everyone else by mountains of plastic rising like the phoenix out of our landfills in the future.

Before leaving our examination of the types of conflict, let us consider one other distinction. Parties to a conflict have a knack for quickly sifting through points of agreement to concentrate on their disagreements. Conflict in these cases often centers on the concrete (who gets the sow, in the initial Hatfield–McCoy confrontation), the *means*. This focus freezes the conflict in a zero-sum confrontation; it overlooks the possibilities that the parties may be in agreement about overall goals, the *ends*. If this agreement about ends were to be used as a starting point, the conflict might be transformed from a zero-sum confrontation into an affair of mutual problem solving. Let us illustrate this point with an example that is all too common to many of us: a couple arguing over child custody as part of a divorce settlement. Both parties begin by taking the position that they want full custody of the child and that the other parent's visitation should be kept to a minimum so as not to upset the child. The conflict swirls around the issue of custody, and compromise appears to be the only solution. The compromise may involve letting each parent have the child half of the time. This compromise will involve the maximum disruption for everyone because the child is constantly shifted back and forth. But this compromise is the middle ground, and this "solution" is often adopted in custody cases.

However, let us now take a step back. Custody of the child may be the means to achieve a number of ends. One goal of the conflict may be to hurt the other party as much as possible. If this is the desired result, we are faced with zero-sum conflicts of both means and ends, and compromise or a third-party ruling may be the only solution. However, to take the more benevolent approach, both parties may be genuinely concerned about the child's welfare, and the conflicting custody proposals represent each party's perception of how best to ensure that welfare. In this case, rather than allowing the couple to become locked on the child custody issue, the mediator may stress the mutual concern about child welfare, and the feuding couple may be presented with the task of considering all aspects of the child's welfare. The question becomes this: "How can we best ensure the child's welfare?" Finding the best solution to this question will involve such issues as neighborhood, schools, finances, friends, and safety, as well as custody. The point of concern here is not to give a lesson on settling child custody issues, but to illustrate that conflicts may involve means and/or ends. It is important to examine the genre of the conflict because of the implications for conflict resolution.

In the tradition of science, we have managed to give a long answer to a short question: What is conflict? We want, however, to stress two important points raised in this discussion. First, conflict occurs in many types and at all levels of human behavior (intrapersonal, interpersonal, and intergroup). Second, in any situation, conflict may be occurring at all levels simultaneously; we have, then, a play within a play. This is an important point to remember, because the tendency of third parties is often to deal with conflict at only one level. Confusion, resistance, and failure may result from not considering the Hydra-like personality of conflict.

THE COURSE OF CONFLICT: JUST A LITTLE
SHOVE GOES A LONG WAY

We now move from defining conflict to developing a better understanding of how conflict develops. One of the most striking aspects of the Hatfield–McCoy feud was its escalation from a disagreement over a sow to a half-century gun battle involving hundreds of people. Although its intensity is unusual, the path that the conflict followed is not. Worchel, Cooper, and Goethals (1988) have compared the path of conflict to a snowball rolling downhill: Both increase in size and intensity. We become entrapped in escalating conflict even when there are rational solutions (Brockner & Rubin, 1985). An illustrative example of this phenomenon is found in the auction experiment (Teger, 1980). In this study, a group of subjects were given the opportunity of bidding for a dollar bill. As in most auctions, the winning bidder would get the dollar. But this differed from most auctions in this respect: Subjects were informed that the next highest bidder must pay the amount he or she bid, and receive nothing in return. After learning the rules of the game, subjects were allowed to choose whether or not they wanted to take part. The bidding began and as the amount approached $1, many of the bidders dropped out. Soon only two bidders remained locked in the conflict, both unwilling to drop out and lose money. In some cases the bidding for the dollar exceeded $20! As the bidding increased, all friendliness and joking ceased. The remaining two subjects grew less concerned about the money and more intent on beating the other person. In the end, both were losers, even the subject who "won" the dollar bill. What is most striking about this demonstration is how the two parties became captured by the conflict, like moths drawn to a light. Even when they saw that their behavior was self-defeating, they could not break off the confrontation. In the normal course of conflict, there are many such factors that entrap people and lead to a spiraling of conflict.

Saving Face

How could a sow be worth 50 years of fighting, over 100 deaths, and the confrontation of the governments of two states? The answer is that the Hatfield–McCoy conflict, like so many others, quickly turned from the issue at hand to the self-esteem of the two parties. The pig was soon forgotten as the parties fought to demonstrate their power and save face. Neither party was willing to suggest compromise or withdraw from the conflict, because to do so would suggest weakness. Not only are signs of weakness a blow to our self-esteem, but embarrassment and distress are associated with the possibility that others may witness our weakness. Along these lines, there is often the concern that others will take advantage of us if they perceive us as weak or too easily yielding. In fact, studies have shown that people are more likely to remain in a self-defeating conflict and to take an unreasonably extreme stand if they feel that others are observing their behaviors or will learn of the outcome of the confrontation (Brown, 1968). Thus, one factor that prolongs and escalates conflict is the concern with saving face.

Threat and Counterthreat

Whether we look at interpersonal, intergroup, or international conflicts, one of the most common and early responses we find is threat. A person watching children at play will not have to wait long before hearing something like this: "You give me the ball or I'll clobber you." Now it is one thing to compromise in the face of a disagreement. In doing so, one can take the position of a reasonable, rational person. However, it is quite another thing to yield in the face of a threat from the other party. To do so is a sure sign of weakness. Therefore, threat leads to counterthreat, which quickly escalates the conflict from one involving a mere disagreement to a question of who is stronger. Thus, instead of settling conflict, threat expands its scope and intensity (Deutsch & Krauss, 1960).

If threats are so counterproductive, why are they so often resorted to? One answer is that they are easy to use and present the opportunity for a swift solution to conflict. In fact, people (groups, nations) feel that conflict will be effective in getting the other party to yield. But this perception is clearly one-sided. In an interesting demonstration of this egocentric bias, subjects in a study (Rothbart & Hallmark, 1988) were asked to play the role of defense minister in a conflict where two nations were developing offensive weapons. When asked to choose a tactic that would most likely get the other nation to settle the conflict, the defense ministers chose to threaten the use of weapons. However, when asked which tactic would most likely lead their own nation to resolve the conflict, the defense ministers suggested that the other nation should make a conciliatory gesture by *reducing* its offensive capability. We see others as responding to threat, while we see ourselves as responding to a reduction of threat! This perception seems to have guided the U.S. approach to world affairs from the beginning of the Cold War until the present day.

Mediators are often faced with parties locked in a cycle of threat and counterthreat. This is a disastrous script and will prolong and escalate the conflict. Even if a solution is reached, negative feelings between the parties will remain.

The Diabolical-Enemy Image

Our perceptions conspire in another way to increase conflict. The effect is most clearly seen in interpersonal relations, but it is also present in international relations. Just before Christmas 1989, 24,000 U.S. troops stormed Panama with the intent of destroying the Noriega regime. In explaining his decision to send troops into Panama, President Bush painted a picture of Noriega as a crazed drug-dealing man who was planning to attack U.S. citizens. Sending troops to Panama was a defensive action to protect U.S. citizens. Weeks before this action, Noriega stated that the United States was planning an offensive attack on Panama, and he justified confrontations with U.S. personnel as defensive maneuvers. History is filled with wars between nations taking "defensive" actions. Indeed, conflict leads us to perceive our opponent as evil and aggressive, while we see ourselves as simply responding to the aggressive actions of the opponent (Sande, Goethals, Ferrari, & Worth, 1989). Conflict escalates as both sides adopt these mirror-image perceptions, seeing the opponent as diabolical and the self as defending against evil.

Another interesting twist in our perceptions also contributes to accelerate conflict. Let us consider two men locked in a confrontation. Most likely, both combatants hurled some thinly veiled threats at each other. Now how does each party perceive the confrontation? One party may suggest that the other one acted because he was aggressive and unreasonable. In other words, the opponent's actions were driven by stable dispositions or traits ("He acted aggressively because he was aggressive"). The same party's explanation for his own actions, however, probably takes a different tone. He, of course, acted aggressively because the situation demanded him to do so. In other words, his actions were a response to environmental demands, not his own traits. There is considerable evidence suggesting that observers tend to see others' actions as motivated by internal and stable dispositions, whereas they perceive their own actions as being responses to situational demands (Jones & Nisbett, 1972). (For a further discussion of this effect, see Cohn & Neyhart, Chapter 11, this volume.)

One reason for this bias is that we have knowledge of our own history, but we lack knowledge about the past action of others. We know that we do not always act aggressively, but we do not know this about our opponent in conflict. A second reason for this bias involves the focus of attention. When we observe the behavior of others, our attention is focused on them. Hence, our explanations for these behaviors include the person. However, when we act, our attention is focused on the situation, not on ourselves. Therefore, our explanation for our behavior includes situational factors. Regardless of the reason for this bias, once we explain others' difficult or aggressive behavior as resulting from a stable disposition, we leave little hope that their actions will change during the course of conflict no matter what we do. Therefore, the best alternative is to beat them into submission.

The Influence of Group Membership

In the dispute that touched off the Hatfield–McCoy feud, one man was a member of the Hatfield family and the other a member of the McCoy family. We might think that this obvious point could hardly be a basis for conflict, yet there is strong evidence that the seeds of conflict may be sown as soon as people are placed into groups. Even more unsettling is the fact that this conflict will occur even when people are randomly assigned to groups, and members of the group have no interaction!

Although this sounds crazy, Henri Tajfel and his colleagues (Tajfel, 1970; Tajfel & Turner, 1986) have argued that we derive an important part of our identity from the groups to which we belong: our social identity. In order to demonstrate this point, one may simply ask a friend to answer the question "Who am I?" Chances are that he or she will include in the self-description information about family, school, church, social clubs, and work group; the person's identity will be closely intertwined with his or her groups. Moreover, most of us want to have a positive image. This desire motivates two behaviors. First, we attempt to join the most attractive groups possible, because being a member of these groups enhances our social identity. Second—and here is the heart of the conflict—we attempt to increase the image of our own groups and to depreciate that of outgroups to which we do not belong. We discriminate against these outgroups in an effort to make our groups seem better. Tajfel demonstrated this behavior when he randomly placed subjects into two groups. The members never interacted with people in their own group or with those of the outgroup. Tajfel then took an individual member and asked him or her to divide money between the two groups. The money could be divided in one of two ways. One involved giving both groups a large and nearly equal amount of money; the other alternative involved giving the person's own groups a moderate amount of money and the outgroup a small amount. The first alternative benefited the ingroup, but it created only a small difference between the two groups. The second alternative gave the ingroup less money, but it created a greater difference between ingroup and outgroup. The majority of subjects chose the second alternative: They gave their own group less in order to hurt the outgroup and create clear differences. It must be remembered that these subjects were randomly assigned to groups and never talked with anyone in their group or the other group.

This suggests that conflict may be inherent in creating groups. But there is more to the story. A number of studies have found that we tend to view our own groups as composed of a variety of different people (Jones, Wood, & Quattrone, 1981; Linville, 1982). However, we see outgroups as being composed of people who are very similar: "They are all alike." This perception reduces our desire to have contact with many members of the outgroup, because we reason, "Met one, know them all." Thus, grouping people sets the stage for conflict, and our perceptual biases ensure that the conflict will have longevity.

Our aim in this discussion is not to ignore the many cases where conflict develops over real issues or competition for scarce goods. The point, however, is that there are many other factors that conspire to ignite and fan the embers of mild conflict into an ever-expanding heated confrontation. Such factors include threat, biased perceptions, and group membership.

TRUST AND DISTRUST: ENGINEERS OF CONFLICT

"The perceptions of the other group (or individual) as untrustworthy are probably a major source of tensions leading to conflict. The history of labor/management strife, interracial violence, war, and revolution demonstrates the significance of distrust" (Webb & Worchel, 1986, p. 213). We might add feuds to this list of examples of the role of distrust. The lack of trust sets the stage for conflict, and conflict increases the distrust between parties.

"Trust" is the expectancy that the word, promise, or written statement of another can be relied on (Rotter, 1971). There is a significant amount of research suggesting that we develop the tendency to trust or distrust others during infancy and early childhood (Ainsworth, 1979). Several scales have been devised to measure individual differences in people's tendency to trust others (Wrightsman, 1964). An intriguing difference between trust and distrust is that the former develops slowly after repeated interactions and demonstrations of trustworthiness. Distrust, on the other hand, may result from only one betrayal, and once aroused, distrust is very difficult to change. Indeed, we have seen lifelong friendships crumble over one incident of betrayal. If the relationship is not completely destroyed after the event, it is changed forever. Distrust leads us to look for the worst in the other person and to suspect the motives behind even the most benevolent actions.

Despite this gloomy picture of distrust, it need not always be a terminal state. There is evidence that the tide can be reversed if the wrongdoer confesses the betrayal and demonstrates that he or she is remorseful. If the wrongdoer has benefited from the betrayal, he or she must make restitution, if possible. Then the wrongdoer must be given the opportunity to demonstrate trustworthiness in an environment where betrayal is again possible. Too often the wronged individual insists on having complete surveillance of the transgressor. Under such conditions, the transgressor can never "prove" worthiness; his or her positive behavior can easily be attributed to the lack of opportunity "to go bad." Without the restoration of trust, however, conflict is exceedingly difficult to resolve. In an atmosphere of distrust, even the slightest event, such as the presence of a strange sow in the pigsty, can ignite conflict.

REVERSING THE TIDE: CONFLICT RESOLUTION

As we have seen, there seems to be a natural tendency for conflict to grow and increase. Even when the parties are separated, absence rarely reduces the conflict; rather, it puts it in cold storage, waiting to intrude upon the parties if they should meet in the future. There has, however, been a great deal of work identifying steps that can be taken to reduce conflict. We can only review some of these steps briefly here. In fact, the mediation process is aimed at reducing conflict. Many of the chapters in this volume identify specific approaches used in mediation that are successful in reducing conflict. We attempt to set the stage for these chapters by examining general theoretical positions on conflict resolution.

An important point to keep in mind, whether a reader's interest is in general theory or in application of the theory in dispute resolution, is that the desired goal is not merely to resolve conflict. Instead, the emphasis must be on finding the fairest possible resolution that leaves neither party feeling that the other has received an unfair advantage. Resolutions that are inequitable set the stage for future conflict that is often of greater intensity than the confrontation at hand. The Hatfield–McCoy feud is a sterling example of this caution: The McCoys felt that they had not received a fair hearing in Anse Hatfield's court, and they vowed to "set things straight."

Contact

Conflict acts like a centrifuge separating the parties and reducing or eliminating the interaction between them. "I don't want to talk to you" may be the first words that reach the lips of many people in conflict. This effect, known as "autistic hostility," generally works against resolving differences. Although separation may cool the fires of anger, it also cements biased perceptions and ensures that there will be no problem-solving efforts. Contact between the feuding parties is a first step to resolution; however, not just any contact will do the trick. There are numerous examples of cases where conflict reignites anger and antagonism. Numerous studies have found that the most effective contact is one that brings the parties together on an *equal basis* (Amir, 1969; Cook, 1985) to *work toward a common goal* (Sherif, Harvey, White, Hood, & Sherif, 1961; Worchel, Andreoli, & Folger, 1977). The "equal-basis" requirement means that the parties have equal power in the interaction to influence decisions. A lopsided power differential may result in increasing conflict because one party feels pressured into accepting an unfair decision. Working toward a common goal encourages the parties to focus on their common interests rather than their differences. Their energy is directed toward solving a problem rather than against each other.

Because the natural tendency in conflict is to reduce interaction, getting the parties together is no small task. Although courts may force the parties to interact, contact under mandate is not most beneficial to finding a satisfactory resolution to differences. Indeed, one of the most valuable roles of a mediator may be to help the parties see that contact is to their mutual benefit. Getting the factions to believe that they have chosen to meet together to find a solution to their differences is a giant step toward conflict resolution. In fact, we might predict that dispute mediation is most likely to have a successful conclusion when the parties have volunteered for mediation rather than being assigned by the court. The choice to participate in mediation not only increases the parties' commitment to the final solution, but may signal the openness to contact of each party.

Reducing Threat

If the first reaction to conflict is not to withdraw, it is likely to be to attack: "You'd better do this, or else." The "or else" may involve anything from veiled threats ("You'll be sorry") to specific references to heinous acts of violence ("I'll cut your ears off and feed them to the dogs"). As we have pointed out, there is a strong belief that amassing power and might is the best way to win in conflict. However, we have also shown that most often threat leads to counterthreat and an escalation in conflict. Even if one party uses sheer might to "win" a conflict, it is unlikely that the resolution will be perceived as fair. There is evidence that the opposite strategy, reducing threat, often opens up opportunities for reducing conflict.

Osgood (1962) offered a plan called "graduated reciprocation in tension reduction" (abbreviated as GRIT) as a way of reducing conflict. His major concern was with conflict between the superpowers in the Cold War. As a first step in the GRIT plan, one party makes an open announcement that it intends to reduce tension, and that party takes the unilateral step of reducing some of its threat potential. The party invites, but does not demand, the other party to make a reciprocal move. The initiating party carries out the threat reduction in open view and announces new steps that it will take toward threat reduction. The steps are graduated so that while vulnerability is increased, the party is not totally powerless. The first announcement of threat reduction will be met with doubt and distrust on the part of the opponent. However, the repeated steps should begin to overcome this distrust.

Osgood's GRIT was only a suggestion in 1962. However, we might wonder whether Mikhail Gorbachev was familiar with this literature when he seized the initiative in 1987 and seemed to follow a similar plan. He began by taking small but significant steps to reduce troop strength in Eastern Europe and dismantle some weapons. His actions were unilateral, but he proposed bilateral steps that could be taken. He offered a new openness and skillfully used the news media to announce his actions. After a period of some confusion and wonder, the United States joined in. By 1989, the race was on to see who could reduce arms and troop levels more quickly and who could make the more dramatic tension-reducing proposals.

Individuals do not have the opportunity to reduce troops or eliminate weapons in their conflicts. Yet they can moderate their demands, change the tone of their rhetoric, and offer concessions; by doing this, they reduce the atmosphere of threat and tension. A mediator may make use of this process by helping each party reduce the level of threat *and* by ensuring that each party is aware of the other's actions to reduce threat.

Depersonalizing Conflict through Norms

One of the impediments to resolving conflict is often the concern with saving face. Neither party wants to appear weak or to seem to be giving in. Concern with self-image will be strong as long as the conflict is personalized and the focus is on the parties themselves. It is, however, possible to reduce conflict by focusing on norms. "Norms" are impersonal rules that dictate how people should respond in a given situation. In most cases, there is general agreement on the content of norms, and people are aware of the norms. For example, three norms can be applied to conflicts involving the division of resources. One is the norm of need, which states that resources should be divided according to the need of the parties. A second norm is equality, which dictates that resources should be divided equally between the parties. And a third norm is equity, which dictates that resources should be distributed according to input. That is, the person who has worked the hardest or contributed the most should receive the largest share of the outcome.

Any of these norms can be used as a guide to resolving conflict. Obviously, there may be disagreement between the parties about which norm should be applied and how much each party has contributed to the relationship or effort. In fact, Deutsch (1973) suggests that equity norms will be preferred by persons concerned with increasing productivity, whereas equality norms will be favored by people most concerned with interpersonal relationships. However, it is important to recognize that these disagreements concern the norms rather than personal characteristics of the parties. It is unlikely that people will feel that their self-image or self-esteem is at stake when the discussion focuses on the merits of norms.

Negotiation

A common means for resolving conflict is negotiation, which often involves a face-to-face meeting between the parties at which each party makes concessions until an agreement is reached. Most of the research on negotiation focuses on identifying effective negotiation strategies. For example, if a party's interest is in achieving the best personal outcome, research suggests that the party should adopt a relatively extreme position and make only small concessions during negotiation (Chertkoff & Conley, 1967). Furthermore, these concessions should be made only when the other party also makes concessions. In other words, the first party should adopt a "tit-for-tat" strategy (Axelrod, 1980). Success may be enhanced if one party can convince the other that he or she is in no hurry to conclude the negotiations (Worchel, Cooper, & Goethals, 1991).

There are numerous strategies that one can adopt to "win" a negotiation. However, caution must be exercised. If the opponent feels that he or she will not achieve a fair solution, the best strategy is breaking off the negotiation. Therefore, too extreme an initial position or too small a concession may result in terminating the negotiation. A second concern is that one party will often be in situations where he or she will have repeated encounters and conflicts with the other. A lopsided "win" in one negotiation may ensure that the other party will not negotiate in the future. In fact, one of the most difficult steps in the negotiation process is getting the parties to agree to meet and work for a solution to their conflict.

A familiarity with the literature on the negotiation process can serve a mediator in many ways. First, the mediator may be able to reduce the likelihood that the parties will break off negotiation because one party has started with an unreasonably extreme position. Second, this knowledge may help the mediator ensure that one party does not gain an unfair advantage over the other.

Mediation and Arbitration

Given that the remaining chapters in this volume deal with mediation and arbitration, we only briefly mention these approaches to conflict resolution.

Mediation usually involves a third party's acting as a facilitator in the negotiation process. A mediator brings the parties together, helps define the issues involved in the conflict, offers a third-party perspective on the problems and solutions, and guides the resolution process. An arbitrator, on the other hand, acts more like a judge, examining each party's side and deciding on a solution.

Mediators and arbitrators can play a valuable role in resolving a conflict. They can help depersonalize conflict, offer an unbiased perspective from a party not involved in the conflict, and help the parties arrive at unique and creative resolutions to conflict. However, there may also be pitfalls to using a third party. First, the involved parties may stray from the issues concerning the conflict and focus on winning the support of the third party. It is indeed very difficult for the third party to avoid getting caught up in the process and expanding the conflict. A second issue involves saving face. As we have pointed out, concern for saving face comes to the fore when the parties of conflict know they are being observed. Finally, it is vitally important for the third party's efforts to ensure that participants in the conflict feel that they have a *voice* in deciding the procedure to be used in resolving the conflict. Regardless of the outcome, research suggests that participants will be satisfied with a resolution to the degree that they have been active participants in the procedure and they have been given ample opportunity to express their views (Folger & Greenberg, 1985).

THE OTHER SIDE OF CONFLICT: ITS GOOD SIDE

It is easy to get caught up in the negative aspects of conflict. The Hatfield–McCoy feud is a story of death and injury. Most of us are in the business of bringing resolutions to conflict. We see the unhappiness and destruction that accompanies conflict. In most cases conflict is associated with bad and evil, and resolution is accepted as a desired goal.

There is, however, another side to this story: Conflict can be very useful. Conflict is part of the process of testing and assessing oneself. Conflict causes us to examine issues more carefully. It challenges us to develop creative responses and solutions. Conflict is at the root of personal and social change (Deutsch, 1973). Conflict helps us recognize important differences between people. In some cases conflict is an enjoyable and exciting experience. Conflict helps us establish a personal identity. Any parent will recognize the use of conflict to this end. During the "terrible twos," children oppose their parents at every turn to demonstrate their independence and establish their position in the family. During the even more terrible teen years, adolescents use conflict to set the stage for greater independence. Conflict helps groups establish their identity by defining ingroup and outgroup boundaries (Worchel, Coutant-Sassic, & Grossman,

1991). In fact, this research finds that a new group often seeks out opportunities for conflict with outgroups as a means of establishing who is a member of the ingroup. Along these lines, conflict increases cohesiveness in groups and helps define who is a friend and who is not.

We could go on listing the benefits of conflict. However, the point should be clear: Conflict has both detrimental and beneficial aspects. A world with no conflict would be as uninhabitable as one that had only conflict. As is true of many a dear friend or intimate relationship, we have a hard time living with conflict, but we would also have a difficult time living without it. Given this dilemma of conflict, we close this chapter with a point for thought: Rather than immediately focusing on *resolving* conflict, perhaps we should direct more effort at *managing* conflict. Conflict management involves understanding the nature of a conflict and attempting to use that conflict to achieve positive goals and avoid the negative outcomes. Clearly, this is no easy task, but then achieving a fair and lasting resolution to conflict is no small feat.

Acknowledgment

This work was supported in part by a research grant from the Texas Coordinating Board, Texas Advanced Research Projects.

REFERENCES

Ainsworth, M. (1979). Infant–mother attachment. *American Psychologist, 34,* 932–937.

Amir, Y. (1969). Contact hypothesis in ethnic relations. *Psychological Bulletin, 71,* 319–341.

Axelrod, R. (1980). More effective choice in the Prisoner's Dilemma. *Journal of Conflict Resolution, 24,* 379–403.

Brehm, J. W., & Cohen, A. R. (1962). *Explorations in cognitive dissonance*. Stanford, CA: Stanford University Press.

Brockner, J., & Rubin, J. Z. (1985). *Entrapment in escalating conflicts*. New York: Springer-Verlag.

Brown, B. R. (1968). The effect of the need to maintain face on interpersonal bargaining. *Journal of Experimental Social Psychology, 4,* 107–122.

Chertkoff, J. M., & Conley, M. N. (1967). Opening offer and frequency of concession as bargaining strategies. *Journal of Personality and Social Psychology, 7,* 181–185.

Cook, S. W. (1985). Experimenting on social issues: The case of school desegregation. *American Psychologist, 40,* 452–460.

Deutsch, M. (1973). *The resolution of conflict*. New Haven, CT: Yale University Press.

Deutsch, M., & Krauss, R. M. (1960). The effect of threat upon interpersonal bargainings. *Journal of Abnormal and Social Psychology, 61,* 181–189.

Festinger, L. (1957). *A theory of cognitive dissonance*. Stanford, CA: Stanford University Press.

Folger, R., & Greenberg, J. (1985). Procedural justice: An interpretive analysis of personnel systems. In K. Rowland & G. Ferris (Eds.), *Research in personnel and human resource management*. Greenwich, CT: JAI Press.

Hardin, G. (1968). The tragedy of the commons. *Science, 162*, 1243–1248.

Jones, E. E., & Gerard, H. (1967). *Foundations of social psychology*. New York: Wiley.

Jones, E. E., & Nisbett, R. (1972). The actor and the observer: Divergent perceptions of the causes of behavior. In E. E. Jones, D. E. Kanouse, H. H. Kelley, R. E. Nisbett, S. Valins, & B. Weiner (Eds.), *Attribution: Perceiving the causes of behavior* (pp. 79–94). Morristown, NJ: General Learning Press.

Jones, E. E., Wood, G. C., & Quattrone, G. A. (1981). Perceived variability of personal characteristics in-group and out-groups: The role of knowledge and evaluation. *Personality and Social Psychology Bulletin, 7*, 523–528.

Jones, V. C. (1948). *The Hatfields and the McCoys*. Chapel Hill: University of North Carolina Press.

Linville, P. W. (1982). The complexity–extremity effect and age-based stereotyping. *Journal of Personality and Social Psychology, 42*, 193–211.

Osgood, C. E. (1962). *An alternative to war or surrender*. Urbana: University of Illinois Press.

Rapoport, A. (1974). Prisoner's Dilemma: Recollections and observations. In A. Rapoport (Ed.), *Game theory as a theory of conflict resolution* (pp. 18–34). Dordrecht, The Netherlands: Reidel.

Raven, B. H., & Kruglanski, A. (1970). Conflict and power. In P. Swingle (Ed.), *The structure of conflict*. New York: Academic Press.

Rothbart, M., & Hallmark, W. (1988). In-group–out-group differences in the perceived efficacy of coercion and conciliation in resolving social conflict. *Journal of Personality and Social Psychology, 55*(2), 248–257.

Rotter, J. B.. (1971). Generalized expectancies for interpersonal trust. *American Psychologist, 26*, 443–452.

Samuelson, C. D., & Messick, D. (1986). Inequities in access to and use of shared resources in social dilemmas. *Journal of Personality and Social Psychology, 51*, 960–967.

Sande, G., Goethals, G. R., Ferrari, L., & Worth, L. (1989). Value-guided attributions: Maintaining the moral self-image and the diabolical enemy-image. *Journal of Social Issues, 45*, 91–118.

Sherif, M., Harvey, D., White, B., Hood, W., & Sherif, C. (1961). *Intergroup conflict and cooperation: The Robber's Cave experiment*. Norman: University of Oklahoma, Institute of Group Relations.

Tajfel, H. (1970). Experiments in intergroup discrimination. *Scientific American, 223*(2), 96–102.

Tajfel, H., & Turner, J. (1986). The social identity theory of intergroup behavior. In S. Worchel & W. G. Austin (Eds.), *The psychology of intergroup relations* (pp. 7–24). Chicago: Nelson-Hall.

Teger, A. (1980). *Too much invested to quit*. New York: Pergamon Press.

Webb, W., & Worchel, P. (1986). Trust and distrust. In S. Worchel & W. G. Austin

(Eds.), *The psychology of intergroup relations* (pp. 213–228). Chicago: Nelson-Hall.

Wicklund, R. A., & Brehm, J. W. (1976). *Perspectives on cognitive dissonance*. Hillsdale, NJ: Erlbaum.

Worchel, S., Andreoli, V. & Folger, R. (1977). Intergroup cooperation and intergroup attraction: The effect of previous interaction and outcome of combined effort. *Journal of Experimental Social Psychology, 13,* 131–140.

Worchel, S., Cooper, J., & Goethals, G. R. (1988). *Understanding social psychology* (4th ed.). Homewood, IL: Dorsey Press.

Worchel, S., Cooper, J., & Goethals, G. R. (1991). *Understanding social psychology* (5th ed.). Monterey, CA: Brooks/Cole.

Worchel, S., Coutant-Sassic, D., & Grossman, M. (1991). A model of group development and independence. In S. Worchel, W. Wood, & J. Simpson (Eds.), *Group process and productivity*. Newbury Park, CA: Sage.

Wrightsman, L. S. (1964). Measurement of philosophies of human stature. *Psychological Reports, 14,* 743–751.

2

Introduction to Community Mediation Programs: Past, Present, and Future

KAREN GROVER DUFFY
State University of New York at Geneseo

Dora, Sandy, and Jayne recently leased an apartment. The apartment was sunny and bright, conveniently located, and affordable. They had an unpleasant surprise, however, when they first left the apartment to go to the grocery store. Dora discovered that the front door wouldn't lock. Sandy stayed behind for safety's sake while the other two shopped. Sandy called their landlord, Nick Holmes, who said he would be over the next day. Next day? The women phoned Mr. Homes for 3 weeks and he never did come over. The tenants then decided to withhold their next month's rent in protest of Mr. Holmes's lack of response. Two weeks after their lack of payment, Mr. Holmes's attorney wrote that he had started eviction proceedings against them.

Bart Montgomery's 4-year-old car was just beginning to show signs of rust, so to prevent further deterioration, he went to Rex's Body Shop. The estimate for preparation, priming, and painting was $723, which at the time seemed reasonable to Bart. When Bart first saw his "new" car, he loved the shiny, uniform appearance.

Three and a half months later, though, the hood of the car faded and began to show telltale, show-through signs of rust. Bart wanted to go to court to recover at least a third of his money. He refused Rex's offer to repaint only the hood for a nominal fee. Rex claimed that he had done an adequate job and that Bart's car had simply been left out in the harsh elements; therefore, the fading was part of the normal aging process for a 4-year-old car under such conditions.

Sue and Jerry did not part amicably. Sue met Jerry through a friend. On the couple's blind date, their first date, it seemed like "love at first sight." After that eventful day, the two spent hour upon hour with each other.

After a year, though, Jerry developed "a roving eye," as Sue called it. After a number of fights triggered by phone calls to Sue's apartment by women searching for Jerry, Jerry and Sue split up. The parting was fraught with tears, anger, and nasty accusations.

Within 3 days of the breakup, Jerry started receiving hangup calls from an anonymous caller. He was sure that Sue was "paying him back" or jealously "checking up on him." When Jerry confronted Sue, she returned his accusation with the comment, "It must be one of your little whores; it's certainly not me." Jerry retorted that he would "see her in court for harassment" after he filed a police complaint.

What do these three seemingly diverse cases—a landlord–tenant dispute, a consumer complaint, and a criminal charge—share in common? The first common characteristic is the element of conflict: a landlord and his tenants disagreeing over terms of the rental agreement; a disgruntled consumer complaining to an entrepreneur; and a former boyfriend and girlfriend embittered against each other. The second common feature is that all three cases are candidates for community mediation.

COMMUNITY MEDIATION: A DEFINITION AND DIFFERENTIATION

"Mediation" is the intervention in a conflict by a neutral third party who assists the conflicting parties in managing or resolving their dispute. The unbiased third party is the mediator, who uses a variety of techniques to assist the disputants in arriving at a consensual agreement to settle their conflict. This agreement is often a mutually negotiated, legally binding contract between the disputants. The word "assist" is important here. Mediators are not supposed to force or coerce settlement. Instead, by facilitating face-to-face discussion, problem solving, and the development of alternative solutions, a mediator enables the disputants to arrive at their own agreement as to how the conflict will be resolved.

For example, in the landlord–tenant dispute, a mediator might point out that simple miscommunication or forgetfulness might have occurred: Perhaps Holmes forgot to respond to the women's call for a lock or misunderstood the urgency with which they made the call. A mediator could also read the lease to help determine whether the lock is the landlord's responsibility and whether rent withholding is a condition approved in the lease, and so remind the parties. In the case of Bart versus Rex's Body Shop, the mediator might test the contention that a 4-year-old, recently painted car exposed to the elements typically fades quickly and shows rust again; the mediator might also test the possibility that the hood might not be one-third of the car. Finally, in the case of alleged harassment between the two former lovers, the mediator might suggest Jerry's placing a trap installed by the phone company on his phone and suggest that Sue might concur with the idea, since she insists she is not making the calls.

Mediation differs from its sister process of "arbitration." In arbitration, the arbitrator (usually after an attempt at mediation that has faltered) hears the facts of the case and renders a legally binding decision, which may or may not satisfy both parties. In mediation, the disputants decide the outcome; in arbitration, the neutral third party decides the outcome. Mediation seems nearly universally preferred to arbitration by neutral third parties, because in mediation the decision or settlement is the product of the disputants, and the disputants are thus more likely to be satisfied with (and hence to comply with) the solution or agreement (Folberg & Taylor, 1984).

Arbitration in some respects may sound like "adjudication," or the resolution of conflict by appealing to the courts for a decision. In some ways arbitration and adjudication are similar, because they involve appeal to an outside authority to make a binding decision. However, the training of an arbitrator generally differs from that of a judge; the judge has obtained a law degree, whereas the arbitrator often has not. Second, in many court cases a judge has to render a verdict of guilty or innocent, while an arbitrator does not. Third, court is not considered to be a forum for exploring underlying psychological issues or for allowing emotional venting by the disputants. Arbitrators (and mediators) often need and want to spend time on each conflict to understand its causes and long-term consequences. However, in court and in arbitration, both authorities can and will decide contract settlements, make monetary awards, and so on. Table 2.1 outlines the similarities and differences among adjudication, mediation, and arbitration.

Data suggest that prehearing conciliation may be higher in mediation or

TABLE 2.1.   A Comparison of Conflict Resolution Processes Utilizing Third Parties: Adjudication, Mediation, and Arbitration

	Adjudication	Mediation	Arbitration
The decision maker	Judge	The parties	The arbitrator
Training of hearing officer	Law degree	Varies with the agency	Varies with the agency
Legally binding solution?	Yes	Usually	Yes
Verdict of guilt versus innocence?	Yes	No	No
Usually explores underlying issues and causes of conflict and addresses them?	No	Yes	Yes

arbitration settings, as compared to situations when the criminal justice system or courts are involved (Harrington, 1985). Many observers have argued that this is an advantage of neighborhood justice programs (which house mediation and arbitration programs) over courts. Moreover, many experts in the justice field perceive court-determined decisions as failing to address underlying issues; they also see courts as delivering justice very slowly (and expensively), and hence as resulting in much citizen dissatisfaction. Several experts (Garofalo & Connelly, 1980; Harrington, 1985; Lempert & Sanders, 1986; McGillis & Mullen, 1977) have declared the courts to be slow, overburdened, and inappropriate for many disputes. Hence attention has turned to methods of alternative dispute resolution (ADR), such as mediation and arbitration.

A BRIEF HISTORY OF COMMUNITY MEDIATION

Mediation and arbitration are fairly recent innovations in communities seeking speedier, more humane, and less expensive alternatives to the courts. The history of use of these two processes in the United States is not long, but their use elsewhere is in fact rather protracted. Readers familiar with ancient Chinese philosophy and custom will not be surprised to learn that the Chinese (and other Orientals) today utilize mediation as a major component in their justice system, just as Confucius suggested should be done hundreds of years ago. Early Christians also adopted peacemaking and the use of third parties to settle their disputes as an acceptable way of life (Folberg & Taylor, 1984).

The history of mediation to settle disputes in the United States relates most specifically to its use in the labor movement. Since the 1888 Arbitration Act, both labor and management have routinely appealed to neutral third parties as a method by which grievances, both contractual and disciplinary, can be heard and reasonably settled (Holley & Jennings, 1980). However, there exist marked differences between mediation as practiced in community justice programs and mediation in labor relations (see Table 2.2 for a summary). The primary difference is that in labor mediation, the parties in the dispute are generally experts; as representatives of labor or management, the parties negotiating in front of the neutral third party are usually well versed in the issues, the laws, negotiation strategies, and so forth. In community mediation—the focus of this book—the parties are often unsophisticated about the law, negotiation strategies, and so forth. Some experts have strongly questioned whether labor mediation techniques are appropriate to community disputes where there already exist rules or laws for decision making (Harrington, 1985).

A second major difference between the brand of mediation practiced in the labor movement and that practiced in communities is that in labor

TABLE 2.2.   Labor Mediation and Community Mediation Contrasted

	Labor mediation	Community mediation
Assignment to case of hearing officer	Usually by agreement between labor and management and/or on the basis of availability	Based on availability, and often on similarity to parties
Level of expertise of negotiators or parties	Expert	Usually nonexpert
Whom do negotiators or parties represent?	Collectives such as unions and management	Themselves
Is a shared future between parties anticipated?	Yes. Parties will generally continue to interact long after the mediation	Yes and no. In certain cases (such as family and neighbor cases) the parties may have an ongoing relationship; in other cases (such as consumer complaints) no long-term relationship is expected

mediation the involved parties are usually representatives of a much larger group. These representatives collaborate with and are answerable to those for whom they negotiate, either labor or management. In community mediation, a party usually represents only himself or herself, or at most the immediate family. This is an important distinction because Bercovitch (1984) has noted that the process and structure of the intervention, as well as the third party's behaviors, are different for interpersonal conflicts compared to intergroup conflicts. Interpersonal conflict, as is often seen in community mediation, tends to be rather emotionally centered, whereas intergroup conflict, as is more typical of labor mediation, tends to be task-oriented.

Fuller (1971) has also suggested that labor mediation differs from community mediation in that the parties of a labor dispute often face a future together, whereas the parties seeking justice through community mediation are experiencing an isolated conflict. At present, Fuller's contention may or may not be true, because some experts are suggesting that community mediation (even of serious offenses) is appropriate when the parties are predicted to have a long-term or ongoing relationship (Vera Institute of Justice, 1977). In fact, published data show that often the parties in mediated disputes do have some ongoing relationship; that is, they are family members, friends, or neighbors (Harrington, 1985). Of course, labor mediation's longer history has given it credibility and acceptance. By contrast, mediation (and arbitration) in community justice programs is a relative newcomer and perhaps encounters more resistance from the public and enforcement or justice system professionals than does labor mediation. Americans have been described as holding much more affection for the older adversarial court system (Lempert & Sanders, 1986), even when mediation services are less expensive or free (Pearson, 1982).

If Americans are so tied to their court system, what motivated the birth and subsequent growth of the community mediation movement? Three movements, two popular and one governmental, probably provided the necessary impetus. In the late 1960s and early 1970s, historical events such as Watergate and the Vietnam War triggered in the populace, especially college students, both a yearning for more self-governance (e.g., the call for lowering the voting age to 18) and less tolerance for injustice (e.g., the reactions to Watergate). The desire for self-governance coupled with the humanistic education movement, which propounded student and citizen empowerment as well as personal relevancy, created a demand for a justice system in which citizens could receive a more expeditious and self-generated form of justice than that provided by the courts. While the public was clamoring for reform, high-ranking government officials and chief justices were promoting a less formal, less cumbersome justice system as well (Harrington, 1985).

CURRENT STATUS

The earliest community mediation programs from the 1960s in Philadelphia and in Columbus, Ohio were developed by local prosecutors and courts in response to the need to speed and improve the processing of minor criminal matters (McGillis, 1986). By the mid-1970s there still existed fewer than a dozen centers, but a surge of growth occurred in the 1980s, the exact reasons for which remain unknown. By the mid-1980s, one author reported the existence of over 180 programs (McGillis, 1986), whereas another claimed that there were as many as 400 programs in nearly 40 different states (Meehan, 1986). In the late 1980s, however, the growth curve appeared to be slowing; whether this slowing will be a permanent phenomenon still remains to be seen (McGillis, 1986).

Programs today are funded by a variety of sources, including (in descending order of frequency) local governments, state governments, private foundations, fee generation, churches, the federal government, and interest on trust funds (McGillis, 1986). This myriad of funding sources has resulted in an equally varied number of programs and philosophies. While apologizing for the parsimony of his system, McGillis (1986) who has conducted extensive studies of programs throughout the United States, classifies most of them into three general types: justice-system-based, community-based, and composite. The justice-system-based programs are usually sponsored by the courts, which refer large numbers of cases to the programs in what McGillis describes as a "coercive" fashion. (This description is controversial, since parties are theoretically supposed to agree voluntarily to come to mediation.) The community-based programs are usually sponsored by a nonprofit agency; their caseloads typically are small, originate outside the courts, and include walk-ins. Composite programs may be sponsored by the government and/or a nonprofit agency. Their caseloads come from a variety of sources, including the justice system. Caseload origins can be important in determining the frequencies of various types of cases, but are surprisingly not as important in determining whether critical parties will appear for a hearing (Harrington, 1985)—a finding contrary to a myth in the mediation field that court-referred cases are often thought to proceed to a hearing more frequently. Readers should note also that this whole discussion of current status does not include parallel programs in school systems and in other community agencies (e.g., Better Business Bureaus) where mediation is offered. Several chapters in this book detail mediation services in these special settings.

THE MEDIATORS

Just who are the third parties, the mediators (who sometimes act as arbitrators), for these programs? First, some agencies utilize one mediator or arbitrator at a time; others provide a panel of from two to five mediators, who may or may not be paid for their services (McGillis, 1986). These hearing officers come from all walks of life: lay citizens, attorneys, academicians, social service professionals, and court clerks. Many of the programs invite participation by a variety of screened volunteers from a myriad of occupations, who receive training in the form of classroom lectures, videotaped role plays with feedback, and apprenticeships under a seasoned hearing officer. New York State, for example, requires a minimum of 25 hours of training plus an apprenticeship and periodic refresher training (Christian, 1986).

Harrington's (1985) research on the Kansas City neighborhood justice project in Missouri indicated that of the 50 mediators, many had work experience in social service and education. Only a few were lawyers. Harrington did not report specifically on the mediators' racial background, but it was noted to be similar to the background of the parties and included most racial and ethnic groups. New York State, a pioneer state with a program in every county, retains a full-time research associate who recently surveyed its volunteer mediators in more depth (Center for Dispute Settlement, Inc., 1987). The survey found that of the responding mediators, 59% were female and 39% were male (a few did not specify sex); 86% were white, 9.5% black, 2% Hispanic, and 1% Native American. The mean age was 46.2 years (with the female respondents being slightly younger), and the mean number of years of education was 16.2. The largest proportion (37%) of the mediators held professional positions and had a mean length of mediation service of 3½ years.

Susan Rogers and her associates (Rogers, Kanrich, & Steinhauser, 1989) have presented preliminary results of survey research on volunteer mediators and their reasons for mediating. The most important reason cited by these volunteers was that mediation provided them with a chance to help others. The mediators also responded that mediation was important because it afforded them new skills and a chance to help build the community. These volunteer mediators also reported that they disliked being underutilized by the mediation centers; in fact, underutilization was the main reason cited by mediators for breaks in service.

The credentialing of community mediators (and arbitrators) is a controversial issue at the moment (Emery & Wyer, 1987; Hartfield, 1988; Shaw, 1988). There are some who believe that specific credentials such as a law degree or a degree in behavioral science would be best; for instance, the Academy of Family Mediators requires such a degree. Others defend the use of lay or nonprofessional mediators who possess adequate empathy, listening, and other interpersonal skills (Bercovitch, 1984; Folberg & Taylor, 1984; Moore, 1986). Some feel that almost anyone can mediate if properly screened and trained (Christian, 1986). The issue of credentialing is explored in depth by Albie Davis later in this book (see Chapter 13).

TYPES OF CONFLICTS HANDLED

The nature of the cases managed by community dispute resolution programs varies widely, depending on a particular program. Some programs handle primarily or only criminal cases, such as trespassing, harassment, assault, and so on. Others handle civil disputes, including breaches of contract, consumer complaints, and neighbor disputes. Some centers manage both criminal and civil matters; still others have expanded beyond the resolution of disputes and, as neutral third-party agencies, manage such activities as housing lotteries, organization elections, victim–offender reconciliation, and other issues. A look at the annual report for New York State (Crosson & Christian, 1990), where many local or county-wide programs are basically of the composite type, shows this breakdown in regard to types of cases processed: harassment (46%), assault (12%), interpersonal disputes (8%), breach of contract (6%), housing (7%), and personal property (3%). An unobtrusive measure of the success of mediation in this pioneer state is that New York has recently passed legislation offering mediation for certain felonies and for conflicts involving larger sums of money than in the past.

In Harrington's (1985) research in Kansas City, disputes referred to the mediation center included harassment (21%), assault (42%), property destruction (5%), neighborhood disputes over children (9%), custody/

visitation (2%), dogs/property (10%), landlord–tenant disputes (11%), debts (9%), and consumer complaints (6%). Unfortunately, each agency classifies disputes differently; thus the New York State and Kansas City data are not strictly comparable. However, it will be noted that in both locations, harassment and assault are the issues most frequently referred to mediation. Both programs rely fairly heavily on court and police referrals, which may slant the data in peculiar ways.

DOES COMMUNITY MEDIATION WORK?

Perhaps a pertinent question to ask at this juncture in the history of ADR is this: "Are these alternative programs doing a good job? Do they seem to work?" An answer would probably begin, "That depends upon whom you ask." A researcher interested in obtaining an answer might ask all or some of the following: the disputants, the hearing officers, the mediation program directors, or sources external to the process (such as prosecutors, judges, or law enforcement officers) who also have a stake in the success of mediation.

Although there appears to be no research on mediators' impression of whether or not they have succeeded, most mediators probably leave each hearing with a healthy impression of whether the dispute has been successfully settled and whether the parties indeed will comply with their consensual agreements. In line with this conjecture is the fact that mediators often attempt to convince parties in certain cases (but not in other cases) that their agreements should contain some form of this caveat: "Should this agreement require modification and/or should further issues arise, the parties will return to mediation." This seems to be a surefire sign that the hearing officer does not expect total compliance or expects further conflict in particular cases. The field might profit from research on mediators' perceptions of the potential for successful settlement and compliance, compared to actual settlement and compliance rates. Such a comparison might yield information about the role of mediator persistence in difficult cases.

The parties or disputants themselves are other possible respondents to the question of whether mediation works. Researchers have queried both the petitioners (the complainants or claimants) and the respondents (or, loosely, "the offenders"). But what to ask? Parties may be satisfied with the process (with perceived fairness or empowerment, perhaps), but not with the actual outcome (provisions in the agreement). The opposite may also be true: Parties may express high satisfaction with the outcome but discomfort with the procedure. Likewise, parties may also profess satisfaction with the outcome and the process, but still may not comply behaviorally with the agreement. We probably all know someone who believes in child support but is delinquent in actual payments.

A researcher might also ask whether, despite professed dissatisfaction

or satisfaction with the process or outcome, the parties have learned anything about each other or about how to manage conflict in the future. This is
a measure of success pertinent to other members of society who may have to
deal in the future with the parties. Such a question is rarely posed by
researchers but is of great social interest.

Researchers have surveyed parties in mediation (but unfortunately have
infrequently compared them to parties randomly assigned to court) concerning their perceived satisfaction with and fairness of the process or its components (such as the mediator). This research has generally found that
mediation is highly rated by clients (e.g., Davis, Tichane, & Grayson, 1980;
Harrington, 1985; Schwartzkoff & Morgan, 1982). It is not unusual in such
studies to find 80–90% of the parties well satisfied with mediation. There is
little research on any other disputant measures.

The mediation program directors who need data to present to funding
agencies probably also collect data on "success." These data are likely to
include settlement and compliance rates, access rates by different groups,
processing time, and cost-effectiveness. Again, mediation fares well in formal studies. Rates for reaching agreement or settlement average 88% of the
cases that proceed to a hearing (McGillis, 1986). In the other 12% of the
cases, not all parties can be reached to schedule a hearing, or will agree to a
hearing or appear for the hearing once it is scheduled.

For purposes of elucidation, let us again turn to some actual data. In
New York State, 51% of the cases after screening went through an ADR
process. In instances where an appropriate case did not reach the process,
the most common reason (21% of these instances) was disputants' failure to
appear for the hearing. In 85% of the disputes that reached mediation,
resolution was attained. On average, 14.9 days passed from intake to final
disposition, and all this took place at an average cost of $25.67 per request for
service (Crosson & Christian, 1990).

Harrington (1985) reports that in Kansas City a hearing was held in 56%
of the cases, and that in 93% of these an agreement was reached. Frequency
data on cases where parties were referred to mediation but refused to
proceed to a hearing were not recorded. Common reasons cited in case files
for no hearing were as follows: Lawyers advised one or both parties against
mediation, either or both parties preferred court, and one or both parties felt
mediation would be a waste of time.

A word about resistance to mediation is merited here. The literature on
resistance (e.g., Volpe & Bahn, 1987) is growing, but appears to be more
impressionistic than empirical or data-based. Paul Olczak's chapter in this
book (see Chapter 10) deals exclusively with this topic.

The question of equal access to justice for the different types of parties
served is more difficult to gauge, but it is of interest to program directors
who need to demonstrate equal access to funding sources (i.e., courts,
legislators, and charitable foundations). Some experts in the justice system

feel, as Fiss (1984) does, that ADR seeks to make wealth irrelevant and to empower equally both parties in the dispute, but that in the end ADR, like its more expensive sisters, suffers from the exact power and wealth imbalances it seeks to make irrelevant. On the other hand, there are those such as Moore (1986) and Murray (1984) who feel that mediators can and should deal with power imbalances and other disputant differences, such as wealth, to hasten the conflict resolution process and ensure fairness.

Rates of use by a variety of ethnic groups are often cited by program directors to indicate equal or at least potentially equal access to justice. Again, let us refer to recent New York State data. Among the complainants, 10% did not report race, but 44% were white, 25% black, and 18% Hispanic. Among respondents, 31% did not indicate race, but 38% were white, 17% black, and 12% Hispanic (those groups representing 1–5% of the population were not included in the data; Crosson & Christian, 1990). Although these percentages do not reflect the New York State population at large, Crosson and Christian believe that these data indicate that the "[c]ommunity dispute resolution centers serve men and women of all races and ethnic backgrounds" (1990, p. 2).

Since Harrington's (1985) Kansas City data have been utilized elsewhere in this chapter for comparison to New York State data, let us turn to her work once again. The percentages reported by Harrington were collapsed across claimants and respondents: blacks (49%), whites (46%), and Hispanics (5%). Again, several ethnic groups are represented, but whether these data indeed support the equal-access concept is debatable.

One final group from whom researchers might elicit responses to the question of whether community mediation works would be those outside of but involved with mediation programs. These individuals include (but are not limited to) judges, police officers, prosecutors, probation officers, and others who refer cases to community justice centers. They, too, are touched in some way by the successes and failures of mediation. These individuals would, of course, be interested in some of the same data generated by program directors, such as settlement and compliance rates, access to justice, and the reduction of their own respective caseloads. However, outsiders might also want addressed the issue of consistency of outcome with similar cases (McGillis, 1986). That is, in similar conflicts, are the outcomes similar? If the outcomes are different despite case similarity, why are the outcomes different? (Uneven justice?) Second, outsiders might ask whether the skills learned in ADR are generalizable to other life situations, thereby reducing disputants' further involvement with law enforcement or justice system officials.

The element of case outcome consistency (similar outcomes in similar cases) is difficult to assess, and little research has been conducted (McGillis, 1986). The same can be said for the learning of conflict resolution skills in ADR and the reduction of future conflicts. There is, however, one study of *prior* involvement with the criminal justice system, which shows that most parties in ADR forums have *not* been involved previously in the justice system (Bridenback, 1979). Perhaps repeat offenders are less likely to be referred to mediation by judges, law enforcement officers, or the like.

What remain, then, for both outsiders and insiders to consider in assessments of community justice programs are compliance rates. Studies on compliance rates are difficult to compare with one another, since each study employs a different dependent measure: perceptions that "all is well" after settlement, perceptions of whether relations between parties are better, or actual behaviors that have changed. Overall, however, McGillis (1986), who has appraised many programs, states that the long-term impact of mediation is very favorable, no matter what measure is employed. McGillis does caution, though, that despite such evidence, community mediation programs still have not significantly lowered court caseloads.

These measures often paint a rather favorable overall picture of community mediation to many interested groups. However, the reader is again reminded of the failure of many disputants to utilize the process; they fail either to volunteer for the process when it is volitional, or to return calls from intake coordinators, or to appear for hearings. Mediation, then, rather than resulting in poor satisfaction or failure to reach agreeable outcomes, seems to falter most often because parties refuse to utilize the process in the first place. Ellen Cohn and Mae Lynn Neyhart's chapter in this book highlights some methods for promoting mediation programs to reluctant parties (see Chapter 11).

SUMMARY AND CONCLUSION

Community mediation involves the use of a neutral third party to assist the disputants in arriving at a consensually agreed-upon settlement in either a civil or a criminal matter. Mediation differs from arbitration and adjudication, in which the hearing officer determines settlement. Research generally shows that parties in mediation are more satisfied with both the process and the outcome, and often are more compliant with the outcome than those parties who seek justice in the courts. Despite the proliferation of community mediation programs and high user satisfaction, such programs appear to be underutilized in comparison to other processes, especially adjudication. More research, particularly on how to promote the use of ADR, would be welcomed by practitioners.

REFERENCES

Bercovitch, J. (1984). *Social conflicts and third parties*. Boulder, CO: Westview Press.

Bridenback, M. (1979). *The citizen dispute settlement process in Florida: A study of five programs*. Tallahassee: Florida Supreme Court, Office of State Courts Administrator.

Center for Dispute Settlement, Inc. (1987, Autumn). Research on New York mediators. *Newsletter of the Center for Dispute Settlement*, pp. 3–4.

Christian, T. F. (1986). A resource for all seasons: A state-wide network of community dispute resolution centers. In J. Palenski & H. Launer (Eds.), *Mediation: Contexts and challenges* (pp. 85–94). Springfield, IL: Charles C Thomas.

Crosson, M. T., & Christian, T. F. (1990). *The Community Dispute Resolution Centers Program annual report*. Albany, NY: Office of Court Administration.

Davis, R., Tichane, M., & Grayson, D. (1980). *Mediation and arbitration as alternatives to criminal prosecution in felony arrest cases: An evaluation of the Brooklyn Dispute Resolution Center*. New York: Vera Institute of Justice.

Emery, R. E., & Wyer, M. M. (1987). Divorce mediation. *American Psychologist*, *42*, 472–480.

Fiss, O. M. (1984). Against settlement. *Yale Law Journal*, *93*, 1073–1090.

Folberg, J., & Taylor, A. (1984). *Mediation: A comprehensive guide to resolving conflicts without litigation*. San Francisco: Jossey-Bass.

Fuller, L. (1971). Mediation—its forms and functions. *Southern California Law Review*, *44*, 305–328.

Garofalo, J., & Connelly, K. J. (1980). Dispute resolution centers: Outcomes, issues, and future directions. *Criminal Justice Abstracts*, *12*, 576.

Harrington, C. (1985). *Shadow justice: The ideology and institutionalization of alternatives to court*. Westport, CT: Greenwood Press.

Hartfield, E. F. (1988). Qualifications and training standards for mediators of environmental and public policy disputes. *Seton Hall Legislative Journal*, *12*, 109–124.

Holley, W. H., & Jennings, K. M. (1980). *The labor relations process*. Hinsdale, IL: Dryden Press.

Lempert, R., & Sanders, J. (1986). *An invitation to law and social science*. New York: Longman Press.

McGillis, D. (1986). *Community dispute resolution programs and public policy*. Washington, DC: National Institute of Justice.

McGillis, D., & Mullen, J. (1977). *Neighborhood justice centers: An analysis of potential models*. Washington, DC: U.S. Government Printing Office.

Meehan, T. (1986). Alternatives to lawsuits. *Alternatives to Legal Reform*, *6*, 9–12.

Moore, C. W. (1986). *The mediation process: Pretrial strategies for resolving conflict*. San Francisco: Jossey-Bass.

Murray, J. S. (1984). Third-party intervention: Successful entry for the uninvited. *Albany Law Review*, *48*, 573–614.

Pearson, J. (1982). Evaluation of alternatives to court adjudication. *Justice System Journal*, *7*(3), 420–444.

Rogers, S. J., Kanrich, S. & Steinhauser, I. (1989). *Understanding our criminal justice volunteers: A study of community mediators in New York State*. New York: Brooklyn Mediation Center.

Schwartzkoff, R., & Morgan, T. (1982). *Final report of the evaluation of three experimental community centres*. Sydney, Australia: Law Foundation of New South Wales.

Shaw, M. L. (1988). Mediator qualifications: Report of a symposium on critical issues in alternative dispute resolution. *Seton Hall Legislative Journal, 12*, 125–136.

Vera Institute of Justice. (1977). *Felony arrests: Their prosecution and disposition in New York City courts*. New York: Author.

Volpe, M. R., & Bahn, C. (1987). Resistance to mediation: Understanding and handling it. *Negotiation Journal, 3*, 297–305.

3

Techniques and Pitfalls of Applied Behavioral Science Research: The Case of Community Mediation

FRANK Y. WONG
Hofstra University

CRAIG H. BLAKELY and STACIE L. WORSHAM
Texas A&M University

> There does not exist a category of science to which one can give the name applied science. There are science and the applications of science, bound together as the fruit to the tree which bears it.
> —Louis Pasteur, *Revue Scientifique*

This chapter is intended to provide individuals in the field with some basic tools for conducting community mediation research. Our goal is not to describe detailed statistical techniques, but rather to provide an adequate overview of applied behavioral science research methods that will enable both practitioners and researchers to appreciate the many interrelated issues involved in evaluating a particular mediation program. We also hope to provide information that will assist individuals in making an educated decision about the types of research methods that can be employed and the advantages and disadvantages of each method. As an aid to readers, Appendix 3.1 at the end of the chapter presents a glossary of important behavioral science research terms that have particular relevance to mediation research. Where appropriate, these terms are also defined and discussed in the text.

THE NATURE OF THE INQUIRY

The multidimensional aspects of applied behavioral science research necessitate attention to two questions. First, what is the goal of the research one is undertaking? Second, can the research be conducted in an ethical manner? We cannot discuss the former question without addressing the latter. Although the two questions also concern basic behavioral science research, they are especially complicated in applied settings. For example, access to personal records, the vulnerability of certain clients, and resource constraints all can be very sensitive issues in applied settings. To that end, the two questions are discussed within the general frameworks of social experimentation and program evaluation.

Social Experimentation

In applied settings, it is not uncommon to find new technologies introduced to satisfy needs. For example, a researcher may begin with the fact that the judicial system is overburdened with the volume of separation agreements, divorce petitions, and custody documents on the docket. Furthermore, knowledge about the social technologies in place to alleviate these backlogs may be scarce or may vary considerably. However, the researcher may believe that a greater number and variety of marital mediation programs are needed to alleviate the burden on the legal system. To find out, a needs assessment should be conducted (see Folger, Chapter 4, this volume, for a detailed discussion of needs assessment strategies). If these suspicions are confirmed, the researcher may proceed to develop and implement various kinds of marital mediation programs in an effort to identify the models that best meet the current needs. The final objectives may range from assuring that the needs are met to evaluating the effectiveness of these programs and incorporating data-based refinements of the programs for future use (Fairweather & Tornatzky, 1977).

Program Evaluation

On other occasions, a viable program may already be in place. However, documentation of the impact of the existing program may be needed. Three sets of questions are basic to all program evaluation research. The first set includes the following: Who are the participants? Where are they located? What are their demographic characteristics? How were they determined to be the target group? The second set consists of these questions: What service is the program designed to deliver? What services did the participants receive? The third set comprises this question: What is the impact on the participants as a function of the services provided?

In regard to the marital mediation program example above, a researcher might ask whether service A is better than service B for resolving disputes. Do well-educated couples make use of such programs more often than less educated couples? What kinds of recommendations can be suggested to policy makers concerning various marital mediation programs as options to the judicial system?

More often than not, the nature of the inquiry will be guided by a series of questions that must be answered following the investigation. At all times, the researcher must retain a focus on those initial research questions. He or she must consider the audience for whom the task is being undertaken and then proceed by following the rational sequences of the scientific method.

Ethical Dilemmas

Having worked out the nature of the inquiry, the researcher must address the question of whether the proposed research approach endangers the welfare of the participants. An ethical issue of critical importance is confidentiality. That is, participants need to feel that their trust will not be violated. However, in some circumstances, a researcher may be faced with situations such that confidentiality may be likely to endanger the welfare of the participants, or of those who are associated with the participants, or of both. For example, an extremely distraught husband confesses that he will kill his wife if she does not comply with his demands. Increasingly, the judicial system is challenging therapists and related professionals regarding their rights to confidentiality, especially in cases like that of the distraught husband, when people who are associated with the participants may be in danger. Although space constraints preclude a detailed discussion of ethical issues here, it is noted that both the intervention (particularly in demonstration project paradigms where a researcher is manipulating service delivery strategies) and evaluation components of a project may adversely affect participants. For a detailed discussion of ethical issues in social science research, see the "Ethical Principles of Psychologists" of the American Psychological Association (1981) or any standard social science research textbook (e.g., Babbie, 1989; Ray & Ravizza, 1988).

TYPES OF BEHAVIORAL SCIENCE
RESEARCH METHODS

Although there are many variations of behavioral science research methods, they can be roughly classified along a continuum ranging from true experimental to correlational methods. Excellent reviews can be found in Campbell and Stanley (1963), Cook and Campbell (1979), and Overman (1989). An overview of several research designs that are relevant for community mediation research is provided here. Table 3.1 presents a summary of

TABLE 3.1. Characteristics of Three Common Behavioral Science Research Methods

	Correlational	Quasi-experimental	Experimental
Type of question	Are the variables of interest related?	Does an independent variable that the researcher does not completely control seem to affect the dependent variable?	Is there a causal relationship between the independent and dependent variables?
When used	Researcher is unable to manipulate an independent variable. Sometimes used in exploratory research.	Researcher wants to assess the impact of a real-life intervention.	Researcher has control over the independent variable and can minimize the number of confounding variables in a study.
Advantages	Convenience of data collection. May avoid certain ethical and/or practical problems.	Provides some information about cause–effect relationships. Permits assessment of more realistic interventions.	Ability to demonstrate cause–effect relationships. Permits control over confounding variables and the ruling out of alternative explanations.
Disadvantages	Cannot establish a cause–effect relationship	Lack of control over confounding variables. Strong causal inferences cannot be made.	Some questions cannot be studied experimentally for either practical or ethical reasons. May lead to artificial procedures.
Mediation research example	Lim and Carnevale's (1990) study analyzing different types of mediator behavior. See Chapter 8, this volume.	Best's report on the impact of the General Motors consumer mediation program. See Chapter 18, this volume.	Duffy and Olczak's (1989) research on perceptions of mediation. See Chapters 10 and 11, this volume.

three of the most common behavioral science research methods and their characteristics.

In general, behavioral science research methods that fall toward the "experimental" end of this continuum are characterized by the use of comparison or control groups. That is, assuming that all other factors are equal, the manipulation of an independent variable leads to the occurrence of an effect in one group or a change in the dependent variable for that group when compared to a similar or control group without the treatment. For example, randomly assigning disputants to either mediation or the regular judicial process and then measuring the disputants' satisfaction with the outcome could be classified as an experimental method.

On the other hand, "correlational" research refers to a finding of a consistent relationship, positive or negative, between two phenomena (or variables) across a number of observations. However, a correlational result does not allow for cause and effect to be clearly discerned, as in the case of an experimental study. For example, divorces are likely to be related to a number of variables in ways that are not clearly understood. Work-related stress may covary with the incidence of divorce. However, without manipulation of an independent variable, one cannot conclude that work-related stress causes divorce or that divorce causes work-related stress. Issues related to experimental and correlational research are further discussed below.

Experimental Method

Two common behavioral science experimental research designs that can be used in assessing the effectiveness of community mediation programs are highlighted here. A common design is the "pretest–posttest control group design." This design involves an assessment of one or more outcomes or dependent variables both prior to and following an experimental intervention. One group of participants is exposed to a change in the independent variable, while another group is not. In addition, assignment to the experimental or control group is random; that is, subjects have an equal chance of being assigned to either group by the researcher.

If the intervention is potent enough to achieve certain desired outcomes, the effect should (ideally) be observable as a change from preintervention to postintervention scores within the experimental group (e.g., those receiving mediation services). In addition, a difference should be noted between the observations or scores derived from the experimental and control groups (e.g., a similar group of clients not receiving mediation services). In other words, the pretest–posttest observations of participants in the control group should remain relatively constant over time, unless some natural maturation occurs or the initial pretest sensitizes all participants to the nature of the assessment being conducted (Campbell & Stanley, 1963; Cook & Campbell, 1979; Overman, 1989). For example, let us assume that a group of couples is being studied before and after their participation in a marital mediation program, while simultaneously being compared to another, similar group of couples who have not participated in the program. In each case, marital disharmony is assessed by observing interpersonal interactions over the course of several observations. We might expect the mediated couples' interactions to improve from preintervention to postintervention, while the control group's do not.

Another common behavioral science experimental research design, the "Solomon four-group design," adds two additional groups that allow direct detection of the influence of familiarity with the assessment process. The inclusion of the experimental and control groups that are not exposed to the pretest is a further investigation of the generalizability or external validity of the experimental manipulations and effect of prior testing (Campbell & Stanley, 1963; Cook & Campbell, 1979). Once again, random assignment of subjects to a condition is used in the Solomon four-group design.

Quasi-Experimental Method

Although experimental manipulations are preferred for causal inferences, there are many variables presented in applied behavioral science research that cannot be manipulated for either practical or ethical reasons. For example, ethnicity cannot be manipulated. Also, length of marriage cannot be ethically manipulated. However, both variables can be controlled for and measured within the context of one's research design.

A common behavioral science quasi-experimental research design is the "nonequivalent pretest–posttest control design," which involves the comparison of a group before and after a certain treatment with another group that has not been treated. However, this design differs from the pretest–posttest design previously discussed, in that subjects are *not* randomly assigned to experimental or control conditions. Group membership is determined not by the researcher, but by the subjects or the mediation center. This allows for a more "natural" or realistic research design, but one in which initial differences between the experimental and comparison groups are not balanced out (Campbell & Stanley, 1963; Cook & Campbell, 1979). In the marital mediation program example given above, the researcher is likely to be bound by program policies to enroll all couples who want to participate in any type of program for which ample resources exist. Consequently, the researcher might decide to study a group of couples before and after their participation in a type of program, while observing another group of couples who have decided not to participate.

Correlational Method

In general, correlational research designs allow one to document the relationship between two variables of interest. However, causal links cannot be confirmed, because correlational designs do not rule out intervening or other unstudied variables that could easily have produced the effects noted. In true experimental research, intervening variables are controlled for through randomly assigning subjects to groups, holding conditions constant, and manipulating an independent variable. In correlational research, these three criteria are seldom if ever met.

An example of a correlational study related to divorce mediation would be examining whether a relationship exists between the length of time a couple has been married and the length or difficulty of the mediation process. The discovery of a correlation between these two variables does not mean, however, that a long marriage produces a long and painful mediation process, any more than such a correlation means that a long mediation process causes a long marriage. All a researcher can infer is that a relationship does exist between the two variables (length of marriage and of mediation), but he or she cannot be sure which variable is the cause and which the effect in the relationship. As mentioned above, what may cause a correlation between a long marriage and a long divorce mediation may be an intervening variable, such as the ages of the divorcing parties. That is, older couples may well have been married longer, but each member of an older couple may also be more self-assured than members of younger couples about what he or she wants to leave the marriage with. Developmental or age-related differences in personal confidence and assertiveness, not the length of marriage per se, may produce the correlation between length of marriage and number and difficulty of medication sessions.

INTERNAL VALIDITY

Having decided on a research method, one must ascertain the rigorousness of the design. The rigor of a given research method is judged in part by "internal validity," which refers to the degree to which an independent variable is responsible for any observed changes in the dependent variable. In rigorously controlled, true experimental methods, internal validity is generally very high and is not an issue of major concern. However, the volatile nature of applied behavioral science research opens the door to a number of factors that have the potential to threaten the internal validity of one's design (Campbell & Stanley, 1963; Cook & Campbell, 1979; Overman, 1989). Some of the more frequent threats to internal validity of which mediation researchers need to be aware are considered below.

Selection Bias

It is not uncommon for the experimental group in applied behavioral science research to be selected through some nonrandom means, because of such real-world constraints as geographical locations, occupations, ethnicity, and the like. That is, not everyone has an equal chance of being selected to participate in the treatment (this is particularly true in quasi-experimental and correlational research designs). Also, there may not be a control group. In regard to the marital mediation program example above, it is reasonable to assume that couples who are under court order to enroll in a program will feel more resentful than those who participate voluntarily. An unbalanced distribution of couples on this dimension could easily distort one's findings.

Compensation

Compensation (not to be confused with monetary reward) becomes an issue in behavioral science research when, for example, participants in the control group who are not selected to participate in a type of marital mediation program may decide to work harder on their marriages; this inadvertently makes it difficult to determine the effectiveness of the program for them.

Diffusion of Treatment

Behavioral science researchers may not have full control of their participants. This becomes particularly problematic when participants in the experimental and control groups are in communication with one another. Those in the control group may thus be indirectly exposed to the experimental treatment(s).

Experimental Mortality

Dropouts are a serious concern in applied behavioral science research, because replacements are usually not easily available. An important consequence is a loss of statistical power. Another is a differential loss of participants in comparison groups. Differences in findings may be linked to differential attrition rates alone, especially in a study over an extended period of time, when attrition is more likely to occur.

Maturation

People change across time as a function of what they are exposed to. Any observed differences between the experimental and control groups may be influenced by the maturation of the participants during the time lag between observations, rather than by the treatment or nontreatment manipulation(s).

Testing

A number of things that have the potential to compromise the experimental manipulations may arise during the initial testing or measurement of the dependent variable. For example, participants may become more sensitive to the instruments used. When a researcher tests for marital discord, those exposed to a pretest may be sensitized to the observtional strategy and may interact differently during subsequent observations.

Instrumentation

A researcher's choice of the outcomes or dependent variables is critical to his or her interpretation of the data. Using an inappropriate metric can easily lead one astray in interpreting the findings of a study. For example, should marital disputes be quantified in terms of complaints from the husbands, wives, or both? Obviously, such a decision can affect one's findings. Also, how should a given dependent variable be measured? Often researchers must choose among many different techniques, including questionnaires/ surveys, interviews, behavioral measures (such as actual payment of child support), and simple observation. The choice of a particular type of measure can greatly influence what a research study finds.

History

Certain historical events that have the potential to confound the results may take place during the course of an experiment. A U.S. Supreme Court decision on abortion during the course of an experiment to investigate divorces would be an example of such an event.

RELIABILITY

In addition to internal validity, scientists are concerned with "reliability," which refers to the consistency of the results (Babbie, 1989). In order to feel confident in the interpretation of his or her findings, a researcher must be comfortable with both the reliability (i.e., replicability) and validity (i.e., accuracy) of the findings. To discuss these topics in adequate detail would require far more space than can be allocated here. However, in undertaking the task of evaluating a community mediation program, the researcher must be aware of these concerns and must ground his or her actions in the fundamental research questions that led to the evaluation effort in the first place.

SOURCES OF DATA

Having decided on the research design and considered the factors that may affect its validity and reliability, the researcher must consider the sources for collecting the data. Data may come from a number of sources (e.g., direct indices, unobtrusive measures, etc.). However, the nature of the data collected is once again determined by the research questions. In the marital mediation program example above, the researcher may choose to survey individuals (i.e., husbands, wives, or mediators) about their knowledge of cases; to seek data from archival records, such as police complaint files on participants from mediated cases; or to do both.

SCIENTIFIC GUIDELINES FOR COMMUNITY MEDIATION RESEARCH

Integrating the issues discussed in the chapter up to this point, Figure 3.1 provides a flow chart of guidelines for conducting community mediation research. In this section, the following example of how to apply these guidelines is used.

The County Board of Directors is preparing the budget for the next fiscal year. The board has asked Ms. Smith, the director of a community mediation center, to conduct an internal programmatic and fiscal audit. The

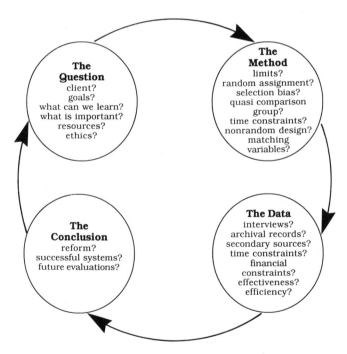

FIGURE 3.1.   Flow chart of scientific guidelines for conducting community mediation research.

members of the board would like to determine the effectiveness of the center. They do not feel as though they can justify spending much money on the center without answering these questions, and they need the answers fairly quickly.

Ms. Smith's staff of eight mediators processes approximately 120 cases a month. The majority of the caseload involves juvenile delinquents who have been referred by the local juvenile court since the establishment of the community mediation program several years ago. The program is limited to those who admit guilt (other cases are processed by the juvenile court), and it excludes individuals who have committed serious crimes against a person. Property crimes are the most common type processed through the program. If Ms. Smith can demonstrate both the effectiveness and efficiency of the program, the County Board of Directors is likely to maintain adequate funding to keep the program in operation for the next biennium.

The Questions

To begin with, Ms. Smith must chart a direction. At the outset, there are four sets of issues she must consider for an adequate evaluation of the community mediation program. The first set includes these questions: Who is the client? What are the major questions to be answered? What are the benefits to be derived from the evaluation? The second set consists of these questions: What would Ms. Smith want to be known about the community mediation process? What would an evaluator want to know? The third set includes this issue: What ethical constraints must be considered in designing an evaluation to address these questions? The fourth set comprises this question: What resources are available?

At first glance, Ms. Smith may surmise that the answers to these questions are not always compatible. Also, the research questions presented may not coincide with what Ms. Smith (or a trained evaluator) might consider most important. Often, compromises must be considered. In this example, the County Board of Directors is considering the community mediation program's future. Should it be re-funded? They have raised issues of effectiveness and efficiency. They have also noted resource constraints. To start with, Ms. Smith may want to consider some strategies that could yield appropriate answers to these questions.

The Method(s)

The issues raised above will dictate the research method(s) to be considered. In the ideal situation, Ms. Smith can randomly assign some juvenile delinquents to the experimental group (i.e., the community mediation program) and some to the control group (i.e., the juvenile court). In this way, the recidivism rates of the two groups can be compared to determine the

effectiveness of the two systems. If Ms. Smith has a large sample of juveniles, she can assume that the two groups will be very similar, and
therefore that the only factor affecting recidivisim will be the systems that
have processed their cases. Although this is an extremely simplistic summa-
tion, the best strategy she can employ to minimize confounding in her
design is random assignment.

However, there are a couple of reasons why random assignment may
not be feasible. Ms. Smith will be limited in the degree to which she can
generalize her findings by the constraints imposed by the system (e.g., only
those admitting guilt for property crimes). Another reason is that juvenile
delinquents may refuse to participate in the community mediation program;
they may opt instead for the juvenile court. This concern (referred to earlier
as selection bias), in particular, causes problems for Ms. Smith's research
method. For example, it is not unlikely that guilty verdicts levied through
the juvenile court may be less severe (in terms of time and resources to the
youths) than mediation outcomes, which typically include restitution and
community service. Street-smart delinquents are often fully cognizant of the
potential costs of different system options. Such a situation may bias Ms.
Smith's findings by limiting the local relevant population to whom she can
generalize the results. Surely it would be a fair relative comparison to look at
only those volunteering for mediation and then randomly assign some to the
court comparison condition. In this case, a nonrandom design may have
more generalizability or external validity to the real-world situation.

On the other hand, to utilize a quasi-experimental research method that
includes these street-smart juvenile delinquents may lead to a liberal test of
the community mediation program if these offenders are differentially habit-
ual. The real constraint on the use of a random assignment design, however,
lies with the fact that the County Board of Directors wants the answer
quickly. By using a quasi-experimental method, Ms. Smith can collect
retrospective archival data that will allow her to determine the impact of
mediation on delinquents who were processed at some earlier time. This will
allow 1-year recidivism rates to be collected without the actual need for a
1-year waiting period to collect the data. Therefore, it is assumed that a
retrospective quasi-experimental method will be most useful in Ms. Smith's
response to the research questions posed.

Ms. Smith is faced with several variables she cannot manipulate, particularly given the time constraints. However, she will be able to measure or
control for many of the potentially confounding variables without the benefit
of random assignment. Some variables she may wish to measure include age,
sex, ethnicity, educational attainment, and offense history. By matching
subjects in her two groups on these variables, she can create comparable
samples of those receiving community mediation services and those processed by the juvenile court during the same time period. That is, Ms. Smith
will try to ensure that both the quasi-experimental and control groups are

relatively similar in terms of age, sex, ethnicity, and other factors, thereby reducing the problem of self-selection mentioned earlier. She must then collect the appropriate information that will allow her to respond to the research questions put before her.

The Data

If Ms. Smith were conducting a prospective research design of more elaborate proportions, she might consider conducting interviews with juvenile offenders, claimants, mediators, prosecutors, judges, and other interested parties. Such a data set would add considerably to her understanding of the complexities or process of the community mediation program in operation. In brief, "process information" refers to the nuts and bolts of an operation. By contrast, "outcome information" is a summary of the impact(s) of an operation. In Ms. Smith's case, time and fiscal resource constraints limit her ability to pursue process data collection and analysis. However, she can still gather data that will allow her to respond accurately to the research questions of effectiveness and efficiency.

Ms. Smith can examine the dimension of effectiveness through comparative means. That is, how do recidivism rates differ between those exposed to the community mediation program and those exposed to the juvenile court? Two archival data sets are the most likely sources of information regarding recidivism. Ms. Smith will also want to review the contact and arrest records at all area police departments. These will include the offices of neighboring cities and counties whose geographic bounds should be based on the community composition and the habits of relevant residents. If possible, a 12-month follow-up period is ideal. The literature suggests that the vast majority of those who are going to commit repeat offenses will do so within a 12-month period (Morash, 1982). If Ms. Smith's sample can be drawn to permit a 12-month follow-up period plus a 4- to 8-week filing period, it will allow for variance in the timeliness of different police department's filing systems. If Ms. Smith does not allow for this variation that regularly occurs in the time it takes various departments to file archival data, it may introduce considerable bias into the data. In other words, if Ms. Smith collects her archival recidivism data in June, she will want to sample juvenile delinquents for some time interval prior to the preceding April. Those processed in the month of March of year n should have the files searched from that date until March of the year $n + 1$. Ms. Smith should not conduct that search until May of the year $n + 1$, allowing 2 months for the archival files to be updated.

Another archival source Ms. Smith will want to check will be the county court records. Although police records are more prevalent, court records do reflect further system penetration. Youths may be diverted from the system at the street level by victims/complainants, at the street level by individual police officers, at the police department level by failure to refer the case formally to the juvenile court, and at the juvenile court level by the choice not to process a referred case formally. Each step along the continuum of system penetration represents some combination of offense seriousness and criminal history or a biased system response. Because of the bias inherent in these systems, both archival police and juvenile court data represent the least costly data available to address the issue of recidivism.

The data addressing efficiency are somewhat more complex and difficult to identify. The data Ms. Smith wishes to obtain involve identifying the costs per unit of all system expenses affiliated with the processing of a case. Many questions must be answered about what costs should and should not be included. For example, what maintenance and utility costs should be included in each question? Some of these questions can be posed to the County Board of Directors; however, that may be inconvenient. What is critical is that all the assumptions Ms. Smith makes about what costs should be included for analytical purposes should be clearly specified in her summary report.

Although this is by no means an exhaustive list, Ms. Smith should include the salaries of mediators and support staff at the community mediator center, facility costs, utility costs, transportation costs, the costs of handling a juvenile court referral, and other such expenses. Salary structure may vary from one mediator to another. It may be more efficient to determine the overall costs associated with running the center for some fiscal period (e.g., 1 year), to determine linkage costs to the court system, and then to determine average costs per participant. Similar costs could be calculated for the comparison group, thus allowing Ms. Smith to determine unit costs for each method of case management.

CONCLUSION

Although a minimal amount of familiarity with behavioral science research methodology has been assumed, this chapter has been written in an attempt to provide practitioners with two skills in particular. First, we hope that readers are now in a better position to evaluate community mediation research. In this way, they may be more critical readers of the reviews of other programs and may do a better job of considering what implications the literature may hold for a particular mediation. A second objective is to help readers develop the skills necessary to assess the benefits of evaluation, and to provide enough of a background for readers to understand the general issues of evaluation research. In this way, they will be in a better position to assess the impact of their own programs. Among researchers and practitioners, there is a strong advocacy for ongoing evaluation in the field of mediation, because only through research can they be successful advocates for service programs such as community mediation programs.

REFERENCES

American Psychological Association. (1981). Ethical principles of psychologists (revised). *American Psychologist, 36,* 633–638.

Babbie, E. (1989). *The practice of social research.* Belmont, CA: Wadsworth.

Campbell, D., & Stanley, J. (1963). *Experimental and quasi-experimental designs for research.* Chicago: Rand McNally.

Cook, T. D., & Campbell, D. T. (1979). *Quasi-experimentation: Design and analysis issues for field settings.* Chicago: Rand McNally.

Fairweather, G. W., & Tornatzky, L. G. (1977). *Experimental methods for social policy research.* New York: Pergamon Press.

Morash, M. (Ed.). (1982). *Implementing criminal justice policies.* Beverly Hills, CA: Sage.

Overman, E. S. (Ed.). (1989). *Methodology and epistemology for social sciences: Selected papers in honor of Donald Campbell.* Chicago: University of Chicago Press.

Ray, W. J., & Ravizza, R. (1988). *Methods toward a science of behavior and experience* (3rd ed.). Belmont, CA: Wadsworth.

APPENDIX 3.1
A Glossary of Key Behavioral
Science Research Terms

Confounding variable: A variable that is not manipulated by the researcher, but that may have an unintended effect on the dependent variable.

Control group: The group that does not receive the treatment(s).

Correlation: A measure of the extent to which two variables are related. It does not allow inference about causation.

Dependent variable: A variable that the researcher measures to examine the impact of the independent variable(s).

Diffusion of treatment: A potential confounding variable that may bias the outcome(s) of an experiment (accidentally exposing participants in the control condition[s] to the treatment[s] may affect the results).

Experimental group: The group that receives the treatment(s).

Experimental method: A research method in which phenomena are examined through the manipulation of one or more independent variables.

Experimental mortality: A potential confounding variable that may bias the outcome(s) of a study (dropouts may affect the results).

External validity: The generalizability of the result(s) of a study.

Independent variable: A variable that is systematically manipulated by the researcher to examine some phenomenon.

Instrumentation: A potential confounding variable that may bias the outcome(s) of a study (different instruments may not measure the same construct[s], and this may affect the results).

Internal validity: The degree to which one or more independent variables are responsible for any observed changes in the dependent variable(s).

Matching: Equating participants of a study on a number of dimensions.

Maturation: A potential confounding variable that may bias the outcome(s) of a study (participants' natural maturation process may affect the results).

Pretest–posttest control group design: An experimental research method that involves an assessment of one or more outcomes or dependent variables both prior to and following an experimental intervention.

Program evaluation: A scientific approach that systematically evaluates an existing program or programs.

Quasi-experimental method: A research method that allows researchers to manipulate some aspects of the independent variables(s).

Random assignment: A procedure used to assign participants to various conditions so that only chance dictates the placement.

Reliability: The consistency of the result(s) over time.

Selection bias: A potential confounding variable that may bias the outcome(s) of a study (failure to select participants on the basis of randomization may affect the results).

Solomon four-group design: An experimental research method that adds two additional groups to the pretest–posttest control group design, to allow researchers to directly detect the influence of familiarity with the assessment process.

Testing: A potential confounding variable that may bias the outcome(s) of a study (participants' sensitization to repeated testing may affect the results).

Assessing Community Dispute Resolution Needs

JOSEPH P. FOLGER
Temple University

In every community, representatives of a variety of public and private agencies act as third parties in attempts to resolve disputes. These groups include the clergy, the police, public regulatory agencies, consumer organizations, and advocacy groups, to name only a few. To the extent that these organizations are successful in resolving disputes, they can relieve part of the courts' burden. But when they lack the ability to provide needed interventions, or are inappropriate resources for the disputes brought to them, they can become frustrating false leads as disputes escalate on their way to the courts (Merry, 1979).

Community mediation services are often established to help resolve disputes that are not adequately addressed by available community forums but need not enter the courts. Mediation programs can be tailored to specific needs of a community if planners obtain information about unaddressed disputes and assess existing dispute resolution forums. Such information can reveal places where disputes first surface; it can suggest why available forums fail; and it can provide valuable links to community members who can refer disputes to mediation programs.

The purpose of this chapter is to report partial results of a study that was conducted to assist the development of a court-sponsored program for alternative dispute resolution (ADR). The study attempted to characterize the range and nature of disputes occurring within a community, to assess the out-of-court options for addressing disputes, and to suggest dispute resolution needs that could be met by court-based mediation services. This study illustrates how court administrators or program planners can turn to one research approach for help in designing and launching mediation services.

THE COMPREHENSIVE JUSTICE CENTER

In 1984, the New Jersey Supreme Court's Committee on Complementary Dispute Resolution chose Burlington County as a site for a pilot program in

ADR in the state. The Burlington County Superior Court established the Comprehensive Justice Center in the following year as an umbrella organization to create and coordinate resources for the resolution of disputes. Broadly modeled after the idea of the "Multi-door courthouse" (Sander, 1976; Ray & Clare, 1985), the center's goals are to "enhance access to justice, to decrease court backlog and to provide alternative methods of dispute resolution" (Kruger, 1987, p. 2).

The center houses a small-claims mediation program that was in existence for 4 years before the center was established. This program is closely tied to the small-claims court (i.e., law clerks trained as mediators help to resolve cases during court sessions). The center expands ADR in the county by establishing municipal court mediation programs staffed by trained volunteers from the community. Mediation programs were initially established in 5 of the 33 municipal courts. These programs address a range of disputes, including domestic, neighbor/community, landlord–tenant, and consumer–merchant conflicts. The center's intake unit also refers disputes to other specialized dispute resolution services, including services for complex cases, ethnic/racial disputes, minor civil disputes, and automobile-related conflicts.

The Comprehensive Justice Center is designed as a hybrid program, one that is court-annexed but has heavy community involvement and support. The center's policies are established by a committee composed of Burlington County Bar Association officers, the County Bar Association trustees, and community leaders. Volunteer mediators are recruited from diverse educational and socioeconomic backgrounds in the communities where municipal court mediation programs are established.

OBJECTIVES AND SCOPE OF THE STUDY

As the Comprehensive Justice Center was started, the planners commissioned a study of existing dispute resolution needs. There were three specific objectives for the research: to characterize disputes that were not being resolved with available out-of-court forums; to map and assess formal and informal channels community members used in addressing disputes; and to identify key community people and agencies that could support intake efforts.

The study focused on providing an in-depth analysis of one township within the county. This township, Mount Holly, was chosen for several reasons. It was one of the five communities targeted for a municipal court mediation program. In addition, it was the county seat. This meant that many of the agencies and individuals who acted as mediators or referral agents would be available not only to members of the township being studied, but to the county as a whole. This township also offered a fair demographic representation of several other municipalities in the county. The population of the township was 11,000 at the time of the study; 16% were black, 4% were Puerto Rican, and there were small communities (under 100) of Native American, Korean, and Japanese residents. The township consists mostly of lower-middle-class working families, with a median household income of $16,967 (1980 census). The township has a council–manager government, one high school (1,300 students), one major hospital, and a police department staff of 21 people. The township is a designated historic district in New Jersey.

METHOD

Rationale

Several different research approaches are available to assess dispute resolution needs. These methods range from legal needs assessments that rely on telephone surveys of households (Miller & Sarat, 1981; Benson & Conway, 1976) to participant/observation studies that offer ethnographic accounts of conflict processes in neighborhoods (Merry, 1979). The method employed in this study provided a detailed, descriptive account of dispute processing from the point of view of third parties who heard about or addressed a wide range of conflicts. The study relied on in-depth interviews with key informants to obtain detailed information about how disputes were addressed within the community (Spradley, 1979; Whyte, 1984). In studying the channels in place outside the courthouse door, the study attempted to profile the conflicts that eluded quantification but had a significant impact on the quality of life for community members. The interviews provided detailed examples of how disputes first surfaced, who responded, and what impeded or enhanced effective intervention.

The study examined disputes between individuals, between individuals and organizations, and between organizations. These disputes fell into the following categories: interpersonal/property (harassment, vandalism, conflicts within households over money or responsibilities); interfamily (children, pets, nuisance); environmental issues (noise, property upkeep); consumer problems (landlord–tenant, products, service contracts); government (entitlement eligibility); and community concerns (racial/ethnic conflicts, youths, changing neighborhoods).

Informants

The individuals chosen as informants for the study included representatives of agencies and organizations who became involved in disputes, acted as third parties in attempts to resolve conflicts, or heard about conflicts that went unaddressed in the community. In addition, individuals who were identified as key community members and were marked as good sources of information about community dynamics were also interviewed. Informants were identified by the center's personnel and through an examination of the census report for the township. In addition, during the interviews, informants were asked whether they could suggest other individuals who might provide useful information. This procedure identified potential informants and also helped validate the initial list, since much overlap and considerable repetition of names were observed in the suggestions made by different sources.

A total of 40 interviews were conducted with agency representatives and community members from May through August 1986. The informants came from diverse groups within the township, including several social service agencies, religious organizations, business and consumer associations, police and hospital personnel, racial and ethnic support organizations, and neighborhood groups (see Appendix 4.1 for a list of these organizations). Eight people who were identified as community leaders were also interviewed. This group included members of the clergy, a physician, a former police administrator, and neighborhood spokespeople.

Pilot Study

A pilot study was conducted to enable the researchers to develop a set of questions that could serve as an effective basis for the interviews, and to evaluate the interviews in light of the study's objectives, making any necessary adjustments before proceeding. Two sets of questions were developed for the pilot interviews (see Appendix 4.2). One protocol was designed for interviews with representatives of agencies or organizations who intervened in particular types of disputes or acted on behalf of a particular subgroup within the community. The second protocol was developed for interviews with key community members who might provide overviews of disputes in the community but who were not speaking for any particular agency or organization. Both protocols were only starting points for the interviews; interviewers pursued ideas and issues as the informants raised them. Six people were interviewed in the pilot study. Each person was interviewed by two members of the research team, and all interviews were audiotape-recorded with permission. The interviews lasted from 45 to 90 minutes.

In general, informants had little difficulty providing the information sought in the interviews. In the case of people speaking as key community members, there was variability in their knowledge of different kinds of disputes. This limitation suggested that a sufficient number and variety of people needed to be interviewed to study a broad outline of disputes. It was apparent from the pilot interviews that some agency officials did not keep records on disputes that arose during their work at the organization. This was the case when disputes were ones that were indirectly related to the agency's work but were not specifically addressed as part of the organization's official function. The disputes were related to counseling or some other function the agency served. Information about these disputes was seen as crucial, because they were disputes that might go unaddressed.

An issue arose in one of the pilot interviews that was recognized as a possible threat to gaining accurate and complete information about disputes in the community. An administrator at one agency questioned how the information obtained from the study would be used. His concern was that the new mediation center might divert cases from his agency; since the agency's funding was contingent upon the number of cases handled, his budget might be jeopardized. This issue was important methodologically, because if agencies feared such an outcome, this fear could influence the type of information their representatives provided. Although informants knew the general purposes of the planned mediation service, it was clear from this pilot interview that informants should be made aware that the center would not replace any current services provided to the community. Rather, its purpose would be (and is) to fill gaps in service or to respond to overflow cases. Folberg and Taylor (1984) make a similar point when they suggest that program developers need to convey to helping agencies and professionals that "mediation is not a duplication of services already being provided by other professions" (p. 308).

FINDINGS

The study provided a wide range of information about the emergence and resolution of disputes in the township. The focus here is on describing (1) possible sources of referrals for unaddressed disputes, (2) constraints on existing dispute resolution forums that limited or impeded their effectiveness, and (3) influences on disputants' willingness to avail themselves of mediation services.

Referral Sources

Many of the community and governmental agencies contacted in this study did not officially engage in dispute resolution, but they became aware of disputes through their relationships with the public. Representatives from various organizations offered first-hand accounts of domestic, neighbor, community, or consumer disputes that came to their attention and were often related to the services they provided but were left unaddressed. Several examples help illustrate how disputes first surfaced through local community organizations and governmental agencies.

A troubling set of domestic disputes between parents and children came to the attention of a community program addressing housing emergencies.

These disputes would arise when a child (or some member of the household) was asked to move out because of unresolved conflicts. A representative of the housing emergency agency reported a large number of calls related to these underlying domestic disputes. She characterized these calls as follows:

> A person has a conflict with his parents. The parents throw him out and he tries to get emergency help. Sometimes he is up for 24 hours. That's about all we can do. Then he's back on the street; the police pick him up, and they try to convince the parents to take him back, and the parents don't want to do that. Or the person will leave when the police are called. And we'll get a call sometimes from the police, sometimes from the person who's been put out. The police will make them leave, and then the police will call us and ask us if there is any way we can help this person out.

> There's a lot of disputes that go on that we hear about through housing calls. People who are living together . . . get into some type of horrendous argument, and somebody is put out. Sometimes it's a young mother with a baby where the parents have been taking care of them, and they just can't tolerate the behavior any more. I think there is a lot of that. We look at it as a housing problem. We send these to Emergency Services or Catholic Welfare. Emergency Services can put people up for 24 or 48 hours, and then [they] are out on the street again. So they have to go back to the family. Some accommodation has to be made so that they have a place to live.

In these instances, domestic disputes triggered the need for emergency housing. However, the housing assistance did little to alleviate the underlying conflict that prompted the call for help.

Neighbor disputes came to the attention of several different agencies. A caseworker from the Division of Youth and Family Service in the county reported, for example, that often complaints about child neglect or abuse proved on investigation to be ploys in ongoing neighbor disputes:

> We get calls from an anonymous neighbor who says, "I saw Mary Jane beat her child." "When did you see this, Miss?" "I saw this 3 weeks ago." "Where were you?" "I was at her house and we were having a fight." Then when I go to the house, either they had borrowed money, or the kid had broken a fence, or there's unpaid drugs or just regular internal neighbor issues that should be resolved among themselves but [aren't], and they use the outside agencies as a means of venting their hostilities inappropriately.

The agency did not intervene in such disputes once the charge of neglect or abuse was found to be unwarranted. Head Start, the Welfare Board, and other agencies working with low-income families reported receiving similar complaints of neighbor disputes, often because the party making the complaint had a relationship with the agency through a counselor or other staff person and perceived that this was a place to turn when a problem arose. Most agencies would not become involved in such disputes. Occasionally, a caseworker would act as an advisor or advocate.

Elderly people maintaining their own homes were sometimes involved in unique neighbor conflicts, according to local agencies providing services to senior citizens. The Office on Aging, and in particular the Bar Association Lawyer Referral Service, responded each year to cases in which formal complaints were filed against elderly homeowners because of their inability to maintain property, do yardwork, or the like. When such a complaint was filed, the senior citizen would often turn to the Lawyer Referral Service for assistance. Sometimes the volunteer lawyers who staffed this program attempted to act informally to settle the problem. In one case, a complaint was filed against a woman because her half of a duplex house was in ill repair and rubbish remained uncleared from the yard and surrounding area. The attorney who took the call cleaned the yard himself as a favor to the woman to get the charges dropped. A spokesperson for the Office on Aging noted, however, that neighbor complaints against the elderly "don't ever seem to get resolved a lot of times," especially when the same neighbors complained repeatedly about the same problems.

Certain juvenile complaints surfaced through specialized agencies in this community. For example, the Family Case Management Intake Office oversees juvenile offenses and routes them into the appropriate channels. An arm of this office is the Juvenile Conference Committee, a set of volunteer panels addressing charges made against young people when the juveniles' guilt is admitted or assumed. The panels try to find a means of restitution for the offense that will be instructional for the offender as well as remunerative. Some cases described by informants from this committee resulted from conflicts between juveniles or between the juveniles' parents. The background dispute would become apparent as the charge was investigated during intake or at the Conference Committee meetings. An administrator offered the following description of a case that she considered to be appropriate for mediation rather than for the Conference Committee:

> I had a case yesterday where an 11-year-old girl was charged with assault. She allegedly hit a 7-year-old boy with an open hand in the back of the head. And it is definitely a neighbor problem. They live across the street. This has been going on for over a year. There's problems between the parents. The parents go home and tell the kids what creeps the other one is. . . . The victim was calling me up the day before, and when I met the child, the way he was describing her was two different kids. . . . And it went back to a thing about the cat was on the neighbor's car a year ago.

Although the problem above was presented as a juvenile offense, it was clearly embedded in a deeper neighbor issue. Juveniles' offenses were often symptoms of broader problems that were usually not addressed by the committee. A minister who sat on the Juvenile Conference Committee noted that such cases were common:

> In some of the cases the problem with the kids was not a problem with the kids; it was a problem with the parents. "I don't like you, so I'm not going to let Johnny play with your child, but Johnny and your child get along fine, but I can't tolerate it, so I make the problem." Yes, there is one type where you'd like to get both parties in, and one time we did. . . . We said to the parents, "Look, you complain about these kids, Let's send these kids into another room and we'll go look behind one-way mirrors, and you watch them play together nicely, but what we sense from both of your children is that you don't get along together, and let's talk about your problem."

One administrator at the Family Case Management Intake Office estimated that about 30% of her caseload (10–15 cases per month) involved ongoing disputes.

Besides domestic and neighbor conflicts, landlord–tenant and consumer disputes also came to the attention of community and governmental agencies. One type of landlord–tenant conflict, for example, was described by a spokeswoman for the Citizen Advocacy Program, an organization that works with disabled and mentally retarded individuals in the county. Renters with physical disabilities sometimes have special needs for adaptive equipment that can result in disputes with landlords over how those needs will be met. The program representative described a situation involving a deaf mother of a 5-year-old child. This woman needed a light indicating when the back door was open, allowing her to keep track of her child. Having the fixture could help prevent the Division of Youth and Family Service from claiming that she was an unfit mother. The landlord refused to provide the equipment.

Similarly, Head Start representatives indicated that landlord–tenant disputes often arose in families of Head Start children and that they would act as advocates in the disputes. A spokesperson for the county Welfare Board noted that the three caseworkers who worked with the elderly and disabled were each involved in three or four landlord–tenant conflicts at any one time.

These examples typify the first-line appeals that disputants made to various government and community agencies as they sought outside help for resolving family, neighbor, or consumer disputes. Many agency representatives believed that unresolved disputes often brought clients to their doors. These cases support previous research by Merry and Silbey (1984) suggesting that disputants know of and attempt to use a wide range of helping and service agencies as they cope with unresolved conflict. Reports from our informants support Merry and Silbey's view that disputants, in effect, shop around and even redefine problems to elicit action from various agencies, which may not in themselves be designed to resolve disputes. The neighbor disputes that went to the Juvenile Conference Committee, and the landlord–tenant disputes that went to the Citizen Advocacy Program, were couched in terms that legitimized bringing them to the attention of a known agency.

In several instances described above, disputants knew individuals at the agency on a personal basis because of an ongoing provider relationship with the organization. In cases such as these, the social service agencies may be approached with disputes because they provide clients with the only known third party who regularly acts on their behalf. This ongoing relationship may play a part in determining who is comfortable bringing disputes to outside intervenors. Merry and Silbey (1984) suggest that, because certain segments of the poor interact on a regular basis with welfare and other public agencies, they may be more comfortable turning to public forums to remedy interpersonal disputes than working-class and middle-class families may be.

Although personal relationships with the agencies are important, it is also true that for some groups of people, particular types of disputes arise because of unaddressed needs that are under a service agency's purview. The needs themselves are not the disputes, but the situation the needs create become the basis for conflict (Sarat, 1988). Neighborhood disputes involving the elderly may surface, for example, because senior citizens are unable to maintain their property to an unsympathetic neighbor's satisfaction. The elderly's need for assistance becomes the basis of a neighbor dispute. Similarly, disputes between landlords and tenants involving nonpayment of rent are often rooted in underlying financial needs that social service agencies address. The link between needs and the emergence of disputes contributes to clients' willingness to bring these disputes to the attention of helping agencies.

A network of channels for referring disputes to mediation can be established once it is recognized that disputes often surface through existing agencies and community service organizations (Beer, 1986). Informants in this study often expressed relief that disputes they became aware of through their work could be referred to an appropriate forum once the mediation program was available. They reported cases of conflicts that escalated severely because disputes continued over long periods of time and were beyond their ability to resolve.

Constraints on Existing Forums

The study revealed three types of constraints on existing, out-of-court forums that limited or impeded their ability to provide effective third-party mediation. The first constraint stemmed from agencies' attempts to provide both advocacy and mediation. Serving both functions could potentially undermine mediative efforts. For example, this community has an active Consumer Affairs Office, which informants felt was generally effective in handling consumer complaints. At the time of the study, this office investigated approximately 100 complaints each month about fraudulent business practices. In the main, the agency viewed itself as an advocate offering assistance to disgruntled consumers who might want to bring cases to court. Representatives from the office reported, however, that they would in certain cases mediate disputes between consumers and merchants over issues related to purchases, product maintenance, or the like. This intervention might not always involve face-to-face meetings, but the goal was to reach a mutually acceptable resolution. The informants could not provide any clear overall sense about the effectiveness of this type of intervention. It appeared to be secondary work of the agency.

Although this agency primarily defended consumers against possible merchant abuses, in its nonadvocacy role it provided a service comparable to mediation. Balancing the two roles, however, was difficult, and several forces worked to undermine the mediative role. Merchants might perceive that agency representatives acting as mediators were biased toward the consumers. The public image of this office was and is primarily that of a consumer advocate. As one community leader said, "All you have to do is pick up the phone and call. . . . Their people will take care of it." A phone call from this office to a merchant typically meant that a complaint had been leveled and that the office was willing to assist a consumer. It was difficult for merchants to assume equitable treatment when advocacy played such a large role in the agency's mandate. This perception could easily deter merchants from participating in the mediation process.

Moreover, the office did not address complaints that merchants leveled against consumers, such as bad checks or customer nonpayment. This limited the office's involvement in consumer–merchant disputes, leaving an important gap in this arena and contributing to an overall sense of partiality.

A second constraint on existing forums stemmed from the extent to which agencies chose or were compelled to work within a set of regulations or statutes to shape agreements. In some arenas of conflict, intervenors act in an adjudicative capacity if they view their role as essentially that of interpreting regulations. More mediative interventions establish broader parameters. Third parties search for resolutions that reside within the disputants' own frame of reference, and at times ignore clear adjudicative options.

One agency's approach to intervention illustrates how mediative intervention can be given priority in a context where adjudication is clearly possible. Environmental concerns produced disputes in this community between homeowners and the Historic Preservation Commission. The commission oversees regulations controlling the preservation and restoration of certain buildings in areas that have been designated as historic districts. Informants indicated that such disputes would often emerge when a homeowner wishing to make renovations applied for a building permit and discovered that he or she could not make alterations at will, but must conform with preservation regulations. The Historic Preservation Commission would determine whether specific changes to the buildings were permissible. The commission met with the homeowner and, in a sense, attempted to mediate between the homeowner and the requirements. Commissioners were sometimes able to convince the homeowner of the desirability of alternative changes to the house, or, more frequently, they negotiated tradeoffs between the requirements and the personal preferences or financial constraints of the homeowner.

The commission found mutually acceptable resolutions in all cases that had been brought to it at the time of the study (i.e., the commission approved all building permits). The law provides for an appeal to the City Council if a homeowner refuses to accept the minimal requirements set by the commission. This procedure, at the time of the study, had not been invoked. The commission made a conscious effort to approach cases from a mediative rather than an adjudicative stance, and thus to remove the need for additional intervention. However, in some instances this meant sidestepping straight-forward interpretations of existing regulations.

Other agencies adopted a much stronger adjudicative stance in their approach to interventions. The Landlord–Tenant Panel in this community attempts to mediate a wide array of housing issues. Their approach is heavily guided, however, by housing codes and other regulations. In some instances, as informants noted, panel members inspected properties and in effect rendered decisions about compliance. Although such adjudicative intervention might be necessary in many landlord–tenant disputes, for some conflicts a more mediative intervention might be overlooked because of the panel's general orientation to disputes.

For example, a tenant might fall behind in rent payments. To pressure the tenant, the landlord might turn off the heat. A mediative forum would allow for a variety of options to be negotiated that would stress the parties' needs rather than the demands of specific regulations. The tenant might agree to perform maintenance work to repay back rent, and, in turn, the heat would be restored. A statute-based approach would be more likely to demand specific outcomes according to the terms of the lease, building code regulations, and so on.

Constraints on the timing of an intervention constituted a third factor that the study found to impede the effectiveness of available dispute interventions. Some existing forums interceded at points where effective, long-term intervention was unlikely. Police officers reported this type of constraint as they attempted to intervene in domestic disputes that caused immediate disturbances or threatened someone's safety. One officer interviewed for this study estimated that he spent 8–10 hours each week answering domestic dispute calls in this community. He indicated that these disputes frequently involved substance abuse and that domestic problems of this type tended to recur within the same household:

> We get to know the addresses over and over again. We go back and it's the same thing, domestic dispute. The same thing. We've had three of them at _____ Street in the last three nights. The same thing over and over again.

As Christian (1986) has previously noted, police officers become frustrated with recurring calls such as these and with their own inability to be effective. A spouse who makes such a call frequently refuses to sign a written complaint, and thus no court referral is possible. The officer can file a complaint on probable cause, but many are reluctant to do so, often because the spouse wants the charges dropped. One officer in this study described spouses' reluctance to carry through with a complaint:

> I've seen a lot of these domestic first-time arguments where the husband threatens the wife and you got to throw someone out. Then all of a sudden comes court night and "Well, I don't want to file a complaint against my husband. I want to drop everything, nothing happened. I want to get back together." What we've done with them up until now is to tell them to get a restraining order. They never get it because next day they're called down and they don't want to get the restraining order. They want their husband back in or wife or whatever.

The informants suggested that any attempts to mediate these disputes when the calls were made were ineffective because the situations were usually quite volatile. Stable resolution of these recurring domestic problems could not be found. Police suggested that the option to mediate should be introduced after the police visit, as a follow-up to the decision not to sign a complaint.

Concerns about the timing of available interventions in other areas, such as landlord–tenant disputes, were raised by informants. Agencies responding to these disputes reported that their assistance was frequently sought at a point of severe escalation in the conflicts. When such disputes escalated and involved rent withholding or eviction, a lack of awareness about legal regulations could cause insuperable problems. A tenant withholding rent with good cause might not understand proper procedures for creating escrow accounts and notifying landlords, so an effort to force a landlord to address some issue might backfire against the tenant. Tenants might ignore eviction notices until they received a summons to appear in court. Informants reported that it was not until this late stage that many individuals involved in housing disputes sought intervention, and, at this point, it was too late to assist successfully. These concerns about the timing of available interventions parallel those reported by Roehl (1986) in her assessment of multi-door courthouses and by Shonholtz (1984) in his assessment of traditional justice systems.

Influences on Community Members' Willingness to Use Mediation

The planners of the mediation service wanted to identify any obstacles that might deter people from using the program once it was established. The interviews revealed several influences on community members' willingness to avail themselves of the mediation service.

There was misunderstanding in the community about the nature of mediation, even among those who worked regularly in conflict situations. In several of the interviews, informants raised questions suggesting that they had obtained misleading perceptions of the process. The misunderstandings existed in part because some informants were familiar with the mediation that had been available for some time in the small-claims court.

The small-claims mediation is conducted in a substantially different way than the planned volunteer mediation program was to be. In the small-claims program, judges read the names of plaintiffs and defendants in the cases to be heard. When both parties are present, the case is assigned to a mediator. Cases that cannot be resolved within 30 minutes go back to the judge for a decision. The mediators in the small-claims programs are law clerks. The procedures followed in these sessions are often markedly different from those that are typically recommended for mediation. One small-claims mediator who was observed by a member of the research team did not explain to the disputants that the goal of mediation is to find a mutually satisfactory resolution. Nor did she encourage disputants to discuss their feelings about the issue or press for closure in the session. Of the five mediation sessions observed in small claims, only one concluded with resolution. The others were referred back to the judge.

Judging from the comments made by several interviewees, first-hand and word-of-mouth experience with small-claims mediation left some community members confused about the nature of mediation in general. Roehl (1986) reports similar misperceptions about how mediation programs function in her analysis of multi-door centers. Unless mediation is understood by those who can refer disputes, there may be some hesitancy to recommend using the service.

Cultural or ethnic differences were also found to be a potential influence on community members' willingness to avail themselves of mediation. Concerns have been raised previously about the ways in which racial or cultural differences can influence conflict and mediation (Donohue, 1985; Gulliver, 1979; Goldstein, 1986). This study corroborated such concerns. Informants from minority groups in the community expressed doubt about whether all cultural or ethnic groups would be equally likely to use a mediation program staffed by volunteer mediators. Representatives from the Hispanic Social Service Center indicated that there was a strong cultural preference in the Hispanic community not to air close interpersonal disputes with a stranger. She felt that members of the Hispanic community might turn to mediation if they had disputes with non-Hispanic persons. In this case, however, language barriers might be a deterrent as well. Members of the Hispanic community would need bilingual mediators or translators so that they would not feel disadvantaged during the process.

Three members of the clergy from this community were interviewed in this study about their role in addressing domestic disputes. Two of the clergy were from white Protestant churches, and the third was from a black congregation. The two white ministers reported being approached regularly by church members for help with domestic conflicts. The black cleric was rarely asked for assistance in such disputes. Although these findings are clearly preliminary, they could be suggestive of differences in the way dispute resolution channels are perceived by different racial groups. Such differences might extend to how receptive various ethnic groups are to employing mediation services. If cultural differences do exist, it is unclear whether volunteer mediation programs would be more or less appealing to people from different racial backgrounds.

Finally, the accessibility of the mediation program emerged as a possible influence on whether community members would use the service. Among the groups of people identified as likely candidates for using the program were those with low or fixed incomes. Representatives of agencies working with these groups expressed a strong concern about the mediation program's accessibility. The court location would restrict access for people of limited mobility, especially because there was minimal public transportation available. For the program to be widely accessible, informants suggested that alternative locations or provisions for transportation be provided. The concerns raised about accessibility support Folberg and Taylor's (1984) call for establishing appropriate environments for mediation programs.

IMPLICATIONS

The results of this study influenced the development of the Comprehensive Justice Center in several ways. First, information obtained in the study prompted plans for responding to disputes that involved different cultural groups in the community. Bilingual mediators were recruited, translators were sought, and special training in cultural and ethnic differences was designed for the volunteer mediators. Second, given the misperceptions found in the community about the nature of mediation, the planners undertook additional outreach and public relations efforts to clarify the program's goals and procedures. Third, the planners took steps to ensure that mediations were conducted in places where disputants of all income and age levels could employ the service. Finally, the study set in place a network of people at agencies and organizations that acted as valuable referral sources for disputes as the program unfolded. Disputes that might not otherwise have surfaced were referred regularly to the center.

At a somewhat broader level, the study also suggests that mediation programs can best supplement dispute resolution needs in a community if the program is based on an examination of the different outcomes that existing out-of-court forums provide. Resolution of a dispute means different outcomes for different out-of-court forums. For most police intervention in domestic disputes, for example, resolution means that no more calls come from the home. Substantive issues prompting the complaint are rarely addressed. For other programs, resolution means addressing substantive issues and constructing an agreement that all parties accept. Other forums, such as the Landlord–Tenant Panel, resolve disputes by reaching settlements that are in accord with a set of statutes (e.g., housing code regulations). For still other agencies, resolution means that parties are referred to another source for possible assistance. Such referrals are considered resolutions because they may be made to an agency that addresses a need related to a dispute (e.g., emergency housing for a young adult who is asked to leave a parent's home). Any assessment of dispute resolution needs must clarify what existing forums consider resolution and assess whether these outcomes supplement, fall short of, or are consistent with the goals of the planned mediation service.

Perhaps the greatest benefit of conducting a needs assessment is that in the process of consulting with key community people and agencies, their awareness and understanding of the program is reinforced. The needs assessment itself becomes an effective way to imbed the program in the community it intends to serve. In offering her assessment of multi-door courthouse programs, Roehl (1986, p. 29) notes, "The means by which citizens come to the Multi-Door Centers have important effects. They determine, in large part, the nature of the caseload, the scope of the centers' services, and the public's and legal community's image and use of the program." A needs assessment study can shape the means by which citizens come to a mediation program. It can establish an effective, community-based network for referring important disputes that often remain unaddressed.

Acknowledgments

I would like to thank the Honorable Martin L. Haines, who initiated the Comprehensive Justice Center, and Judith Kruger, the first director of the program. Michel Avery, Patricia Foley, and Patrick McLaurin deserve special thanks for their valuable contributions in conducting the study and writing the initial project report.

REFERENCES

Beer, J. E. (1986). *Peacemaking in your neighborhood*. Philadelphia: New Society.

Benson, D. K., & Conway, R. (1976). *Patterns of legal needs in the Columbus metropolitan area: A report to the Columbus Bar Association*. Columbus, OH: Columbus Bar Association.

Christian, T. F. (1986). A resource for all seasons: A state-wide network of community dispute resolution centers. In J. E. Palenski & H. M. Launer (Eds.), *Mediation contexts and challenges* (pp. 85–94). Springfield, IL: Charles C Thomas.

Donohue, W. (1985). Ethnicity and mediation. In W. B. Gudykunst, L. P. Stewart, & S. Ting-Toomey (Eds.), *Communication, culture and organizational processes* (pp. 134–154). Beverly Hills, CA: Sage.

Folberg, J., & Taylor, A. (1984). *Mediation: A comprehensive guide to resolving conflicts without litigation*. San Francisco: Jossey-Bass.

Goldstein, S. (1986). *Cultural issues in mediation: A literature review* (University of Hawaii Program on Conflict Resolution Working Paper, 1986, No. 1). Honolulu: University of Hawaii Program on Conflict Resolution.

Gulliver, P. H. (1979). *Disputes and negotiation: A cross-cultural perspective*. New York: Academic Press.

Kruger, J. A. (1987). *Comprehensive Justice Center Summary of Accomplishments May 1985–December 1986*. Unpublished manuscript, Burlington County Superior Court, Burlington County, New Jersey.

Merry, S. E. (1979). Going to court: Strategies of dispute resolution in an American urban neighborhood. *Law and Society Review, 13*, 891–925.

Merry, S. E., & Silbey, S. S. (1984). What do plaintiffs want? Reexamining the concept of dispute. *Justice System Journal, 9*(2), 151–178.

Miller, R., & Sarat, A. (1981). Grievances, claims and disputes: Assessing the advocacy culture. *Law and Society Review, 15*(4), 525–565.

Ray, L., & Clare, A. L. (1985). The multi-door courthouse idea: Building the courthouse of the future . . . today. *Ohio State Journal on Dispute Resolution, 1*(1), 7–54.

Roehl, J. A. (1986). *The Multi-Door Courthouse Project of the American Bar Association Special Committee on Dispute Resolution: Phase I. Intake and referral assessment* (National Institute of Justice Grant Executive Summary). Washington, DC: National Institute of Justice.

Sander, F. (1976). The multi-door courthouse: Settling disputes in the year 2000. *The Barrister, 3*, 18–21, 40–42.

Sarat, A. (1988). The "new frontier" in disputing and dispute processing. *Law and Society Review, 21*(5), 695–715.

Shonholtz, R. (1984). Neighborhood justice systems: Work, structure and guiding principles. *Mediation Quarterly, 5,* 3–30.

Spradley, J. P. (1979). *The ethnographic interview.* New York: Holt, Rinehart & Winston.

Whyte, W. F. (1984). *Learning from the field.* Beverly Hills, CA: Sage.

APPENDIX 4.1
Community Organizations and Agencies Contacted in the Needs Assessment

American Association of Retired Persons
Animal Control Office
Bar Association Lawyer Referral Service
Better Business Bureau
Caring Center
Children's Home
Christian Retirement Center
Citizen Advocacy Program
Community Action Program
Community Nursing Association
Consumer Affairs Office
CONTACT of United Way
Department of Human Services
Division of Youth and Family Service
Downtown Business Association
Family Case Management Intake Office
Head Start
Hispanic Social Service Center
Human Services Agency
Juvenile Conference Committee
Landlord–Tenant Panel
Legal Services
Mount Holly Police Force
National Association for the Advancement of Colored People
Neighborhood Watch
Office on Aging
Preservation Commission of Historic Mount Holly
Prosecutor's Office Victim–Witness Assistance Unit
Retired Senior Volunteer Program
The Well (a religious counseling service)
Volunteers in Probation
Welfare Board

APPENDIX 4.2
Question Protocols for Open-Ended
Needs Assessment Interviews

AGENCY AND ORGANIZATION INFORMANTS

1. How did the agency get established? What prompted its development?
2. What types of disputes/problems does your agency address?
3. Out of the general areas covered by the agency, what cases would not be addressed?
4. Are there records available summarizing: the number of cases addressed, the outcomes of the cases, participants' satisfaction with the outcomes?
5. Does the agency address certain subgroups in the community? What other agencies address similar groups?
6. Describe the process that is followed in addressing cases. Are forms used? Are face-to-face meetings held? How long does it take to resolve cases?
7. How is the organization perceived in the community? How effective is the agency in addressing disputes it handles or hears about? What improvements do you see as critical? What might prevent the agency from making these improvements?
8. Does the agency have links with other services in the community? Is there overlap with other services?
9. In what ways could the proposed mediation service assist in this area?

KEY COMMUNITY MEMBER INFORMANTS

1. Where do people in this community bring problems/disputes for out-of-court help in the following areas: interpersonal disputes, property disputes, interfamily conflicts, environmental issues, consumer disputes, problems with government agencies, community or neighborhood conflicts?
2. Have there been any key incidents that triggered the development of conflict-focused agencies or services?
3. Which available services do you see as most successful? Why? Which have been least successful? Why?
4. Do any out-of-control forums for settling disputes have particularly positive or negative reputations in the community? Why?
5. What disputes are not addressed by available forums? Are any particular subgroups of people not well attended to?
6. Who else do you know in the community who might be knowledgeable about disputes and dispute resolution channels?

Note: These protocols were only general guides for interviews. Specific topics were pursued as they arose in each interview.

Marketing Mediation Programs

LISA HICKS
Center for Dispute Settlement, Inc.
Lyons, New York

LETITIA J. ROSENTHAL
Center for Dispute Settlement, Inc.,
Geneseo, New York

LYNNE STANDISH
Lifeline, Inc.,
Rochester, New York

Mediation, ancient as a skill, is a relatively new concept as it is offered to the general public. Although superior to many of the existing ways of dealing with interpersonal problems, it can be ineffectual unless those in need of it are aware of its availability and understand what it is. Implementation of a marketing strategy can help alleviate much of the uncertainty associated with both the service and the service provider when a program is introduced to a new area.

WHY MARKET?

Nearly every activity undertaken by a service-oriented program will have an impact on its acceptance and success. The whole area of human services is often closely scrutinized because of its dependence on outside funding sources. This scrutiny makes it imperative that a marketing plan be considered at an early stage in the evolution of a new service. Kotler and Andreasen (1987) advise that marketing is not something that happens on the periphery of an organization, but grows out of the organization's mission to serve some human need. Many marketing strategies are planned and carried out without ever being labeled as such by program directors who are attempting to encourage members of their community either to support or to use their service.

MARKETING DEFINED

"Marketing" is that practice of communication that enables service providers to link certain designated groups (publics) with available services and/or products for which they have a want or need. The publics that need to be considered when a program director is planning a marketing strategy for alternative dispute resolution (ADR) are (1) the agencies whose services the ADR program will be augmenting (i.e., potential referral sources such as the courts), (2) the parties who will make use of ADR's services (i.e., the general public), and (3) those groups within the community from whom ADR staff and volunteers will solicit financial support for the program's endeavors.

The observations and practices described in this chapter have been gleaned primarily from our 15 years of collective experience in managing county-wide programs in ADR for a nonprofit organization based in western New York. Most of what is contained herein is applicable to any similar organization that provides a mediation service for its community.

BUDGETING CONCERNS IN MARKETING

Now that the necessity for marketing has been determined, it is essential to point out the budgetary concerns that must be taken into account in an effort to make the public aware of a community mediation program's existence.

Many community mediation centers are operating on limited budgets because of funding constraints. McGillis (1986) cites three distinct types of dispute resolution programs: justice-system-based, community-based, and composite programs. Most community-based and composite programs are not-for-profit organizations that expend the greater portion of their budget on personnel, office rental, and needed support equipment. It is evident, then, that the ordinary methods of marketing (e.g., paid newspaper advertising, radio and television advertisements, posters, and billboards) are less affordable methods of program promotion for most ADR centers. Many offices are understaffed and often are run by one person. It is rare that these small operations can afford the luxury of hiring a public relations expert to promote a program in a professional fashion over a long period of time.

Effective marketing is often accomplished through personal contacts with referral sources, such as local town and village justices. However, because many centers are located in rural areas with considerable distances to travel, budget constraints make this mode of program promotion difficult and costly.

Professional printing costs, as well as lack of funds to hire artists and layout designers, make if difficult to print pamphlets, newsletters, and posters. Staff members must find the time to design and lay out these promotional items themselves. Furthermore, the costs of postage to send program updates, newsletters, and pamphlets become prohibitive for smaller programs.

It is our experience that in order to use any of the above-mentioned marketing methods on a regular basis, one must borrow from another line item in the budget in order to make up for the lack in the public relations area. Moreover, because of the additional burden that marketing puts on the one-person office, it is often an area that is direly in need of attention.

The remainder of this chapter, therefore, is intended to aid programs with similar budget concerns. It is our aim to assist readers in setting up a marketing program, to indicate the necessary tools for marketing, and to share our ideas for cost-effective marketing.

INITIAL MARKETING STRATEGIES

The decision to begin a community mediation program must take many factors into account. As with any concept that is referred to as an "alternative," it may be difficult breaking ground and marketing the idea. For this reason, it is of utmost importance to research the need for the service.

Generally, the mediation program will be relying on the law enforcement and judicial branches of the criminal justice system for initial as well as long-term referrals to the program. Our experience has shown that in order to pursue these areas effectively, the program director must show that the mediation process will complement rather than hinder the procedures already in place. For instance, the process of making a referral should be as painless as possible. If the program staff inundates other agencies with multiple forms and paperwork, and complicates the work of the referring officer, judge, or human service worker, the "alternative" does not seem as attractive.

Researching the Need

Statistics are available through local police agencies and the state judicial districts that detail the number of complaints, the number of arrests, and court caseloads each year. The breakdown of these caseloads is helpful to the professional who is beginning a mediation program. It is necessary to examine the number of violations and misdemeanors handled by the courts in the target area. Once the extent of criminal activity is understood, the next step is to examine the disposition of these cases. The mediation professional should be aware of the length of time each case has been pending (number of days to disposition), as well as what the exact disposition of the case was. Was a defendant fined or given community service? Was the matter simply adjourned by the court? Research into the operation of the local courts and law enforcement agencies can readily be translated into data demonstrating the need for a mediation program.

It is important to stress that a thorough exploration of existing systems must be completed before local officials are contacted.

Preparing an Introduction

The mediation professional must be aware of who the organization's relevant publics might be and determine how best to communicate with these specific groups (Lauffer, 1984). Since it has been determined that the mediation program will probably be relying on law enforcement officials as well as criminal court judges for referrals, we describe how to organize a presentation for these officials.

The mission of the mediation program, and specific ways in which it will benefit existing programs, constitute a good place to start. Mediation can be very successful. It can be the basis for achieving new understandings, finding common ground, and developing win–win solutions; this notion must be relayed during these discussions. The mission of mediation, it must be stressed, is to offer a successful alternative form of conflict resolution by gaining the disputing parties' agreement to participate in a nonthreatening, neutral, and fair forum that will assist them in reaching a successful resolution of their dispute.

The benefits of the mediation process are many, and exploring these thoroughly is crucial to the success of the marketing package. The program director should be specific in one-to-one situations with potential referral sources: He or she should ask about their caseloads and be quick to point out those situations where mediation might help them to bring about quicker and more peaceful justice.

For example, it is well known that law enforcement agencies must respond to many "callbacks" regarding neighbor disputes. The police officer becomes a short-term mediator who may quell a disturbance for a day or a week, but before he or she knows it, the conflict has erupted once again. After several return trips, it becomes evident that the problem is not going to go away. Does the officer now make an arrest? If the officer does have sufficient reason to make an arrest, is a fine or jail time going to resolve the problem between these neighbors? Probably not. Has the real problem even been addressed? Probably not. If an officer can identify with the problem as outlined so far, the mediation professional can take the matter one step further: What would happen if the case were referred to mediation? First, the session would be confidential, so the parties could maintain their community standing and dignity. The hearing would also be scheduled much sooner in most cases than a trial date would be. Moreover, both parties would have an opportunity to tell "the whole story" (a luxury our courts cannot afford). And finally, the parties would have input into any agreement that came out of the session, and would therefore be more personally invested in it.

The same kind of scenario can be utilized in speaking with judges and court clerks. Violations such as harassment and aggravated harassment take up a good deal of court time and make excellent cases for mediation. Parties who are truly committed to their dispute find much satisfaction in discussing their problem with a neutral third party in a private forum, rather than in front of a judge in a public courtroom. It is important for a program director to stress to judges (especially in smaller town and village courts) that he or she is not suggesting taking their cases away from them, but is merely asking them to adjourn some matters for a set period of time so that the parties may attempt to resolve their disputes in a nonadversarial forum.

One drawback to being a new mediation professional attempting to expand a program is that the professional probably does not have overall program success stories and compliance rates to quote during the presentation. If such information can be requested from an umbrella agency, it will help validate the proposal. Also, the professional should not be afraid to ask for assistance from a program that is already operational. Everybody loves to share success stories.

Now, with the mission outlined, the benefits of the mediation program detailed, and successful examples and compliance data in tow, the program director is ready to make the crucial contacts in the target area.

Making Contacts

The discussion so far has concentrated on the research and preparation of the program's presentation to officials, specifically those in the law enforcement and judicial areas. A telephone call to schedule a meeting is the first step. The program director should not take it upon himself or herself to "drop in" on very busy people. The message to be relayed is an important one, and the director needs to ensure that he or she will have time to present it in its entirety.

The director should make every effort to meet with the top official, as well as with anyone else necessary. It has been evident time and time again that the top official (i.e., the police chief or sheriff) is not necessarily the individual with whom all future contacts will be made. The reason for contacting law enforcement and court officials is to gain support for the program to move into their area. These people will be the life or death of the program with regard to referrals; however, there are many other crucial contacts to be made. If the targeted area has a county administrator or manager, a board of supervisors, or other named administrative body, these persons are of utmost importance as well. Generally, a mediation program is operating on a shoestring budget—one in which no budget line exists for office rental space—and these officials can often be instrumental in finding a spot for a program that they feel will benefit their community. Making a well-researched, concise presentation of the ADR program's goals and objectives will move the director closer to the possibility of seeing the program begin.

There is nothing harder than being the "new service on the block" and asking for money for the program. If obtaining money is difficult, the program director may consider requesting in-kind office space and the use of a copying machine and telephone. It is often easier for a county to shuffle the office space issue in order to get a program off the ground than it is to guarantee a set start-up dollar amount. Very often, a board of supervisors will pass a resolution that outlines the points agreed upon with the mediation program regarding this start-up. This resolution is also a confirmed, written recognition of the target area's genuine support for the program.

Now that the groundwork has been laid and a top official has granted his or her support for the mediation program, many logistics need to be worked out.

Developing Marketing Tools

Once the office location has been determined, the total marketing package moves to the next step, which is the representation of the program through stationery, brochures, and business cards. The color and logo for the office stationery must be considered carefully, as these choices will reflect the image of the program. All other printed materials should be consistent in color and bear this logo. The mission at this point is to "get the message" out to many other contacts than have been previously noted. The program director's personal appearance and knowledge of the subject, as well as the information sent on stationery with a brochure enclosed, will certainly be the keys to those contacts remembering the director and the message.

Let us examine the subject of brochures in more detail. The program director has established the colors the office will be noted for; he or she has developed a logo that is uniquely the program's and reflects the mediation process; so he or she must now carefully consider the contents of the brochure. The first and most important question is this: "Who needs to read these brochures?" It may be a referral source, it may be the prospective parties in the program, or it may be both. If it is assumed that a person reading the brochures takes at most a few minutes to decide whether or not to make use of the program, what things should be stressed?

The office brochure must be clear, concise, and interesting, whether a client or a judge is reviewing it. It must explain how the process of mediation works, what the cost of the program (if any) is, how an individual can obtain the service, and what the outcome of the service is intended to be. Some programs' brochures note case examples or scenarios that would be appropriate for the service of mediation.

The program budget will probably reveal that there are very limited funds for printing; therefore, a well-thought-out single brochure is essential. If the director has initial input into the budget, he or she should be sure to target funds for ongoing advertising and updating of program literature.

If the budget will allow it, a poster should be printed as part of a successful marketing package. If there is a college or university in the target area, the program director might consider contacting the graphic arts department in the fall, when there may be students interested in a class project. The program may be lucky enough to receive some creative talent for next to nothing. The director should keep options open and should always be thinking of what resources are at hand.

Now that an impressive array of marketing tools has been assembled, the program director's best friend becomes the telephone. The director must be aggressive and assertive in making contacts in the community. Some suggestions for contacts would include the district attorney's office, local courts, police and sheriff's departments, state police, the department of social services, probation officers, school counselors, the local bar association, and area clergy. After each scheduled appointment with local contacts, a letter thanking them for their time is a necessary and very professional touch. The closer the program office is to the county seat (or the local circle of criminal justice professionals), the better. It is good for these contacts to see the director and the office, and to know that the director is busy. This is how additional referrals come about, because once the groundwork has been established, the service itself must be proven to be effective, expedient, and inexpensive.

Media Involvement

Each of the aforementioned tools is basic to the marketing package, but the program director must take extra steps to promote the newborn service whenever possible. Being "the new kid on the block" can be used to advantage. The local media (television, radio, newspapers) can become involved in the new venture in several ways.

An open house can be used as a way to get the entire community to focus on the new service. Invited guests can include all of the local judges, police, human service representatives, and community leaders. The director should contact radio stations about the time of the open house, and should send a press release to the newspapers prior to the event. If a news conference can be organized, all local officals should be aware of this; they rarely miss an opportunity for publicity. The director should take advantage of this event to *shine*—to talk about the program and its benefits, and to discuss with those present other ways to gain support and acceptance. There are no better contacts for good ideas than the people who have been working in the system, especially if they believe that the new program will be making their job easier. These contacts should always be asked whether they know of other areas in which the program might be promoted. The director must be persistent if the message is to be heard and the mission to be realized.

Advisory Board

As the mediation professional is making various contacts in the community, it is helpful to keep in mind the idea of an advisory board for the program. The members of the board will bring credibility to the program, but, beyond that, will offer advice and support to the staff. Since many mediation programs can be sorely understaffed, this support is vital and can be a real source of encouragement to the program director. The board should be composed of individuals representing various branches of the criminal justice system (e.g., a probation officer, a state trooper, the sheriff, a local attorney, a local justice), someone from the school community (e.g., a school counselor, the superintendent, a school psychologist), and a representative of the business community, as well as one or more of the mediators. The board members will help the staff identify new areas of referrals and funding and will go back to their respective offices promoting the program.

Public Education

Because the whole concept of mediation may be unfamiliar to the people who reside in the area the program serves, they may need to be educated about its many benefits. Many community groups, such as the Kiwanis, Rotary, and Lions Clubs, have weekly or biweekly meetings and are always looking for informative and interesting presentations. Church groups, women's circles, and senior citizens' gatherings are all places where people will be interested in the new program and eager to carry the message further into the community.

Contact should also be made with educators and guidance counselors. A mediator can offer to make presentations to social studies classes or to work with small groups on problem-solving skills. The local youth bureau should not be overlooked when exploring youth programs, as they are often a source of inspiration, additional contacts, and funding. Mediators should let the youth bureau director know that they are available for local youth conferences and as a resource for any ongoing teen programs.

Almost all professionals who have coordinated a community mediation program will admit to times when they felt they were operating in a vacuum—when the program's survival seemed to depend solely on their efforts. For this reason, it is very important for a program director to become part of a professional association in the community, such as a criminal justice council. Meeting regularly with other human service providers will allow the director to update the program by keeping it current to the needs of the community, to make new contacts, and to continue to strive for the program's acceptance as the "new service on the block."

ONGOING MARKETING STRATEGIES

Maintaining Credibility

It is important to maintain the reputation and character of the established ADR program by providing services of the quality that the program initially undertook to deliver. It is helpful in this respect to keep all agencies and individuals who refer matters for mediation apprised of the overall success of the program. In the instance of a court-supported program, this can be done by participating in the local magistrates' association and by providing prompt feedback to all individuals who refer cases. If there is a video or slide show available that demonstrates the mediation process, this should be shown to justices so that they have a clearer expectation of the service being offered. In some instances, and with the consent of the disputing parties, it may be possible to allow referral sources to observe the mediation process.

Case Examples

Whenever a program director has an opportunity to address either funders or parties who refer matters to mediation, it is a good practice to present several case examples. These examples should be modified to protect the anonymity of the participants, but should include reasons for referral, a capsule version of the dispute, underlying issues that surfaced during the mediation, a condensed version of any agreement, and an opinion as to why mediation was important in that instance. It makes the program more "real" for those supporting it if they can see how its efforts are affecting people in the community.

Program Feedback

Several areas of interest can be monitored for program feedback and used in most discussions of the program. A chart or graph can demonstrate the disposition of all matters referred to mediation in a given time period. Individual reports can be made to local justices and other human service agencies detailing the number of cases they referred; the number of cases successfully resolved; and the ways in which the disposition of their referrals measure up to those of referrals from other courts, agencies, and so on. Local funders are also interested in knowing the effect their money is having and enjoy getting feedback on office activities.

The mediation process itself can also be monitored to determine its effectiveness. The questionnaire shown in Appendix 5.1 was developed by one of our advisory boards as a check for program effectiveness and has been used to ascertain how individuals who have gone through the mediation process perceived both the process and the mediator.

Visiting and Contacting Referral Sources

Most parties who refer cases to a mediation center have already made a commitment to the process. Individual meetings provide the time for a mediation professional to share any feedback information, discuss cases for possible referral, and put a face behind the service. When a service such as mediation is offered, there is something intangible about what the person is receiving. It differs from buying tires or groceries in that there is nothing solid to show for the effort, at least not immediately. Often, the service provider and the service are linked in the minds of referral sources, and this makes frequent and regular contact with these individuals very important. Successful program directors will soon find that they have made so many contacts that they have a network of support, which will continue to expand as their service gains acceptance and respect.

Professional meetings provide a means of networking among human service providers. It is very important that a program director have a strong sense of all of the services that are available in the area, and that all other human service agencies understand the scope of the services the ADR program offers. Mediation can often provide the impetus for individuals to accept referrals for other necessary assistance, such as counseling or preventive services.

Surveys are useful in determining the effectiveness of the program's efforts, but can also be invaluable in finding out how the service is perceived by the general public and in assessing the need for new programs. A marketing class can be a great deal of help in conducting such a survey, and may be able to give a program director insight into the data collected. The director should be sure to share survey results with staff members and the advisory board, who can help with future goal setting.

Effective Use of Media

A media list is an important tool. If a program does not have one, it would be a worthwhile use of an afternoon for a mediator or a local college student intern to compile one. A media list should contain all of the information needed to contact any and all radio and television stations and print media in the area. This list should give the name of the contact person for each medium and any deadlines that should be taken into account in submitting information.

Radio

Radio can be the most effective way to reach large numbers of residents of a particular area. Most stations will run a free public service announcement (PSA) for a nonprofit service agency. The PSA must make it clear what service the agency is offering, who is eligible to receive the service, and how to contact the agency. An example follows:

> If you are having a problem with a neighbor or friend and can't seem to resolve it, why not call the Center for Dispute Settlement? We have experienced mediators who can help the two of you talk through your problem and come up with solutions. Call 243-4410 today. We can probably help.

This can be submitted on a 3" × 5" index card, with the organization's full name and mailing address on the reverse side of the card. Usually new PSAs should be sent out every 6 months or so, but this time period varies with the station. Many stations do interview programs to familiarize the community with locally available services. To arrange to participate in this type of show, a program director should contact the station manager. It is a good idea to let the station know that the mediation program staff would appreciate a second airing of the show once it has been released.

Cable Television

Some areas have access to cable television stations that provide free air time for not-for-profit agencies. This is a valuable resource if it is available in the area.

Newspapers

Every opportunity should be taken to get the name and mission of the ADR program before the public, and newspapers can offer this opportunity in a number of ways. News releases on any and all activities, profiles of programs and funders, reports on year-end statistics, and thank-yous to volunteers are just some instances of articles that can be submitted for publication. Of course, along with any of these public relations items, a review of the services offered should be submitted. Newspapers can also be used to announce searches for volunteers and training sessions that are to take place.

Posters

Posters and fliers can be made up rather inexpensively and are good ways of keeping the name and purpose of the organization before the public. If possible, separate posters should be used for each specific service. These can be hung in local courtrooms, store windows, supermarkets, churches, and community centers. These posters should be checked periodically to see whether they need replacing. If a poster is tattered and faded, it will not represent the program very well.

Use of Human Resources

Professional Contacts: Networking

One of the least costly yet most effective methods we have found for marketing is networking. Often, in areas where community mediation centers exist, there are committees operating that promote the use of alternative programs in the criminal justice system. Examples of these committees include criminal justice councils, PINS (persons in need of supervision) diversion committees, youth bureaus, and jail advisory committees. If program coordinators and directors take an active part in these committees, other agencies and referral sources become aware of the advantages offered through participation in a community mediation center. It is a direct, inexpensive, and informative way to promote an ADR program.

One can also be instrumental in forming a committee with other not-for-profit agencies for the purpose of discussing similar operating concerns, such as marketing and budget restrictions. Programs can be encouraged to work together by informing their respective clients of the advantages of one another's services. At times, one program may have access to marketing equipment or materials that another may not, and they can thus help one another to obtain these items.

If forming a committee or becoming part of one is too time-consuming, arranging to meet for lunch with agency executives can obtain the same results.

Advisory Board

A previously mentioned marketing strategy is the formation of an advisory board. An important factor to keep in mind in forming this board is to ask someone from the business community whose background is in marketing or public relations to become a member. Such an individual may also have easy access to donations of goods and services.

Volunteers

Another way of using human resources for marketing is the use of volunteers. Most community mediation centers would not be able to operate their programs without the use of volunteer mediators. There are many ways in which these volunteers can assist in marketing the ADR program. Prospective volunteers may be employed in the business community and may be able to lend time and advice in their areas of expertise. They can assist in laying out and printing an agency newsletter, designing an agency pamphlet or poster at little or no cost, obtaining access to free printing, or soliciting donations for printing and paper.

Community mediators, as noted earlier, can be very effective speakers for these organizations such as Rotary, Lions, and Kiwanis Clubs; enthusiastic volunteers can perform this function, in addition to those on staff. The volunteers may live in different geographic areas and have better access to police departments, local magistrates, businesses, and social service agencies in their respective locales. Periodically, they may be willing to make these direct contacts with referral sources, in order to save on the mileage costs and time involvement necessary for a staff person to make these contacts. Volunteers may also be interested in making appearances on television talk shows or on radio interviews, and their respective business connections may afford them easier access to the media.

If a program has a community volunteer who works for a local newspaper, this would be an ideal way of obtaining low-cost or free advertising. Other volunteers may be willing to make the contacts or write the articles for this form of public relations.

Volunteers can be asked to participate in "mock" mediation sessions, which can be videotaped as another marketing strategy. For example, the Tri-County Office of the Center for Dispute Settlement, Inc. (Geneva, New York) coordinated efforts with the audiovisual department of the Community College of Finger Lakes (Canandaigua, New York). Volunteer mediators participated in role play for a video titled *The Mediation Session*. Exchange of services resulted with little or no cost to either organization. Also, a videotape could be developed as an educational tool that would be used both in the classroom for criminal justice training and in the community for public education in ADR. Videotapes are publicly appealing and a quick way of demonstrating visually the advantages of community mediation.

Centers may wish to pool their financial resources and work together to make a single, professional tape. An example of this is the videotape *Mediation: A Better Way*, designed by various mediation center directors and financed by the New York State Office of Court Administration. All of the community mediation centers in New York State have access to this tape to assist them in their public relations efforts.

Drama Clubs

Aside from networking and the use of volunteers, some program directors have used drama clubs within school systems to help act out scenarios of conflict and the use of mediation to resolve them. Program promotion therefore has a dual effect, in that it reaches its targeted audience and also teaches young people that conflict can be resolved in a constructive manner.

College Students

Local college students have been another resource for marketing for community mediation centers. Often a center is located in the same area as a college. Two such programs are the Livingston County Office of the Center for Dispute Settlement, Inc., located near the State University of New York at Geneseo, and the Ontario County Office of the Center for Dispute Settlement, Inc., located near the Community College of the Finger Lakes. Student interns from these colleges, anxious to complete courses in criminal justice, communications, psychology, and marketing, are invaluable resources for marketing the mediation program. Laying out and editing newsletters, designing pamphlets, contacting people and writing articles for local news media, and developing and distributing posters are all ways that these young people can be involved in a marketing effort.

The Aging Population

Finally, we cannot complete this chapter on marketing strategies without mentioning utilizing one of our nation's most valuable resources, the aging population. The Office for the Aging, the American Association of Retired Persons, and similar groups have many older persons who want to make use of their time and contribute their experience to worthwhile agencies. If a program director is fortunate enough to find senior citizens with background or talent in any of the areas we have mentioned previously, their years of experience will be an asset to the program.

CONCLUSION

This chapter has provided an introduction to various marketing strategies that have been successful when money and time are at a premium. Through individual experimentation, mediation professionals will find which of these strategies serve them and their programs most effectively.

In conclusion, the reason for marketing a mediation program is to generate and to fill a demand for services. When more costly methods are not feasible, there are many viable alternatives. Time and money limitations are shortcomings to marketing efforts, but if program directors take the opportunity to analyze their goals and their audiences, and to use the resources that are available, their public relations efforts will be very effective and rewarding.

REFERENCES

Kotler, P., & Andreasen, A. (1987). *Strategic marketing for non-profit organizations*. Englewood Cliffs, NJ: Prentice-Hall.

Lauffer, A. (1984). *Strategic marketing for not-for-profit organizations: Program and resource development*. New York: Free Press.

McGillis, D. (1986). *Community dispute resolution programs and public policy*. Washington, DC: National Institute of Justice.

APPENDIX 5.1
Sample Satisfaction Questionnaire
for Mediation Parties

It is our belief at the Center for Dispute Settlement that the people who use the Center are best equipped to render an opinion of how effective our work is here. We would appreciate your filling out the questionnaire below to give us an idea of how *you* feel about the process.

1. I am here (check one)
   _____ as the person who filed the original complaint.
   _____ because a complaint was filed against me.

2. If this case had been handled in the courts, I think there would have been (check as many as you think apply):
   _____ a fine.
   _____ restitution to the offended party (money, return of property, etc.).
   _____ a warning from the courts.
   _____ a sentence of:
   _____ time in jail   _____ how long
   _____ community service
   _____ probation
   _____ other (explain) _____

3. When I came to the Center for Dispute Settlement, I expected the outcome to be _____.

4. I am satisfied that the case was handled fairly and professionally by the mediator: (explain) _____

5. Were you satisfied with the process of mediation? _____yes _____no

6. Do you think the problem you came with has been resolved? _____yes _____no

7. If any other problems were to arise, would you consider mediation as a way of handling them? _____yes _____no

8. If you have any other comments about your experience with mediation, please note them here:

PART II

THE PROCESS
OF MEDIATION

There are many ways of understanding the process of mediation. One way is simply to think of mediation as the road to managing conflict, with the mediator as the guide and the disputants as the sojourners. The guide, the mediator, also steers the travelers down other subsidiary routes that converge on or are fostered by mediation, such as interpersonal communication and trust. On the other hand, mediation can be examined in terms of its destinations or outcomes rather than as the road upon which we travel. For instance, at the end of mediation the parties have usually successfully navigated the conflict, mapped out a consensual resolution, and perhaps come to appreciate each other's viewpoint. Mediation, then, can be examined in terms of both its processes and its outcomes.

Another way of looking at mediation is as an art form. Just as an artist via training and instinct paints a shaded path on a canvas, mediators as artists develop case intuitions and strategies via some training interwoven with lots of personal savvy. In contrast to this view is the notion that, much as a surveyor uses certain tools in combination with science to plot a roadway, a mediator armed with appropriate tools such as caucusing and reality testing—and perhaps given adequate training in relevant research—can better chart the course of a case.

In this section of the book, we explore mediation procedures in terms of processes and outcomes—as art and as science. First, Melinda Ostermeyer, a highly experienced program manager, takes us through the stages of a typical hearing, from case intake to agreement writing. Ostermeyer's commentary about the art of the mediation process challenges both practitioners and researchers to design, use, and assess the best possible dispute resolution techniques.

We next venture into the science of the mediation process. In Chapter 7, Gary Welton steers us through his and others' research on the parties to the dispute. Specifically, he examines the role of disputant power imbalances, types of relationships, conflict styles, and other factors in influencing the course of the mediation session. In Chapter 8, Peter Carnevale and his fellow researchers map out how mediator behavior and characteristics affect mediation. As they make clear, some mediator tactics (such as neutrality and focusing) are positively related to the course of mediation, while other strategies (such as pressure tactics with nonhostile parties) are negatively related.

Finally, Neil McGillicuddy and his colleagues lend cohesiveness in Chapter 9 by discussing how all components of mediation (the mediator, the parties, and the process itself) interact with one another and affect its outcome. For example, when third-party power varies, so too does disputant and mediator behavior. These researchers examine variables affecting both short- and long-term success.

In this section, then, we explore the art and science of the mediation process itself. We hope to inspire future collaborative efforts by mediation practitioners and scientists, in the belief that refinements to the process will improve it.

6

Conducting the Mediation

MELINDA OSTERMEYER
Superior Court of the District of Columbia

This chapter discusses general methods of program administration and principles of mediation at a typical mediation program that accepts referrals from civil and criminal courts and prosecuting organizations. All programs, however, are not the same, and therefore generalizations are made. For example, dispute resolution programs throughout the country, whether court-sponsored, community-based, or a combination of both, have established policy and procedures based on local norms and political realities. However, some similarities may be found, particularly on a regional basis.

As a former director of the Dispute Resolution Centers in Houston, Texas, I believe that Texas is one of the best examples of a state that works to achieve statewide consistency in the delivery of dispute resolution services. Although all of the dispute resolution programs in the state of Texas are independent, the centers coordinate efforts to standardize the gathering of statistics and the training of mediators. Most of these organizations have adopted a uniform center name, to promote statewide recognition of services. However, the dispute resolution centers in Texas, like programs in other states, vary regarding criteria for case selection and procedures for case management.

A second example of program differences from one locale to another is that of the mediation model used as the basis of training. A "mediation model" consists of the stages of the mediation process, together with specific rules or the "dos" and "don'ts" of conducting a mediation session. One model may stress private sessions between the mediator and individual parties, whereas other models may expressly prohibit the mediator from caucusing with one party out of the presence of the other. The model may encourage interaction between the parties, with little intervention by the mediator, or may advocate that the mediator serve as the sole conduit of information between the parties. Whatever model is used, basic principles of mediation are always incorporated. This chapter provides a framework of those basic mediation principles, and it sets out for consideration various systems of case administration.

INTAKE AND REFERRAL

The method by which a case is selected for mediation, and prior contact with the parties (if any) by the program or the mediator, are important. With growing frequency, dispute resolution programs are taking the "multi-door" approach to case screening. The multi-door concept provides for a coordinated system of referring citizens to various dispute resolution processes during the citizens' initial contacts or intake interviews. Instead of discussing the dispute with the complaining party strictly to determine whether mediation alone is appropriate, the professional doing the intake interview analyzes the dispute with the thought of selecting various processes appropriate to resolving the dispute.

This multi-door system offers an information and referral network, linking the small-claims, misdemeanor, city, state, and federal courts; mediation and arbitration programs; volunteer lawyer and legal aid offices; lawyer referral; district, county, and city attorneys' offices; and other governmental and private service agencies, including those for mental health. Consequently, citizens avoid the frustrating and usually unproductive sequence of multiple referrals to varying services.

Through the multi-door system, the intake specialist conducting the intake interview examines "case type" characteristics, such as the history and dynamics of the conflict and the possibility of physical threat or loss of property. Questions of principle or of fact and the complexity of issues are determined. The intensity of the relationship between the disputing parties and the number of parties involved in the dispute are likewise considered. Neither the citizens' financial status and emotional support systems, nor the parties' willingness to participate actively in the resolution of their dispute (which is pivotal in selecting a viable dispute resolution option), can be overlooked. Furthermore, it is important to explore any consequences relating to action taken by the parties.

After clarifying the issues and analyzing "case type" characteristics, the intake specialist attempts to match the dispute with "process" characteristics of a referral agency. Process characteristics include factors such as financial eligibility requirements or the immediate availability of services; these factors most commonly preclude referral to many organizations.

The citizen seeking assistance and the intake specialist jointly decide the best course of action. Before leaving the intake interview, the citizen may be scheduled for an appointment with the referred agency, and he or she is given extensive information about each of the recommended approaches, including any associated costs. Subsequently, if the dispute is not resolved through one resource, the citizen is armed with sufficient information to continue with his or her pursuit. An attempt at voluntary mediation may be the first step. If mediation is unsuccessful, the second recommendation may be to file a suit in small-claims court. In some instances, a supplementary referral to a lawyer or counselor is given to assist with ancillary problems arising from the dispute.

The justice system is often perceived by the general public as an overwhelming and confusing maze of bureaucracy. Citizens can easily find themselves at the door of a criminal justice agency, only to learn that prosecution of the matter necessitates evidence and witnesses. Furthermore, prosecution is not likely to secure financial compensation. Prior to directing the citizen to a criminal justice agency, the intake specialist will have explored issues of evidence and compensation and contacted the agency to inquire about the appropriateness of the referral. This network results in cooperative working relationships between personnel across agency lines, and it also consolidates resources.

REFERRAL TO A MEDIATION CENTER

Once a dispute has been referred for mediation, a telephone call is made or, more often, a notice is forwarded to the responding party about the complaint and scheduled hearing. This notice sometimes indicates the organization referring the case to the dispute resolution program, and possible ramifications (if any) of declining to mediate.

By talking with dispute resolution professionals around the country, one can surmise that the degree of persuasion used to encourage people to mediate, referred to by some as "coercion," will be a continued issue for debate. Often, mediation programs receiving referrals from civil and criminal courts issue a judicial order to mediate. Participation by all relevant parties is ensured, and noncompliance can be sanctioned. In some instances, prosecuting entities may consider the result of mediation, prior to making a final decision about prosecution. The exchange between the parties during mediation is considered to be confidential. But it is common practice for mediation programs to report to the referring agency basic information, such as whether an individual agreed to mediate and whether an agreement was reached.

Kressel, Pruitt, and Associates (1989) found that across domains of mediation, a conservative estimate would place the median settlement rate at about 60%. Therefore, mediation more often than not is successful; yet parties do refuse to engage in mediation, or they are sometimes unable to reach an agreement. Subsequently, the mediation program may advise one or both parties about the mechanics of processing their dispute through the traditional justice system. The program serves as a neutral source of information.

Premediation Contact with the Parties

Parties may be notified that a mediation has been scheduled in as early as 1 week or as far away as several months. Neighborhood disputes are typically mediated immediately, whereas court-referred civil matters involving deadlines for discovery may receive extensive notice. Prior to the mediation, the parties may be asked to submit documentation about the dispute or to complete financial reporting forms. They may be advised of their right to secure legal counsel and then are given ample time to do so.

Programs differ as to the efforts taken to contact the parties before the mediation. Contact may be initiated by the parties—for the most part, through the complaining party, who was spoken with at the time of intake. Other programs aggressively contact all parties to the dispute. For example, the Multi-Door Dispute Resolution Division of the Superior Court of the District of Columbia requests parties involved in mediating their pending civil litigation to submit confidential settlement statements. These statements include information about the nature of the case and its status in litigation, as well as the parties' respective settlement positions. The statements are forwarded to mediators, who contact the parties or their attorneys several weeks in advance of mediation. During these telephone calls, issues are clarified and the parties are encouraged to exchange documents, to complete relevant discovery, and to begin to consider possible settlement options.

Selection of the Mediators

The process by which mediators are matched to cases may be a relatively routine and random assignment: The first mediator arriving on any given day may automatically mediate the first case for which all parties have arrived. Or it may include an analysis of the case type and special factors in an attempt to select a mediator with specific training or expertise.

Programs often provide advanced training to those mediating cases segregated from the general caseload. An understanding of the effects of divorce on children and a command of local legal guidelines are required when mediating matters involve divorce-related issues (e.g., child custody, support, and property division). Mediators who conduct sessions with juvenile offenders must have an ability to balance the negotiation between a youth and an adult or institutional representative, while striving for a fair and equitable agreement for restitution. Serving as the neutral third party in a technical contract matter or a highly emotional personal injury suit can require knowledge of current law and likely disposition of the case if decided by a judge or jury.

Policy regarding the number of mediators selected to conduct a session may be dictated by the type of case or may simply be a result of limited or plentiful mediator resources. Often domestic cases are comediated by a male and a female to offset concerns about gender bias. Program policy may require that more than one mediator be used in the interests of quality control and monitoring. Other programs simply do not have an abundance of volunteer resources, and therefore all cases are facilitated by a single mediator.

OBJECTIVES OF MEDIATION

Communicating rationally in the midst of a disagreement is difficult. When communication between two people becomes strained or nonexistent, the intensity of the conflict is heightened. The mediator seeks to improve the ability of the parties to communicate and to explore each other's attitudes and positions. Once this barrier against exploring options is broken, the parties can proceed toward joint problem solving, with everyone's interests of equal priority.

Figure 6.1 shows a basic model of the mediation process. The stages provide a framework for communication. By using such a framework, the mediator assists the parties in informal yet structured communication. Assumptions are tested and perceptions are put into words. The mediator is aware of body language and voice tone, while encouraging honesty and disclosure of important facts. Above all, mediation provides a neutral forum in which valuable information is shared. It allows a person to "save face" or to rectify past words and deeds with what he or she is about to say and agree to do.

CONDUCTING THE MEDIATION

A mediator must be flexible and patient. Less experienced mediators are cautioned against "rushing the process." If during the mediation the parties are having difficulty bargaining, it is probably due to the circumvention of a previous stage. That is, the mediator did not gather sufficient information to identify the issues underlying the dispute, or to bring to light everyone's ultimate interest. It is impossible to generate solutions to satisfy interests that are not clearly understood by all.

It is often frustrating to be discussing possible solutions to one problem, only to have additional problems reveal themselves. The mediator must be quick to decide whether to address the new problem, or to set it aside for the moment and remain focused on the previous issue at hand.

The mediator prepares for transition between stages by summarizing the basic agreements reached thus far and gently moving the parties to

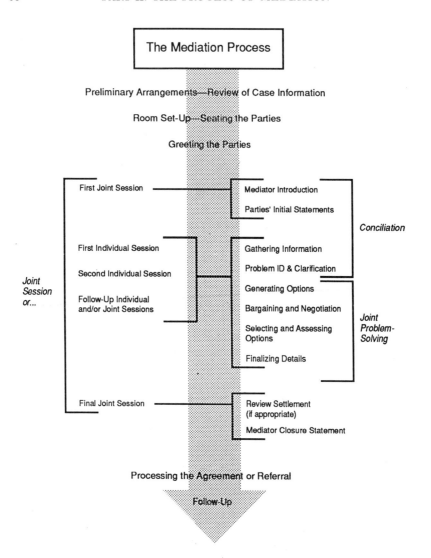

FIGURE 6.1. A model of the mediation process.

another task. The mediator ensures that all parties have an understanding of what is to be accomplished in the next stage of discussion, and gains their commitment to work to achieve these goals. At all times the mediator is the "keeper of the process," redirecting the discussion and rephrasing statements in more positive and productive terms. Individual feelings are validated, while at the same time common interests are emphasized. Areas of agreement, no matter how small, are reinforced throughout each stage of the mediation.

Bringing the Parties into Contact

It is safe to assume that before the mediation begins the parties are reluctant to talk to each other. During the introductory statement by the mediator, the parties feel uncertain as to what is about to happen and what they will be called upon to do. As each party proceeds with an initial statement, the party wishes to make the best case possible to prove to the mediator that he or she is right and the other party is wrong. At this time, the parties may ventilate emotions, and the conflict may intensify. As information is gathered, the parties (one hopes) are becoming less defensive, and trust is being generated with the mediator. A new understanding of circumstances or perceptions leads to an atmosphere of decreased tension as the parties move toward joint problem solving and consideration of solutions.

The mediator should be aware of the level of interdependence and especially of possible power disparity between the parties, which may result from an imbalance of knowledge or from a prior relationship of authority. The physical presence of one party as exhibited in body language may overpower the other. One party's willingness to mediate may also inhibit the other party, if he or she is not so inclined. All of these factors can affect the ability of the parties to negotiate effectively and should be kept in mind as the mediator facilitates the discussion.

Introductory Statement by the Mediator

The room in which the mediation is to be conducted should be comfortable, with sufficient chairs, and a private waiting area. Paper and pens for note taking should be available for everyone. From the moment the parties are greeted, the mediator should have a good command of their names and roles so that initial perceptions can be noted. The introductory statement by the mediator establishes the relaxed atmosphere of the session. The mediator's role is explained as one of a neutral facilitator, not an advocate or decision maker. So that there is a clear understanding of what will be expected of the parties and what they can expect from the process, the purpose and procedures of mediation are outlined in detail. All parties are guaranteed an opportunity to share information and told that the success of any mediation is contingent upon their active participation. However, instructions are given that only one person should speak at a time, and the taking of notes is encouraged. It is helpful for the mediator to stress that the parties listening to each other does not indicate agreement with what is being said.

The parties are asked whether a conflict of interest exists with the mediator, or whether they can foresee any reason why the mediator would not be fair or impartial. The mediator may ask whether any of the parties knows him or her, as a way of further establishing neutrality. In addition, any special requirements involved in processing the agreement are reviewed, such as the approval of a court of law, or (in restitution agreements) the approval of a probation department or district attorney's office. The mediator provides assurances that nothing said in a private meeting with one party will be shared with anyone, unless permission is given to do so. Privacy of the entire proceeding is discussed, with reference to any statute or case law that expressly guards the confidentiality of mediation. Many dispute resolution programs require the parties to sign a "statement of understanding" that the mediation is confidential and that the neutral third party will not voluntarily testify in a subsequent legal action. It is becoming more common for mediation programs to secure mediator liability insurance. Insurance carriers may require written confirmation that confidentiality was explained and that the parties were advised to consider whether a lawyer should review any agreement prior to its signing.

Before proceeding to the parties' initial statements, the mediator allows for questions. The opening remarks may be brief, but they are vital. A rapport between the mediator and the disputants is established, and the ground rules for negotiation are defined.

Initial Statement by Each Party

Programs differ as to which party begins the session with an initial statement. Often, the party who brought the complaint to the attention of the program is the first to offer his or her comments. In mediation involving a juvenile, the juvenile may be asked to speak first, to assure him or her of equal status with the adult. The person who is to begin should be asked to provide a brief statement of his or her understanding of the situation. If possible, events should be presented in chronological order. Parties who talk nonstop may be asked to summarize.

At this point in the process, it is best for the mediator to ask as few questions as possible. Extensive questioning may entrench the parties in their positions or alienate one party. However, broad clarifying questions, such as "Could you tell me a little more about . . .?", are appropriate. The mediator provides an opportunity for venting emotions, and reflects his or her understanding of feelings. Some exchange of dialogue between the parties is permissible, but it should be remembered that the purpose of this stage is to provide everyone with the opportunity to speak uninterrupted.

At the conclusion of one party's initial statement, the mediator may ask, "If you could draft an agreement right now, what would it say?" or "What is it that you would like to see accomplished in this mediation?" Important points are summarized by the mediator in neutral, non-negative terms, and the parties are asked to correct any misrepresentation. A transition is made to the other party, again with an open-ended question, such as "Now, if we could hear from you?"

Joint or Individual Sessions

Typically, it is some time following the initial statements that the first individual session will occur. Bethel (1986) indicates that private sessions should be considered a routine part of the process, but he cautions against calling a separate meeting as a tactic to avoid conflict. Direct confrontation of the parties allows for a release of pent-up frustration, and therefore is good. However, sensitive information, such as whether a spouse has been physically abused, is better shared in a private session. Information can be more easily gathered from one party without risking estrangement of the other. Particularly in divorce mediation, the opportunity for total disclosure between each individual party and the mediator is important.

However, Folberg and Taylor (1984) feel that meeting with one party alone makes it more difficult to maintain the appearance of absolute impartiality. All people come to mediation with basic fears. One such fear is that the mediator will favor the other party and find his or her story more believable. The use of individual sessions may exacerbate this fear. An immediate counter to one person's version of the story cannot be offered by the other, and the mediator's reaction to both stories cannot be observed and therefore confirmed as neutral. The fact that one party is not privy to information can be detrimental to the mediator's ability to guide the parties toward joint problem solving. Individuals participating in mediation benefit from learning conflict resolution skills. Working through mediation without separating the parties often reinforces a cooperative approach to resolving future problems, particularly for those individuals with an ongoing relationship.

In addition, a concern arises regarding the inadvertent disclosure of information learned during a private session. If the mediator cannot convince the party of the importance of sharing the confidential information with everyone, then is the information of any real value to the mediator? Most mediators say that it is—that at least one brief meeting with each party alone provides the mediator with an advantage. Positions and true interests can be explored that might not be readily disclosed in the joint session.

Before the first individual session, the mediator should review notes taken earlier, decide which party to see first, and outline the questions to be asked. The mediator may wish to meet with one party before the other for a variety of reasons. In some instances, the mediator will wish to gather crucial information or to address the emotional needs of one party. Regardless of which party is met with first, the mediator should begin to develop a sense of the areas of agreement and impasse, as well as individual interests and positions. Discussions during a session with one party should always begin by addressing the needs of that party; beginning with the other person's agenda will only reduce trust in the mediator.

Information Gathering

Whether in a joint or individual session, the mediator should begin gathering information, building upon the perceptions indicated during the initial statements. The use of open-ended, closed-ended, and focused questions is of paramount importance; the mediator controls the flow of information through these questioning techniques. Open-ended questions are best used early in the mediation, unless the party's comments are disjointed and the mediator must continually clarify facts as the story unfolds. In this instance, questions that allow for short answers direct the party to a specific topic. The mediator should be cautious about eliciting information that would be damaging to the negotiations. The old adage "Timing is everything" is certainly appropriate in mediation. The mediator should not interrupt to ask a question unless it is absolutely necessary, as issues are more often clarified by allowing the parties to finish their dialogue. A quick series of questions will be received as intrusive, and questions phrased by the mediator in an accusatory manner are disastrous to the mediator's credibility.

During this stage of mediation, information given by one party is used to correct false assumptions by another party. The events that led to the dispute are reviewed, as are any previous efforts of the parties to resolve the dispute between themselves. Information should be gathered about all participants with direct involvement in the controversy; inquiries may be appropriate about emotional and financial resources. It is important to consider the history of, or desire for, an ongoing personal or business relationship between the parties. As the mediator gathers information, he or she begins devising a strategy to enhance the opportunities for settlement.

Problem Identification and Clarification

As relevant issues are discussed, the mediator continually rephrases negative comments in more positive terms. As the issues are defined, the parties begin to make a distinction about their importance, based on interests. Issues are the questions being posed by each side going into the negotiation. The parties' positions are the answers initially offered to remedy those issues, and their interests are the fundamental needs or the "whys" behind the issues and positions.

Before options can be generated that focus on interests and not positions, the mediator must find out the "why" behind each stated position. This technique can best be exemplified in a short story. Sandy and Megan share a small office. Sandy wants the window open and Megan wants the window closed. To identify their interests, they are asked why they want the window open or closed. Sandy responds that she wants fresh air, while Megan's concern is exposure to a draft. One possible solution is to open a window in an adjoining office, which will provide fresh air without a draft. This technique seems simple enough when summed up in a short story.

However, mediators can fall short when differentiating between parties' issues, positions, and interests.

Furthermore, the mediator's ability to restate the parties' positional statements into a statement of joint interests is crucial. For example, one party states, "I want the money right now, because he's not going to come through with it," and the other party responds, "I won't give him the money now, because he won't give me the radio once he has the money," can be restated by the mediator as follows: "It seems that you both have concerns about the arrangements for this exchange. Let's see what we can figure out that makes everyone feel comfortable."

It is important for the mediator to outline the list of issues and interests clearly, so that everyone has a clear understanding of what concerns have priority. The mediator assists the parties in organizing the list, in terms of personal value and in terms of what issues might be discussed first. The mediator may focus on that issue for which consensus will be reached most easily. Once consensus is reached about a few issues, it is easier for the mediator and the parties to build momentum toward agreement about more difficult points.

The term "hidden agenda" refers to those issues that may be revealed indirectly, usually much later in the mediation. The hidden agenda includes the underlying, fundamental issues that may be at the root of the problem. The hidden agenda often becomes the focus of the mediation, and minimizes the importance of the other issues being discussed. For example, in the story about Megan and Sandy, a possible hidden agenda may surface regarding their prior working relationship. It may seem to Megan that Sandy always gets her way, and Megan resents this. Therefore, Megan's real concern is not the exposure to draft, but her wish that a fair system for decision making be established in the office so that Megan's feelings are taken into account as well. The mediator must be sure to explore the possibility of any undisclosed issue. However, the mediator should not create issues that do not exist; not every case turns on a hidden agenda.

Bargaining and Negotiation

Once information has been gathered and the interests are defined, the objective of the mediation becomes the generation of options and solutions. Kressel et al. (1989) indicate that despite a persistent ideology that mediators ought to refrain from pushing their own ideas, it is quite evident that they are often a primary source of settlement proposals and that they are not at all shy about playing such a role. Several techniques for assisting the parties to generate settlement proposals exist, such as brainstorming options, no matter how unrealistic they may seem. The parties should not be allowed to accept or reject options one at a time as they are offered. The parties often will need assistance with this exercise, and therefore the mediator should provide a few suggestions to get the ball rolling. The mediator must be sure to offer more than one suggestion and to preface suggestions with such phrases as "What if . . ." or "Others in similar situations have tried . . ." Another technique is to offer a solution that will not be accepted by either side; this sometimes motivates the parties to consider proposals more to their liking. If one party is consistently negative toward suggested options, he or she should be asked to replace a rejected option with another option. Once several options are on the table for consideration, the mediator must again make sure that the parties are evaluating solutions to interests, not positions.

It is important for the mediator to deflect negativism about an inability to settle the case. The mediator may wish to take a moment to reinforce the fact that a very high percentage of those individuals participating in mediation are able to resolve their disputes. This may also be an appropriate time to discuss the alternatives to no settlement. Questions that lead the parties to verbalize the weaknesses of their positions or their ability to "win" if they should go to court are effective. If the parties seem to have reached an impasse with one issue, redirecting the focus to another issue may restore a more positive atmosphere.

The mediator must be careful in the framing of proposals. Depending on the circumstances, it may be better either to develop agreements based on general principles and then work out the details, or to first break issues into smaller problems and discuss solutions to subissues. Throughout the bargaining and negotiation stage, the mediator redefines stated positions in broad or narrow terms. For example, if a specific amount of money is mentioned, it may be wiser to phrase the statement thus: "So you would like a significant increase." On the other hand, if general terms are used, the mediator may need to encourage the party to attach a specific monetary amount to the demand, and therefore should say, "We need to understand the amount of money you feel is fair." At all times, the mediator attempts to develop proposals that are comprehensive and that satisfy both parties' interests.

The mediator must determine the appropriateness of individual or joint sessions. Typically, if the parties can agree on most issues, it is advisable to meet jointly. However, individual sessions may help the parties consider options on their merits, without playing to the other side. The mediator may claim a suggestion as his or her own idea, so that it is not rejected simply because it is thought to have come from the other side. It is sometimes effective to present a worst-case settlement offer first, and then to present a more favorable offer. Individual sessions are useful in exploring with one party all of the possible reactions to an offer that might be received by the other party. The mediator can assist the parties to develop rational and logical arguments behind the settlement offer, thereby helping them to "save face" in offering or accepting a settlement. However, if the mediator meets with one party separately, it is advisable for him or her to meet separately with the other party as well.

As points of agreement are clarified, it is important to consider any positive or negative consequences of the agreement. In other words, the mediator must explore with the parties whether the agreement will withstand the test of time and whether it can realistically be implemented. For example, it is the mediator's responsibility to ascertain the feasibility of one party's paying $100 per week, if the mediator has learned during the sessions that this party's income is $200 per week.

Agreement Writing

The agreement is important, because typically it is the only document that results from the mediation. The written agreement may be viewed as a contract, and therefore as legally binding on the parties. However, the specifics of writing an agreement vary, depending on program procedures. Agreements that must be approved by some other individual, such as a judge or prosecutor, may need to be drafted in a specific format. In some instances, the details are agreed upon by the parties in mediation; however, the actual contract is drafted by their respective attorneys. Agreements should not incriminate either party. For example, an agreement should not contain any subtle or explicit admission of guilt. It should indicate what the parties agree to do, rather than what they agree not to do (e.g., "John Doe agrees to walk on the sidewalk in front of Sally Rogers's yard" rather than "John Doe agrees not to walk in Sally Rogers's front yard again").

Generally, it is important to specify the who, what, when, where, and how of the plan of action. The agreement should be balanced, with fairly equal responsibility outlined for both parties. For example, an agreement between Sandy and Megan might include the following factors:

> Sandy agrees (1) to consult with Megan before she rearranges the office furniture and (2) to keep the office window open only when Megan is at lunch. Megan agrees (1) to eat her lunch outside of the office and (2) to consult with Sandy before ordering office supplies. Megan and Sandy agree to abide by the decision of the office manager when they are unable to reach consensus on work-related issues.

A "what-if" clause that outlines what will occur if any portion of the agreement is not upheld is wise. As appropriate, mediated agreements should provide for the future, particularly when the parties maintain an ongoing relationship. Their patterns of communication should be discussed so that any new conflict can be remedied before it escalates. For instance, if two neighbors have been fighting over a barking dog, the agreement should specify how the dog owner will be notified if in the future the neighbor is disturbed by barking.

CONCLUSION

This general model of the mediation process should provide a framework for discussion. As mentioned in the beginning of this chapter, not all programs or mediators view the process in the same way. The stages of mediation are fluid, and transitions are subtle. The techniques suggested are not appropriate for every case, because mediation is often an art, not a science. Mediators come to the table with a sincere desire to help people resolve conflict. This desire is coupled with the use of a few good tricks and a lot of luck. Not every case should be mediated, and not every case mediated will be resolved. The process of mediation empowers individuals to determine their own destiny. The mediator guides the parties through the process, keeping them focused on and positive about their ability to make informed choices.

REFERENCES

Bethel, C. A. (1986). The use of separate sessions in family mediation. *Negotiation Journal: On the Process of Dispute Settlement, 2*(3), 257–271.

Folberg, J., & Taylor, A. (1984). *Mediation: A comprehensive guide to resolving conflicts without litigation.* San Francisco: Jossey-Bass.

Kressel, K. & Pruitt, D. G., (1989). Conclusion: A research perspective on mediation of social conflict. In K. Kressel & D. G. Pruitt (Eds.), *Mediation research: The process and effectiveness of third party interventions.* San Francisco: Jossey-Bass.

7

Parties in Conflict: Their Characteristics and Perceptions

GARY L. WELTON
Tabor College

In the final analysis, community mediation exists for the benefit of the disputants. Their use of and experience with community mediation are influenced by the nature of their relationship, their conflict management styles, and their perceptions about each other and about the mediation process. Hence, this chapter analyzes the characteristics and perceptions of the parties in conflict.

THE NATURE OF THE RELATIONSHIP
BETWEEN THE PARTIES

The disputes that are considered most appropriate for community mediation involve parties with an ongoing relationship, who are thought to have fairly equal power. These two requirements are analyzed in this section.

The Requirement of an Ongoing Relationship

Community mediation programs have been designed primarily to handle conflicts that occur between people who are interdependent as a result of some type of ongoing relationship (Underhill, 1981). Typical mediated disputes involve current relationships (e.g., neighbors, coworkers, landlord and tenant, family members, etc.) or recent relationships (e.g., former lovers). It is argued that individuals in these types of relationships have the most to gain from mediation services. Because of the nature of their interdependence, they are most likely to experience continuing difficulties, leading to ever-increasing levels of conflict. Hence, they will be more motivated to seek a mutually satisfying agreement (Levine, 1986).

Acceptance of the premise that mediation is most effective for those with continuing relationships, however, does not necessarily rule out the possibility that mediation might also offer significant benefits for individuals

105

in other types of relationships. For example, victim–offender mediation (Umbreit, 1985) is one model that has broadened the use of mediation. Certainly victims need to be protected, and this protection will often require litigation. However, there are benefits of including mediation as part of such cases.

In victim–offender mediation, there is no requirement of any ongoing relationship. Two parties, who are interdependent as a result of some criminal act, appear to benefit from the mediation process. After the offender has been convicted in the courts, but prior to sentencing, the victim and offender are brought to mediation. The victim, often motivated by stress, anger, and a sense of vulnerability, seeks a chance to vent his or her emotions in a protected environment, and perhaps to negotiate a plan for the recovery of (or compensation for) certain losses. The offender is motivated by a desire for a lighter sentence. That is, if he or she can convince the judge of future cooperative intent, based on his or her behavior within the mediation hearing, the judge may suspend a part of the sentence.

This mediation process offers a critical benefit beyond these personal advantages. It is an educational process, through which the parties come to some mutual understanding—the victim and the offender become much more personalized to each other. The parties come to recognize the critical interdependence that exists within the community at large. In light of the apparent success of victim–offender mediation, it behooves us to redefine mediation not only as an alternative to litigation, but also as a tool that may be used in conjunction with litigation.

Although the victim–offender mediation process differs in some respects from typical community mediation, it serves as a demonstration that the benefits of mediation can be generalized beyond those cases involving ongoing relationships. The benefits of investigating underlying emotions and interests, as well as the advantages of learning and applying problem-solving techniques, may prove to be valuable in a broad array of conflict situations. As such, it seems arbitrary to require tangible interdependence before offering mediation.

The Requirement of Equal Power

Community mediation has been built upon the assumption of relative equality between the disputants and is thought to be most effective in such situations (Riskin, 1982). When relative equality does not exist, less powerful disputants are disadvantaged. For instance, if the difference is one of economic resources, poorer parties may be disadvantaged in comparison to richer parties in three ways (Fiss, 1984/1986). First, they may be less able to gather and evaluate the information needed to predict the outcome of litigation, and hence may have less information about their best alternative to a negotiated agreement (Fisher & Ury, 1981). Second, they may need the damages immediately, and may thus be induced to settle as a way of accelerating payment, though they may realize that they will get less now than if they awaited judgment. Third, they may not have the resources to finance the litigation. These sorts of disadvantages tend to put such disputants in a disadvantaged bargaining position. The resulting inequality produces unequal agreements (Levine, 1986), because, with few exceptions, a mediated settlement reflects the pre-existing inequalities between disputants.

The problems surrounding inequality are especially acute in divorce mediation. Discrepancy in relative bargaining power has been identified as the most important reason for excluding divorce cases from mediation, as it is thought that there are some cases in which power imbalances are so great as to make fair negotiation impossible (Emery & Wyer, 1987). In these cases, the wife is generally seen as less powerful because of her relative lack of experience in bargaining, limited access to financial documents, and increased anxiety related to postdissolution financial outlook.

The obvious solution is to exclude cases from mediation in which power differences are thought to be sufficient to create unequal bargaining positions. This solution is too simplistic, however. As noted by Levine (1986), either the definition of "sufficiently unequal" would become too broad, and hence would not solve the problem at all, or it would become too narrow, and thus would considerably limit the application of mediation.

There is, in fact, recent evidence that meaningfully unequal bargaining positions may actually be very common in community mediation. There appear to be significant inequalities between complainants and respondents—inequalitites that may be built into the very nature of the mediation process. Research by Castrianno, Pruitt, Nochajski, and Zubek (1988) has demonstrated that there are significant differences in mediation behavior and outcomes between the disputant who filed the complaint (the complainant) and the disputant named in the complaint (the respondent). Evidence from 73 mediation hearings coming from two mediation centers revealed that complainants are more demanding during their hearings, engage in less problem-solving behavior, and achieve better outcomes than respondents.

This can be interpreted in two ways. First, there may be naturally existing differences favoring complainants. Complainants may feel they have more legitimate grievances than do respondents; this may reflect the reality that, on the whole, they do have stronger cases. Also a complainant may be the party who feels more strongly about the case, which may have motivated him or her to file the complaint in the first place. At any rate, there may be a natural power inequality favoring complainants.

A second interpretation is that there may have been existing inequalities in a subset of these particular cases, for which those cases should have been excluded from mediation. Once all such cases are excluded, however, the application of mediation would become so limited and the caseload so small as to make it unfeasible except in the largest of metropolitan areas. Most scholars and practitioners are unwilling to accept that conclusion.

Either interpretation leads to the same conclusion: that inequalities do exist and must be handled, and that the solution of excluding all such cases is not adequate. A second solution that has been suggested is to ask the mediator and the mediation process to empower the weaker party so as to create a situation more closely approximating equality. Although this may be feasible in some situations, it has been suggested that to ask mediation itself to equalize an unequal relationship is asking too much of the process (Levine, 1986). It may not be possible for mediators, who play an impartial role, to actively support a weaker side without damaging the mediation process as a whole.

A third solution, which has been employed in divorce mediation, seems to be the most appropriate. This solution recognizes that, whereas there may be some extreme cases that should not be mediated, the typical case will still include meaningful though often subtle power differences. To handle such differences, many divorce mediators require their parties to retain independent counsel as a prerequisite for mediation (Emery & Wyer, 1987). Such an attorney, who can help to empower a weaker party, need not be present during the long hours of the mediation process, but must be available to discuss likely outcomes of litigation and to review the mediated settlement.

This solution would increase the price of mediation for many disputes, but not prohibitively. Also, it does not guarantee equality of outcomes, but neither does litigation. The solution does, however, create an opportunity for the less powerful party to obtain empowerment apart from the mediator and the mediation process. Although it is standard policy in many mediation centers to inform disputants that they have the right to bring attorneys to the hearing, it may be more appropriate to inform parties that it is often helpful and sometimes necessary to retain legal counsel. This suggestion leads us back to the earlier proposal—that mediation need not be thought of as an alternative to more traditional forms of settlement and litigation, but may be used in conjunction with them.

THE NATURE OF THE DISPUTES

As long as we define mediation as an alternative to litigation, there will be certain necessary limitations on the types of disputues that are referred. Our court system serves a critical role as an arm of justice and is essential for certain forms of conflict.

The cases that are now generally referred to mediation programs are those that fit a specific definition as declared by a particular state. Disputes concerning money typically involve less than $1,500; disputes dealing with harassment generally include situations that are annoying rather than life-threatening; disputes involving custody often deal with implementing a court custody decision. Hence, the typical case involves minor amounts of money, behavioral issues, implementation of interdependent roles, or some combination of these.

If the proposal were more generally accepted, however, that community mediation can be used in conjunction with litigation, then the types of cases that could be served by mediation programs would be greatly increased. Mediation could be used increasingly, in diverse cases, as a means of complementing and implementing court decisions.

CONFLICT MANAGEMENT STYLES

Community mediation is primarily devised as a voluntary program. Although some disputants may be strongly encouraged or even pressured to take their cases to mediation instead of using the court system, and although some disputants do not recognize that they have the right to do otherwise, technically disputants use the service because they have chosen to do so. (There are, of course, exceptions, such as mandatory divorce mediation in some states.) This leads to several unanswered questions. Do those who choose mediation differ from those who choose litigation? (For example, Duffy & Olczak, 1989, found that persons who use mediation are perceived as being more likable than those who choose litigation.) If so, how might this difference affect the mediation process?

Research on personal styles of conflict management has demonstrated consistently that there are strong individual differences in approaches to conflict (Kramer, McClintock, & Messick, 1986; Kuhlman & Marshello, 1975; McClintock, 1977; Psenicka & Rahim, 1989). Some individuals tend to approach conflict situations with a competitive motivation, in which they try to do better than the other party. Others tend to approach conflict with an individualistic motivation, in which they try to do as well as possible for themselves, without regard for the welfare of the other. Still others tend to approach conflict with a cooperative motivation, in which they attempt to develop the best alternative for all involved. Additional research has demonstrated that people are fairly consistent in their aproach to conflict (Sternberg & Dobson, 1987; Sternberg & Soriano, 1984). That is, those who approach conflict with a cooperative motivation tend to do so consistently across time and across situations.

Although research findings have often questioned whether people act with predictable consistency from one situation to the next (Mischel, 1984), the evidence cited above does give some credence to the notion that there are important general differences in individual levels of cooperation that may play a significant role in a mediation setting. First, it may be that cooperative

individuals are more likely to choose mediation, whereas competitive individuals are more likely to choose litigation. If so, evidence supporting
mediation as being more effective than litigation may be a result of the
self-selection process involved. If competitive individuals were also channeled into the mediation process, perhaps the mediation picture would
appear much less successful (see Vidmar, 1985).

A second implication is that mediators may need to be aware of the
types of persons with whom they are dealing. For example, an individual
may be unwilling to compromise on a demand for one of two very different
reasons. First, the individual may be a competitive person who rarely agrees
to compromises. Alternatively, the individual may be a cooperative person
who is hesitant in this particular situation. If the mediator can determine
whether the competitive behavior is properly attributed to a global trait of
competitiveness or to a specific instance of suspicion, it may assist him or her
in deciding how best to handle the impasse. In the latter case, the disputant
may only need concrete assurances from the other party in order to make
agreement possible. In the former case, however, progress may be much
more difficult.

PERCEPTIONS OF THE PARTIES

To understand the parties' experience in mediation, one must comprehend
the benefits and difficulties that often result from the parties' perceptions of
each other and of various components of the mediation process.

Perceptions of Each Other

In their description of the escalation and persistence of conflict, Pruitt and
Rubin (1986) discuss the vital role of negative perceptions. According to
their analysis, the relationship between conflicting parties often develops
through a series of psychological changes, including the development of
negative attitudes toward the other, and attributions of blame and other
negative traits (e.g., being self-centered, morally unfit, or perhaps even
diabolical). Emotions become dominated by anger, fear, and wounded
pride. Competitive goals develop in which one desires to look better than,
punish, discredit, defeat, or even destroy the adversary, regardless of personal costs associated with these goals. Empathy becomes unlikely or even
impossible. Disputants forfeit their ability to solve problems creatively as
each becomes increasingly convinced of the other's malicious intent. In
short, one party develops negative perceptions and expectations about the
other party.

These negative perceptions and expectations are very difficult to
change. A number of mechanisms serve to increase a person's confidence in

the accuracy of his or her (often erroneous) perceptions. First, when a person tests his or her expectancies, the testing tends to follow a confirming process. That is, instead of asking questions that might lead to disconfirmation, the tendency is to ask questions that are likely to provide supportive arguments (e.g., to ask "What behaviors can I recall that would prove that Joe is a troublesome neighbor?" rather than "What behaviors of Joe's can I recall that represent some positive intent?"). The result is an expectancy confirmation process (Cooper & Fazio, 1979; Jussim, 1986; Snyder & Swann, 1978). Second, whenever positive or neutral behaviors do occur that might disconfirm the expectancies, the tendency is to misperceive such behaviors as having negative intent—as being a part of some plan devised to harm in some way (e.g., upon learning that Joe has recently obtained a bug exterminator, the person assumes that he deliberately put it near the shared property line so the noise would be irritating). Third, a person's negative perceptions and expectancies tend to cause him or her to act in negative ways toward the other party, which tends to elicit the very behavior that was expected (e.g., confronting Joe about his intentional placement of the bug exterminator, which may well lead to future intentional harm on his part), hence creating a self-fulfilling prophecy. The results, then, are persistent negative expectancies that produce escalation and persistence of the conflict (Kulik & Brown, 1979; Pruitt & Rubin, 1986), making cooperation less likely (Braver & Barnett, 1974). Altering these negative perceptions may be a critical goal of the mediator as he or she attempts to affect change.

Hence, it is not sufficient merely to generate a creative solution that is tolerable to both parties, for a party will not agree with a reasonable alternative if convinced that the other will not follow it. The lack of trust makes it extremely difficult to work through the underlying problems and to produce an agreement. Because these negative perceptions are an important part of the escalation process, any technique by which the perceptions can be altered will be a valuable tool to the mediator.

One suggestion for altering perceptions is to teach each disputant the ability to understand the emotional (Johnson, 1975) and cognitive (Carroll, Bazerman, & Maury, 1988) perspective of the other party. Carroll et al. (1988) demonstrated that negotiators have a systematic tendency to ignore the cognitions of the other party. Neale and Bazerman (1983) provided evidence that those individuals who had high perspective-taking ability were more successful in their negotiations than those with low perspective-taking ability. This suggestion relates to the earlier discussion about power equality, since more powerful persons tend to be less interested in taking the perspective of the less powerful other (Tjosvold & Fabrey, 1980; Tjosvold & Sabato, 1978). Future research should address whether mediators can teach those with low perspective-taking ability (which is likely to include many disputants) to develop this ability, with the desired results of generating more accurate perceptions and a de-escalation of the conflict.

A second suggestion is to inform each party about the other's expectancies. When one is told about inaccurate expectancies that another holds about him or her, one becomes better able to overcome the false beliefs (Hilton & Darley, 1985). Recognition of these expectancies may enable the parties to negotiate their identities and motivations (Swann, 1984, 1987; Swann & Hill, 1982).

A third alternative is suggested by the research of Swann, Pelham, and Chidester (1988). They demonstrated that a counselor could change a client's self-conceptions (perceptions about the self) through the use of a paradoxical strategy. By advocating even more extreme negative viewpoints than those held by the client, a counselor could create a denial and resistance that would encourage movement in a positive direction. A colleague and I (Welton & Miękisz, 1990) investigated whether perceptions in conflict might be altered by a similar strategy, in which the mediator suggested that the other party was much worse than the disputant currently perceived. This suggestion should elicit a denial by the disputant ("No, Joe is not that bad"). This rejection should result in a softening of the perceptions held about the other, and hence should facilitate the change process.

Results from this laboratory study provided evidence that the paradoxical strategy can be effective in changing the expectancies held by conflicting parties. In those cases in which mediators employed a paradoxical strategy, subjects were less likely to attribute blame to the other party than were subjects in those cases in which the mediators used a nonparadoxical (reflective) strategy. The application of this to actual cases, however, presents some intriguing empirical and ethical questions. To what extent would genuine disputants be affected by the use of a paradoxical strategy? Under what conditions might the strategy backfire? Also, is this sort of manipulative strategy even appropriate in a mediation hearing?

If it is accurate that negative perceptions lead to the escalation and persistence of conflict, practitioners and researchers must be concerned with testing current strategies and developing additional strategies for altering these perceptions.

Perceptions of the Mediation Process

The effectiveness of community mediation is ultimately dependent upon the improvement of interpersonal relationships. This improvement is often judged by the criteria of outcome quality and compliance (though it obviously includes much more than these, as the relationship can improve even in the absence of an agreement). The outcome quality and subsequent compliance are largely determined by the parties' perceptions of the mediation process and outcome.

Perceived Procedural Justice

Procedural justice theory (e.g., Lind & Tyler, 1988) has emphasized the importance of disputants' perceptions of the quality of the resolution process. The evidence supporting this emphasis on process rather than just outcome is derived from research on trials and police actions. Individuals who thought they had a fair hearing—one in which their concerns were voiced and considered—were more likely to endorse the decision, the individual making the decision, and the justice system as a whole (Lind, Kurtz, Musante, Walker, & Thibaut, 1980; Tyler, 1984; Tyler, Casper, & Fisher, 1987; Tyler & Folger, 1980). Tyler (1987) has speculated that similar results might be obtained in mediation.

Research on community mediation (Pruitt, Peirce, Zubek, Welton, & Nochajski, 1990) has supported this analysis. We examined the relationship between (1) the beliefs that the basic issues of the dispute had been aired, that the mediator had understood what was said, and that the hearing was fair; and (2) both short-run success (goal achievement, short-run satisfaction with the agreement, support for the mediation service) and long-run success (compliance as reported by the other party, long-run quality of the relationship, development of new problems, long-run satisfaction with the agreement) of the hearing. Results indicated that respondents' perceptions that the basic issues had been aired and that they had received a fair hearing were related to respondents' compliance and good relations between the parties, as reported by the complainants.

Two reasonable explanations for these findings were offered (Pruitt et al., 1990). First, parties may view the agreement as more just because of the perceived fairness of the process that produced the agreement. In support of this interpretation, perceptions of fairness were related to increased compliance, even though the outcome was not rated any more favorably by the parties. Second, better procedures may serve to directly improve the relationship between the parties, which would then enhance the likelihood of success. In support of this interpretation, there was a relationship between the parties' perceptions of fairness and their predictions that the relationship would improve. Hence, either or both of these explanations seem possible. What is clear is that the mediation process itself, which provides both parties the opportunity to express all of their concerns, and endeavors to consider all underlying issues, is a therapeutic process that can assist in reaching potentially higher-quality and longer-lasting agreements.

Perceived Mediator Impartiality

Mediator neutrality is often considered to be an important component of procedural fairness. It is often argued that the mediator must be perceived as neutral. This point is emphasized so strongly in mediator training that a newly trained mediator I observed was devastated when informed that one of the role-playing disputants felt she was biased against him. Indeed, one manual recommends that a mediator who is either a landlord or a tenant should consider disqualifying himself or herself from serving in a landlord–tenant dispute (Underhill, 1981). Just how far should this thinking go? Should a female mediator disqualify herself from hearing a case between a man and a woman because she might be more closely affiliated with one party than the other? If so, there would be many cases for which an acceptable mediator could not be found.

This emphasis is misplaced, however, because the critical component is *perceived* impartiality. Whenever a disputant perceives partiality—whether real or imagined—perceived fairness may be affected. Lehmann (1986) cites an example in which both parties perceived that the mediator favored the other side. The male considered the mediator to be the female's advocate, whereas the female thought that the mediator was not forceful enough with the male, favoring his arguments. Vallone, Ross, and Lepper (1985) demonstrated that when viewing televised news coverage of the Beirut massacre, both pro-Israeli and pro-Arab partisans rated the programs as being biased against their side. This evidence implies that to a large extent perceived neutrality is beyond the control of the mediator, because a given neutral action can be perceived by both sides as indicating favor for the other party.

Fortunately, however, perceived partiality is not as critical as has been supposed (Welton & Pruitt, 1987; Zartman & Touval, 1985). Certainly, if a mediator works actively to advance the cause of one party to the detriment of the other, the mediation process will be seriously affected. Hence, mediators should always be aware of potential biasing factors that might cause them to prefer a certain outcome for a certain party at the expense of the other.

On the other hand, the fact that a mediator has closer ties to one party than to the other does not imply that he or she will not maintain high concern for the outcomes of both sides. Rather, the mediator may still conduct the hearing in such a way as to foster cooperation between the parties. Research evidence indicates that as long as the mediator is able to demonstrate that he or she is concerned for and values the outcomes of both parties, in spite of some personal preferences that might indicate bias, disputants are likely to be willing to work with and be influenced by the mediator (Welton & Pruitt, 1987).

The issue is not that of absolute neutrality between the parties or the groups they represent. Rather, the issue is whether the mediator is concerned about the outcomes of both sides and can demonstrate that concern to the disputants. As long as this is accomplished, the mediator has fulfilled his or her role as a neutral third party.

Perceived Fairness of the Outcome

The final agreement in mediation is generally a result of a series of compromises and a search for creative alternatives. Whereas procedural fairness may often be more critical than the perceived fairness of the outcome, the latter is still significant. One primary mechanism that endangers the problem-solving process and the perceptions of the agreement requires consideration here.

Reactive devaluation (Stillinger, Epelbaum, Keltner, & Ross, 1988) can make the difficult task of reaching agreement even more monumental. "Reactive devaluation" is the process by which a party tends to devalue concessions made by the other party in relation to his or her own concessions. That is, there is an egocentric bias that causes each party to overvalue his or her own concessions in relation to the other's, and hence to perceive unfairness.

Negative perceptions about the other party cause an individual to distrust any concessions the other might make. The interpretation is that if the other is conceding on some issue, he or she must not feel strongly about that issue, and hence is not truly conceding. At the same time, one tends to overlook this reasoning in regard to one's own concessions. The result is that each party tends to think that he or she has made more significant concessions during the hearing than has the other. Hence, each side may conclude that the final agreement favors the other party.

Certainly mediators are often able to overcome this problem, as they often achieve agreements that produce compliance and satisfaction. Nevertheless, reactive devaluation is a mechanism of which mediators need to be aware. It may indicate that mediators need to use more caucusing to help parties better understand each other's position and concessions. Also, it may be necessary for many concessions to come as suggestions from the mediator rather than directly from the disputants (Stillinger et al., 1988).

SUMMARY

Mediation is flourishing in many parts of the United States because it is meeting the needs of conflicting parties as well as, or better than, litigation alone. This trend can gain additional momentum as we continue to understand the mediation process in general and the disputing parties in particular. In this chapter, three primary issues have been raised for further consideration. First is the possibility of broadening the use of mediation by applying it to cases that do not include a continuing relationship between the parties. This may require our redefining mediation as a complement of litigation rather than solely as an alternative to it. Second is the possiblity of requiring certain parties to retain legal counsel as a means of approximating equality between the parties. Third is the critical task of altering the parties' negative perceptions, with three possible suggestions: the teaching of skills in perspective taking to disputants, the overt discussion of expectancies, and the use of a paradoxical strategy involving the exaggeration of negative expectancies. Further consideration of these issues will better enable us to serve the parties in conflict.

REFERENCES

Braver, S. L., & Barnett, B. (1974). Perception of opponent's motives and co-operation in a mixed-motive game. *Journal of Conflict Resolution, 18,* 686–699.

Carroll, J. S., Bazerman, M. H., & Maury, R. (1988). Negotiator cognitions: A descriptive approach to negotiators' understanding of their opponents. *Organizational Behavior and Human Decision Processes, 41,* 352–370.

Castrianno, L. M., Pruitt, D. G., Nochajski, T. H., & Zubek, J. M. (1988). *Complainant–respondent differences in mediation.* Paper presented at the annual meeting of the Eastern Psychological Association, Buffalo, NY.

Cooper, J., & Fazio, R. H. (1979). The formation and persistence of attitudes that support intergroup conflict. In W. G. Austin & S. Worchel (Eds.), *The social psychology of intergroup relations* (pp. 149–159). Monterey, CA: Brooks/Cole.

Duffy, K. G., & Olczak, P. V. (1989). Perceptions of mediated disputes: Some characteristics affecting use. *Journal of Social Behavior and Personality, 4,* 541–554.

Emery, R. E., & Wyer, M. M. (1987). Divorce mediation. *American Psychologist, 42,* 472–480.

Fisher, R., & Ury, W. (1981). *Getting to yes: Negotiating agreement without giving in.* Boston: Houghton Mifflin.

Fiss, O. M. (1986). Against settlement. In J. E. Palenski & H. M. Launer (Eds.), *Mediation: Contexts and challenges* (pp. 15–32). Springfield, IL: Charles C Thomas. (Original work published 1984)

Hilton, J. L., & Darley, J. M. (1985). Constructing other persons: A limit on the effect. *Journal of Experimental Social Psychology, 21,* 1–18.

Johnson, D. W. (1975). Cooperativeness and social perspective taking. *Journal of Personality and Social Psychology, 31,* 241–244.

Jussim, L. (1986). Self-fulfilling prophecies: A theoretical and integrative review. *Psychological Review, 93,* 429–445.

Kramer, R. M., McClintock, C. G., & Messick, D. M. (1986). Social values and cooperative response to a simulated resource conservation crisis. *Journal of Personality, 54,* 576–592.

Kuhlman, D. M., & Marshello, A. F. J. (1975). Individual differences in game motivation as moderators of preprogrammed strategy effects in Prisoner's Dilemma. *Journal of Personality and Social Psychology, 32,* 922–931.

Kulik, J. A., & Brown, R. (1979). Frustration, attribution of blame, and aggression. *Journal of Experimental Social Psychology, 15,* 183–194.

Lehmann, H. J. (1986). Mediation and domestic violence. In J. E. Palenski & H. M.

Launer (Eds.), *Mediation: Contexts and challenges* (pp. 77–84). Springfield, IL: Charles C Thomas.

Levine, M. I. (1986). Power imbalances in dispute resolution. In J. E. Palenski & H. M. Launer (Eds.), *Mediation: Contexts and challenges* (pp. 63–76). Springfield, IL: Charles C Thomas.

Lind, E. A., Kurtz, S., Musante, L., Walker, L., & Thibaut, J. W. (1980). Procedure and outcome effects on reactions to adjudicated resolutions of conflicts of interest. *Journal of Personality and Social Psychology, 39*, 643–653.

Lind, E. A., & Tyler, T. R. (1988). *The social psychology of procedural justice*. New York: Plenum Press.

McClintock, C. G. (1977). Social motivations in settings of outcome interdependence. In D. Druckman (Ed.), *Negotiations: Social psychological perspectives* (pp. 49–78). Beverly Hills, CA: Sage.

Mischel, W. (1984). Convergences and challenges in the search for consistency. *American Psychologist, 39*, 351–364.

Neale, M. A., & Bazerman, M. H. (1983). The role of perspective-taking ability in negotiating under different forms of arbitration. *Industrial and Labor Relations Review, 36*, 378–388.

Pruitt, D. G., Peirce, R. S., Zubek, J. M., Welton, G. L., & Nochajski, T. H. (1990). Goal achievement, procedural justice and the success of mediation. *International Journal of Conflict Management, 1*, 33–45.

Pruitt, D. G., & Rubin, J. Z. (1986). *Social conflict: Escalation, stalemate and settlement*. New York: Random House.

Psenicka, C., & Rahim, M. A. (1989). Integrative and distributive dimensions of styles of handling interpersonal conflict and bargaining outcome. In M. A. Rahim (Ed.), *Managing conflict: An interdisciplinary approach* (pp. 33–40). New York: Praeger.

Riskin, L. L. (1982). Mediation and lawyers. *Ohio State Law Journal, 43*, 29–60.

Snyder, M., & Swann, W. B., Jr. (1978). Behavioral confirmation in social interaction: From social perception to social reality. *Journal of Experimental Social Psychology, 14*, 148–162.

Sternberg, R. J., & Dobson, D. M. (1987). Resolving interpersonal conflicts: An analysis of stylistic consistency. *Journal of Personality and Social Psychology, 52*, 794–812.

Sternberg, R. J., & Soriano, L. J. (1984). Styles of conflict resolution. *Journal of Personality and Social Psychology, 47*, 115–126.

Stillinger, C. A., Epelbaum, M., Keltner, D., & Ross, L. (1988). *The "reactive devaluation" barrier to conflict resolution* (Stanford Center on Conflict and Negotiation, Working Paper No. 3). Stanford, CA: Stanford Center on Conflict and Negotiation.

Swann, W. B., Jr. (1984). Quest for accuracy in person perception: A matter of pragmatics. *Psychological Review, 91*, 457–477.

Swann, W. B., Jr. (1987). Identity negotiation: Where two roads meet. *Journal of Personality and Social Psychology, 53*, 1038–1051.

Swann, W. B., Jr., & Hill, C. A. (1982). When our identities are mistaken: Reaffirming self-conceptions through social interaction. *Journal of Personality and Social Psychology, 43*, 59–66.

Swann, W. B., Jr., Pelham, B. W., & Chidester, T. R. (1988). Change through paradox: Using self-verification to alter beliefs. *Journal of Personality and Social Psychology, 54,* 268–273.

Tjosvold, D., & Fabrey, L. (1980). Effects of interdependence and dependence on cognitive perspective-taking. *Psychological Reports, 46,* 755–765.

Tjosvold, D., & Sabato, S. (1978). Effects of relative power on cognitive perspective-taking. *Personality and Social Psychology Bulletin, 4,* 256–259.

Tyler, T. R. (1984). The role of perceived injustice in defendants' evaluations of their courtroom experience. *Law and Society Review, 18,* 51–74.

Tyler, T. R. (1987). The psychology of disputant concerns in mediation. *Negotiation Journal, 3,* 367–374.

Tyler, T. R., Casper, J. D., & Fisher, B. (1987). *Maintaining allegiance toward political authorities.* Unpublished manuscript, American Bar Association.

Tyler, T. R., & Folger, R. (1980). Distributional and procedural aspects of satisfaction with citizen–police encounters. *Basic and Applied Social Psychology, 1,* 281–292.

Umbreit, M. (1985). *Crime and reconciliation: Creative options for victims and offenders.* Nashville, TN: Abingdon.

Underhill, C. I. (1981). *A manual for community dispute settlement.* Buffalo, NY: Better Business Bureau of Western New York.

Vallone, R. P., Ross, L., & Lepper, M. R. (1985). The hostile media phenomenon: Biased perception and perceptions of media bias in coverage of the Beirut massacre. *Journal of Personality and Social Psychology, 49,* 577–585.

Vidmar, N. (1985). An assessment of mediation in a small claims court. *Journal of Social Issues, 41*(2), 127–144.

Welton, G. L., & Miękisz, A. (1990). *Conflict de-escalation: Using expectancy confirmation to alter beliefs.* Paper presented at the annual meeting of the Midwestern Psychological Association, Chicago.

Welton, G. L., & Pruitt, D. G. (1987). The mediation process: The effects of mediator bias and disputant power. *Personality and Social Psychology Bulletin, 13,* 123–133.

Zartman, I. W., & Touval, S. (1985). International mediation: Conflict resolution and power politics. *Journal of Social Issues, 41*(2), 27–45.

8

Mediator Behavior and Effectiveness in Community Mediation

PETER J. CARNEVALE
University of Illinois

LINDA L. PUTNAM
Purdue University

DONALD E. CONLON
University of Delaware

KATHLEEN M. O'CONNOR
University of Illinois

Community mediation programs often rely on the generosity of a large cadre of volunteers who meet with disputants and assist them in reaching agreements. One court-affiliated community mediation program tells its volunteer mediators that the goals of mediation are "1. To assist parties in creating reasoned, workable solutions to their problems; 2. To model good conflict management behavior; and 3. To expand options to formal court proceedings, thereby enhancing the overall effectiveness of the judicial process" (Neighborhood Justice of Chicago, 1987, p. 2). These goals are explicitly tied to behavior—to what the mediator says and does in mediation. The issue of mediator behavior is central to understanding the process. Kochan and Katz (1988), in a discussion of the determinants of successful labor mediation, state that "[p]erhaps the most difficult determinant to study is the very heart of the process itself: what a mediator does to help produce a settlement" (p. 271). We believe, along with McGillis (1981), that community dispute centers provide a natural laboratory for the study of mediator behavior and the outcome of disputes.

The purpose of this chapter is to describe several recent studies that have addressed mediator behavior and the settlement of disputes. We review research on the structure of mediator behavior, with an emphasis on mediator strategies, tactics, and taxonomies of behavior. We present in some detail the results of several studies that have addressed the situational contingencies of mediation tactics. Our discussion of contingencies in mediator behavior considers distinct types of disputes, as well as different types of mediation outcomes. We present the results of a recently completed survey of 34 community mediators, with an emphasis on behavior that distinguished successful and unsuccessful mediation. We conclude with a discussion of communication patterns of successful and unsuccessful mediation, and with a consideration of possible issues for further study.

THE STRUCTURE OF MEDIATOR BEHAVIOR

Strategies, Tactics, and Taxonomies

In training, community mediators are often given specific directions on how to conduct a mediation hearing. This includes instructions on where to position disputants around a table, and a standard opening statement that explains the nature of mediation, confidentiality, and the neutrality of the mediator. Specific procedures are also emphasized (e.g., having disputants take turns in an initial statement about the issues), and even specific nonverbal behaviors (e.g., "Incline your head slightly forward in a 'listening' attitude"; Neighborhood Justice of Chicago, 1987, p. 30).

The literature on mediation clearly acknowledges the tremendous variety of activities in which mediators can engage, and sometimes emphasizes roles and characteristics of mediators (Pruitt & Rubin, 1986; Rubin, 1981), as well as specific behaviors and the organization of these into a taxonomy (Keltner, 1987; Kressel & Pruitt, 1989; Womack, 1985). Perhaps the best-known taxonomy of mediator behavior is the one by Kressel (1972), which was recently updated by Kressel and Pruitt (1989). Kressel and Pruitt have identified three basic types of tactics: "reflexive," "substantive," and "contextual." Reflexive tactics are designed to orient mediators to the dispute and to create a foundation for their future activities; substantive tactics deal directly with the issues in the dispute, such as suggestions for settlement; and contextual tactics involve facilitating the dispute resolution process so that the parties themselves are able to discover an acceptable solution.

In a recent study (Lim & Carnevale, 1990), an effort was made to verify Kressel and Pruitt's (1989) taxonomy empirically. The participants in the study were 255 members of the Society for Professionals in Dispute Resolution (SPIDR), an international organization of professionals involved in community, labor–management, and other kinds of disputes. The mediators responded to a survey that asked them to recall their most recently completed mediation case. They rated the extent to which 24 potential sources of dispute were a problem in that case, the extent to which they used 43 different mediation tactics, and the extent to which 19 outcomes were attained. The sources and tactics were derived from the mediation literature and interviews of labor and community mediators.

To test the Kressel and Pruitt (1989) factor structure for mediation tactics, confirmatory factor analyses were conducted on mediators' ratings of their usage of tactics. Confirmatory factor analysis is a statistical technique in which many different tests and measures are administered and intercorrelated, in order to discover what measures tend to "go together" and thus appear as "factors" that support some theoretical prediction or prior research.

In addition to the Kressel and Pruitt categories of tactics, several other categories were examined, including three subcategories of substantive tactics described by Carnevale (1986): (1) the mediator's use of outcome suggestions designed to aid negotiators in impression management and face saving (cf. Stevens, 1963); (2) mediator tactics designed to move a party onto a new position; and (3) mediator tactics designed to move a party off a currently held position. The latter two types were identified in case analyses of mediation, where mediators frequently developed arguments in favor of possible outcomes, and frequently against positions that they viewed as untenable.

The results (Lim & Carnevale, 1990) were generally supportive of the Kressel and Pruitt (1989) taxonomy: The three general types of mediator behavior (reflexive, substantive, and contextual behavior) proposed by Kressel and Pruitt were identified. The analyses also uncovered the three substantive factors (the coercive type designed to move a party off a position, the more positive type designed to move a party onto a new position, and the face-saving type). However, the analyses also indicated that contextual tactics should be subdivided into two types. The first one emphasized activities important in building trust among the parties and the mediator; it included tactics such as "Formulated clear goals prior to and during mediation" and "Developed trust between the parties." The other contextual factor involved tactics designed to control the issue agenda; tactics that loaded on (or were highly correlated with) this factor included "Helped establish priorities among the issues" and "Arranged agenda to cover general issues first, specific issues last."

Given that mediator behavior can be systematically indexed, the next question concerns usage. Do mediators use different tactics in different situations, and, if so, does it matter for the likelihood of agreement?

Contingent Use of Mediation Tactics

Most authors acknowledge that mediators often make contingent use of strategies and tactics in a particular dispute situation (Carnevale, 1986; Kochan & Jick, 1978; Kolb & Rubin, 1989; Kressel & Pruitt, 1989; Rubin,

1981; Wall, 1981). It is generally assumed that the contingent use of tactics is likely to lead to successful outcomes. Mediator tactics that lead to successful conflict resolution in one dispute may be seen as irrelevant or even detrimental in a different dispute.

The "contingent use" of mediator tactics refers to the mediators' use of different tactics in dissimilar dispute situations. Evidence that mediators use tactics contingently has been found in several studies, including that by Carnevale and Pegnetter (1985). In this study, 32 professional labor mediators rated the extent to which 24 sources of dispute were a problem for a recently mediated case (e.g., the extent to which "a key issue was at stake"), and also the extent to which 37 mediation tactics were used in that case (e.g., "suggested a settlement"). A correlation analysis revealed that the use of some mediator tactics was contingent upon the problems that produced or contributed to the dispute. For example, when bargainers were hostile to each other, mediators reported using substantive tactics, such as trying to change bargainers' expectations and mentioning the costs of continued disagreement; when bargainers brought too many issues to the negotiation, mediators reported using issue-related contextual tactics, such as devising a framework for negotiations and creating issue priorities.

Communicative Aspects of Mediation Tactics

The use of particular tactics also hinges on the way in which mediators communicate with the disputants. Communication researchers focus on three aspects of mediator–disputant interaction: the timing of interventions, the phases in which they are used, and the language intensity of the mediation. The nature of the disputants' behaviors serves as a cue for timing mediator interventions. That is, mediator tactics must be viewed within the ongoing interaction of disputants and mediator. As Kressel (1985, p. 196) contends, "it is important to measure not only what the mediator does at critical moments, but what the parties are doing when the mediator intervenes and what they are doing after an intervention."

For example, Zappa, Manusov, Cody, and Donohue (1990) observe that a mediator needs to intervene immediately following a disputant's attack on the other party. If the mediator waits and the attack–defense spiral builds, the conflict can escalate out of control. If a disputant's attack violates the procedural rules for mediation, the mediator needs to act quickly to control the interaction and to facilitate the dispute resolution process.

The term "interaction phases" refers to the cluster of tactics that move mediation through global stages. Most mediators recognize the need to keep mediation moving through systematic stages of development; however, the type and number of mediation phases vary from source to source. Thoennes and Pearson (1985) posit four phases of mediation: orientation, information gathering, issue processing, and proposal development. In the first stage, mediators orient disputants to the interaction rules, the mediator's role, and issues of confidentiality. In this phase mediators employ such reflexive tactics as establishing protocol for the sessions, setting timetables and deadlines, and clarifying ground rules. The second stage of mediation, gathering background information and obtaining disputants' objectives, is characterized by the use of such contextual tactics as questioning the disputants, paraphrasing and clarifying responses, converting accusations to requests, bridging and integrating statements, and providing reflection and summary (Putnam & Poole, 1987).

In the third phase, mediators help disputants disclose and process issues through such substantive and contextual tactics as narrowing topics of discussion, clarifying positions, reducing unnecessary repetition of arguments, and regulating the affective tone of the meeting with humor and deflection. Finally, the fourth stage, proposal development, entails preparing and selecting specific alternatives for the issues that surface in the mediation. Mediators employ such substantive tactics as creating and initiating alternative proposals, giving opinions about positions, assessing the costs of alternatives, reframing utterances as proposals, identifying points of agreement, synchronizing concessions, and inducing compliance (Donohue, in press; Kolb, 1983).

Mediators rely on language intensity and the wording of disputants' messages to judge the timing and the development of the mediation process. Specifically, the use of qualifiers, pronoun referents, and ambiguous language conveys tacit messages about disputants hostility and competitiveness and about their receptiveness to mediation. Qualifying words such as "I may," "sometimes," or "in most cases," rather than absolute statements such as "always" or "never," serve as verbal codes to signal relational closeness and to mark a readiness to negotiate (Donohue, Weider-Hatfield, Hamilton, & Diez, 1985). Use of particular pronoun demonstratives, such as "I am speaking about this [as opposed to that] agreement that we signed," brings disputants psychologically closer to each other and to the mediation process (Donohue, in press). Ambiguous wording of tactics stems from the abstractness of the language used and the absence of specificity in a message. A statement such as "I feel some sort of monetary compensation is important" not only targets a monetary alternative, but opens the discussion to "what sort of" compensation is appropriate. Disputants often employ ambiguous language to "hint at" alternatives for a settlement and simultaneously to save face in the process (Putnam, 1990). Mediators use ambiguous language to initiate proposals without controlling the specific parameters of an outcome (Donohue, in press).

In effect, the nature and flow of communication in mediation are important factors in deciding when and how to intervene. Determining when to use a particular tactic requires monitoring the disputants' patterns of interaction in light of the overall objectives of the mediation. In addition, mediators use tactics to move the mediation process forward. In particular, nondirective and reflexive tactics may be appropriate for the early stages of mediation, whereas substantive tactics may be more useful in the latter stages of the process (Hiltrop, 1985).

CONTINGENT EFFECTIVENESS OF MEDIATION TACTICS

Few studies have examined the "contingent effectiveness" of mediation tactics—the degree to which the tailoring of tactics to certain types of dispute situations is effective in bringing about settlement. This refers to a change in the relationship between the use of a tactic and an outcome, from one dispute situation to another.

Hiltrop (1985, 1989) conducted two studies that examined contingent effectiveness. In the first study, he found that in disputes where there were high levels of hostility, the use of forceful, substantive tactics was positively associated with settlement; in disputes where there was low hostility, the use of substantive/pressure tactics was negatively associated with settlement. Results of the second study were consistent with these findings, and also showed that the use of contextual tactics (e.g., "Help the parties understand the other side's position" and "Act as a communication link between the parties") was positively associated with settlement when perceived hostility was high and when positional differences were large. Thoennes and Pearson (1985) reported similar results: Mediators who facilitated communication and provided clarification and insights were most likely to achieve settlement. In sum, Hiltrop's (1985, 1989) findings indicate that some mediation tactics are likely to be associated with settlement in some circumstances and not in others, supporting the notion that mediator behavior can be contingently effective.

Dispute Types and Mediation Outcomes

The analysis of contingencies in mediation requires not only a discussion of types of tactics, but also a discussion of types of disputes (in which the tactics are used) as well as types of outcomes. The study by Lim and Carnevale (1990) identified five basic types of disputes:

1. "Hostility," which involved such items as "Interparty hostility," "No interest in settling," and "No trust in the other party."
2. "Internal party problems," which included such items as "Parties lacked leadership" and "Parties not prepared for negotiations."

3. "Comparison problems," which included two items, "Held to a comparison position" and "Broke from a comparison pattern." (These problems refer to an agreement reached in a comparable dispute that serves as a precedent and thus influences subsequent negotiations, and is found in labor disputes more often than in community disputes.)

4. "Resistance to mediation," which involved such items as "No trust in the mediator" and "Wanted control over the proceedings."

5. "Single important issue," which involved two items, "Key settlement issues involved" and "Major principle at stake."

Lim and Carnevale (1990) identified three basic types of mediation outcomes. The first was labeled "general settlement" and represented such aspects of mediation as reaching a settlement, especially one that was mutually beneficial and lasting, and in which nothing ambiguous was stated. The second factor was labeled "mediator outcomes" and reflected outcomes relevant to the mediator, such as feelings of trust toward the mediator, satisfaction of the mediator's needs, and the parties' satisfaction with mediation. The third factor was labeled "improved relationship" and involved an improved relationship and better communication between the parties.

Contingent Effectiveness

Lim and Carnevale (1990) reported that the effectiveness of substantive/pressure tactics depended on the characteristics of the dispute. When the dispute was high in conflict intensity, the use of pressure tactics (such as mentioning that the parties' position was unrealistic) was positively associated with settlement; however, when hostility between the parties was relatively low, the use of pressure tactics was negatively associated with settlement. This finding is consistent with the observation that mediators are advised not to apply a heavy hand when dealing with disputants who might resent the intrusiveness of a forceful mediator (see Rubin, 1980, for a theoretical discussion of this).

The Lim and Carnevale study also found that mediator attempts to help the parties save face were especially likely to promote positive outcomes (general settlement, mediator outcomes, and improved relationship) when there was high hostility. Also, when there was high hostility, and when the parties were resistant to mediation, the use of contextual tactics that affected the agenda of issues (i.e., the order in which the issues were discussed) was especially likely to promote positive outcomes; this finding was consistent with the results of Hiltrop (1989). And when resistance to mediation was high, the mediators were more likely to produce positive outcomes when they relied on reflexive tactics, such as working on the development of a rapport with the parties.

SUCCESSFUL AND UNSUCCESSFUL MEDIATION

Recently, we conducted a study that extended the procedures used by Lim and Carnevale (1990), but employed a sample of 34 community mediators at Neighborhood Justice of Chicago, a court-affiliated dispute resolution center. Neighborhood Justice of Chicago is a not-for-profit organization with a full-time staff of about 7, as well as 105 volunteer mediators, and the organization is still growing. The disputes generally involve people who have some sort of ongoing relationship, such as neighbors, landlords and tenants, consumers and merchants, and family members. Typical disputes involve noise, damage to property, theft, assault and battery, harassment, and the like. In fiscal year 1989, the center resolved 579 cases involving 1,280 individuals and 76 businesses and organizations. More than half of the cases came from 15 misdemeanor branch courts in Cook County's First Municipal District or were mediated on site in the Forcible Entry and Detainer (Eviction) courtrooms of the First Municipal District (see Neighborhood Justice of Chicago, 1990).

The 34 mediators in this study had a mean age of just under 40, and the majority of the mediators were female (23). The average number of cases handled a year by a mediator was 14, and the average number of years of experience in mediation was just under 3. Almost all of the mediators had advanced graduate degrees, with about two-thirds of them having JD degrees and full-time occupations as attorneys.

The mediators were asked to complete a questionnaire that began with the following instructions:

> This questionnaire will ask you to answer questions about two of your (most recent) mediation cases. The questions for both cases are the same. We would like you to report on one mediation that you feel was very successful, and then on one mediation that you feel was very unsuccessful (or one that compared to the first but was not so glorious).

For each case, the questionnaire had three parts. In the first part, there was a list of 17 possible sources of impasse or problems in the mediation case. The mediators were asked to indicate the extent that each was a problem, using 5-point rating scales (1 = "not a problem," 3 = "a moderate problem," 5 = "the greatest problem"). In the second part, they rated the extent to which they used 43 different mediation tactics (1 = "no use," 3 = "moderate use," 5 = "the most use"). In the third part, they rated the extent to which 19 outcomes were attained (1 = "not at all," 3 = "to a moderate extent," 5 = "completely"). They did this for both the successful case and the unsuccessful case.

Criteria of Success

An initial question that was addressed in this study pertained to the criteria mediators use for defining whether a mediation case was successful or unsuccessful. To answer this question, the ratings of the outcomes for the successful and unsuccessful cases were compared. Table 8.1 presents the analysis of the differences between the successful and unsuccessful mediations on the 20 measures of dispute outcome, presented in order of most to least important in distinguishing between successful and unsuccessful mediations. This is useful for telling what aspects of dispute outcome the mediators used in interpreting whether or not a given mediation case was "successful" or "unsuccessful."

The analysis revealed that all 20 scales distinguished the successful and unsuccessful cases. The scale that distinguished them best was "A lasting agreement was reached, i.e., the parties will comply with it over a long period of time." It should be noted that some items were rated relatively high for both the successful and unsuccessful cases (e.g., the measure "The parties were satisfied with your mediation efforts").

Characteristics of Disputes

Table 8.2 presents the analysis of the differences between the successful and unsuccessful mediations on the measures of dispute characteristics, presented in order of most to least important in distinguishing between them. This is useful for telling what dimensions the mediators used in characterizing the features of disputes that were successful and unsuccessful.

The analysis revealed that 12 scales distinguished the successful and unsuccessful cases. The scales that distinguished them best were "The parties were not interested in settling" and "There was a strong-willed person who obstructed movement." The latter variable was rated particularly high in the unsuccessful cases, indicating that one problem in mediation may be having to deal with asymmetries in disputant intransigence (i.e., one person's being more contentious than the other).

Mediator Behavior in Successful and Unsuccessful Mediation

The analysis of mediator behavior revealed that 12 mediation tactics distinguished the successful from the unsuccessful mediation cases. These are listed in Table 8.3 in order of most to least important in distinguishing successful from unsuccessful cases (in terms of variance accounted for).

TABLE 8.1.   Features of Dispute Outcomes in "Successful" and "Unsuccessful" Mediation

Feature	Case type	
	Successful	Unsuccessful
A lasting agreement was reached, i.e., the parties will comply with it over a long period of time.	3.61	1.22
All issues in the dispute were settled.	3.79	1.25
The dispute was resolved within a reasonable amount of time.	4.00	1.41
The relationship between the parties was improved.	3.17	1.18
All issues in the dispute were settled to the mutual benefit of all.	3.78	1.15
The distance was narrowed between the parties' positions.	3.97	1.70
The underlying core conflict was resolved.	3.58	1.09
An agreement was reached that the negotiators felt was their own.	3.70	1.33
An agreement was reached that did not have adverse political ramifications for either side.	3.96	1.17
The number of unresolved issues was reduced through mediation.	4.05	1.81
The parties were satisfied with the procedure of mediation.	4.05	2.28
The parties gained or recovered important, valued resources.	3.34	1.29
The parties learned to communicate and negotiate better with each other so that they could handle future disputes by themselves.	2.93	1.28
The *mediator's* (i.e., your) needs, goals, and interests were satisfied during the mediation process.	3.85	1.75
Feelings of goodwill and trust were created toward the mediator.	3.79	2.48
An agreement was reached that left nothing ambiguously stated.	3.78	1.43
The parties were satisfied with your mediation efforts.	4.11	2.70
The parties held back when they could have made concessions.	1.78	3.61
New problems between the parties are unlikely to arise in the future.	3.10	1.53
The settlement succeeded in averting physical violence.	3.77	2.25

Note. All characteristics of the dispute outcomes distinguished the successful and unsuccessful mediations (*t* test with $p < .005$).

TABLE 8.2. Dispute Characteristics of Succesful and Unsuccessful Mediation

	Case type	
Characteristic	Successful	Unsuccessful
The parties were not interested in settling.	1.93	3.75*
There was a strong-willed person who obstructed movement.	2.14	4.09*
One or both parties were unreceptive to mediation.	1.50	3.18*
One or both parties became committed to a position.	2.20	3.89*
One or both did not trust the other party.	2.94	3.83*
The parties did not seem to place full trust in the mediator.	1.23	2.40*
One or both wanted substantial control over the proceedings.	1.55	2.50*
One or both parties saw a major principle at stake.	2.63	3.53*
There were key "settlement issues."	2.70	3.58*
One or both sides were not well prepared for negotiations.	1.34	2.13*
One or both parties were very hostile to the other party.	2.85	3.65*
The parties had unrealistic expectations.	2.18	3.45*
One or both parties brought too many issues to mediation.	1.47	1.83
One or both parties had internal disagreements about the issues.	2.03	2.26
One or both parties lacked leadership.	1.41	1.72
One or both backed off an initial proposal/agreement.	1.87	1.77
The parties went to mediation without really bargaining beforehand.	1.82	1.71

*This characteristic distinguished successful and unsuccessful mediation (t test with $p < .05$).

As can be seen, some tactics were reported as being used quite often, and as being used more in the successful case than in the unsuccessful case (e.g., "Kept negotiations focused on the issues"). Other tactics were reported as less frequently used, yet also distinguished the two cases (e.g., "Expressed displeasure at their progress in negotiations"). Some tactics were used frequently, but did not distinguish the successful from the unsuccessful cases (e.g., "Tried to gain their trust and confidence"). This latter effect may indicate that mediators do some things in mediation noncontingently—for instance, that they strive to gain trust regardless of the characteristics of the dispute.

The data on the use of expressing displeasure and expressing pleasure at the parties' progress in negotiations, which both distinguished the successful

TABLE 8.3.   Use of Mediation Tactics as a Function of Successful and Unsuccessful Mediation

Tactic	Case type	
	Successful	Unsuccessful
Expressed displeasure at their progress in negotiations.	1.17	1.80*
Tried to change their expectations.	2.08	3.03*
Developed rapport with them.	3.52	3.23*
Kept negotiations focused on the issues.	4.00	3.58*
Expressed pleasure at their progress in negotiations.	3.05	2.60*
Pressed them hard to make compromise.	2.08	2.43*
Attempted to move one or both parties off a committed position.	3.00	3.59*
Made substantive suggesstions for compromise.	2.17	2.74*
Discussed other settlements or patterns.	2.09	2.70*
Avoided taking sides on important issues in joint sessions.	3.94	3.45*
Discussed the interests of all parties affected by the dispute.	3.14	2.77*
Told them the next impasse step was not better.	1.37	1.83*
Attempted to "simplify" agenda by eliminating/ combining issues.	2.91	2.76
Clarified the needs of the other party.	3.51	3.50
Discussed the "costs" of continued disagreement.	3.08	3.48
Controlled their expression of hostility.	2.76	2.84
Suggested a particular settlement.	2.14	2.53
Suggested proposals, helping them avoid appearance of defeat.	2.36	2.58
Helped one or more parties "save face."	2.47	2.48
Suggested that they review their needs with their constituency.	1.39	1.32
Educated them to the bargaining or impasse process.	1.82	2.09
Tried to gain their trust and confidence.	3.50	3.59
Called for frequent caususes.	2.00	2.06
Helped devise a framework for negotiations.	3.36	3.09
Helped the negotiators deal with problems with constituents.	1.58	1.55
Controlled the timing or pace of negotiations.	2.58	2.86
Kept the parties at the table and negotiating.	2.85	2.81
Kept their caucus focused on the impasse issues.	2.69	2.80
Argued their [one party's] case to the other party.	1.88	2.23
Used humor to lighten the atmosphere.	2.00	1.72
Let them blow off steam in front of me.	3.17	3.35
Helped establish priorities among the issues.	3.23	3.22
Took responsibility for their concessions.	1.35	1.46
Suggested tradeoffs among the issues.	2.09	2.40

Attempted to "speak their language."	2.38	2.36
Assured them that the other was being honest.	1.75	1.63
Used late hours, long mediation, to facilitate compromise.	1.32	1.48
Attempted to settle simple issues first.	2.85	2.56
Told them their position was unrealistic.	1.50	1.93
Arranged agenda to cover general issues first, specific last.	1.67	1.78
Allowed the parties to initiate and maintain momentum	2.88	2.58
Formulated clear goals prior to or during mediation.	2.73	2.58
Attempted to develop trust between the disputants.	3.00	3.06

*This mediation tactic distinguished successful and unsuccessful mediation (t test with $p < .10$).

and unsuccessful mediations, suggest that mediators use both approval and disapproval in their efforts to facilitate cooperation. It should be noted that the expression of pleasure at the parties' progress was relatively high in both the successful and the unsuccessful mediations.

It must be emphasized that the data of the present study are correlational in nature. In interpreting the differences in behavior between the successful and unsuccessful cases, one should be careful not to make causal inferences. For example, in Table 8.3, one can see that the tactic "Developed rapport with them" was reported to be used more in cases that were successful than in cases that were unsuccessful. This should not be interpreted as indicating that rapport will cause success in mediation. There could be some other variable, such as a characteristic of the case (e.g., the parties really wanted or needed an agreement), that both led to rapport with the mediator and also led the mediator to consider the mediation a success. This type of third-variable interpretation problem is something that must always be kept in mind when interpreting correlational data.

The same point should be made about the data on expressing displeasure at progress in mediation, which was greater in the unsuccessful mediations than in the successful mediations. It is unlikely that this behavior caused a mediation to be unsuccessful. Rather, it is likely that some other process, such as a lack of real interest in settling in mediation, led the mediator to express displeasure at the parties' progress and also led the mediator to label the mediation as unsuccessful.

Communication Patterns in Successful and Unsuccessful Mediation

Research on mediation in domestic disputes has also demonstrated differences in behaviors of successful and unsuccessful mediators, particularly in the communication between mediators and disputants. Studies on the timing of tactics revealed that mediators initiated structuring statements to exert procedural control when the disputants became defensive (Donohue, in press). Disputants typically responded to these tactics by giving more information and clarifying their positions. In the unsuccessful mediations, however, disputants became increasingly competitive and defensive after these interventions, particularly in the second and third phases of mediation.

Mediators also used fewer structuring statements and rule enforcement behaviors (contextual tactics) in the latter part of mediation. For the successful sessions, fewer contextual tactics resulted in increased cooperation among disputants; however, for the unsuccessful mediations, this change combined with an increase in conflict intensity led to destructive attack–defend cycles. Although mediators in these unsuccessful sessions increased their use of rule enforcement tactics later in the fourth phase, the disputants typically ignored these interventions and continued with their defensive spirals (Donohue, in press).

Surprisingly, there were no differences in the use of proposal suggestions or reframing tactics between the successful and the unsuccessful mediations in the Donohue study. However, these tactics played different roles in the mediation. In the successful sessions, mediators focused almost half of their substantive tactics on identifying and reinforcing points of agreements and on reframing disputants utterances, whereas mediators in the unsuccessful sessions centered their substantive tactics on negative evaluations of disputants' proposals and on creating alternative proposals for them. The former tactic reinforces disputants' progress by using their ideas, while the latter tactic aims for control over the outcome rather than the process of mediation.

Research on phase differences between successful and unsuccessful mediations has uncovered similar patterns. Jones (1988) found that in successful sessions, disputants moved through the following phases: (1) information exchange, (2) dealing with solutions and agreements, and (3) working out specifics of agreements. Disputants in the unsuccessful mediations, in contrast, engaged in competitive information exchanges dominated by attribution statements. These sessions failed to evolve into a problem-solving process that typified the second and third phases in the successful mediations. Jones (1989) also noted that mediators in the successful sessions elicited information about the circumstances of the dispute, used extensive summaries to create momentum in the mediation, and redirected defensive reactions of disputants. In effect, successful as opposed to unsuccessful mediation sessions differed in the amount, type, and timing of substantive and contextual tactics. Maintaining control of the mediation process was particularly critical in the second and third phases of the interaction.

Mediators who use a fairly standard set of strategies and tactics without adjusting them to the disputants may experience problems in dealing with emotionally laden, relationally determined disputes. If mediators de-emphasize contextual tactics and allow the rules to slip in the second phase, disputants in high-conflict situations may pull the mediators into their process of interaction. This pattern typically forms when mediators ask for more details of disputants' stories rather than summarizing, redirecting utterances, requesting proposals, and controlling the process of the interaction.

CONCLUSIONS

Can we make any general statements about the process of mediation and about what is likely to lead to success? Psychological research on mediation, which typically focuses on process and the relationship between tactics and outcome, can offer immediate practical advice (Kolb & Rubin, 1989). The data reported in this chapter are very clear in showing that some mediator behaviors are more likely to be associated with successful mediation than other behaviors, although we can make no claims for a causal connection. Nevertheless, the data suggest that several mediator behaviors are positively associated with success in mediation. These include developing rapport with the parties, keeping the negotiations focused on the issues, expressing pleasure at their progress in negotiations, avoiding taking sides on important issues in joint sessions, and discussing the interests of all parties affected by the dispute. These are all reasonable things to do in mediation (see Neighborhood Justice of Chicago, 1987).

One conclusion from the community mediation study reported in this chapter, and also from our previous work, is that success in mediation is more complex than simply whether or not agreement is achieved. As can be seen in Table 8.1, this sample of community mediators recognized that the nature of an agreement, such as whether or not it was likely to hold up over time, was an important feature. Another important feature was whether or not disputes were resolved in a reasonable period of time. In addition, mediator outcomes were an important part of successful mediation (e.g., whether or not feelings of goodwill and trust were created toward the mediator). The role of mediator interests in dispute settlement is a rich topic for further study.

Another area that calls for further study is mediator gender. In the Lim and Carnevale (1990) study described earlier, one interesting finding was that mediation tactics were used differently by male and female mediators. That study had a sample of 255 professional mediators, and male mediators reported being more likely to use forceful, pressuring tactics than female mediators. Additional analyses indicated that this gender difference was not due to a possible difference in the types of disputes that males and females were likely to mediate (e.g., community vs. labor).

We examined differences due to mediator gender in the present sample of 34 community mediators. The gender of the mediator was used as a predictor of the overall reported use of tactics in both the successful and unsuccessful cases. Consistent with the past research on gender in mediation, male mediators were more likely than female mediators to use forceful mediation tactics. Compared to female mediators, male mediators were more likely to express displeasure at the parties' progress, to try to change the parties' expectations, and to suggest specific tradeoffs among the issues. Males also reported using caucuses more frequently than females.

However, it should be noted that Lim and Carnevale (1990) did not find any differences between male and female mediators on measures of dispute outcome. Male and female mediators were equal in achieving successful outcomes, but apparently achieved those outcomes by way of distinct styles of mediation.

We conclude this chapter with a statement about the positive aspects of conflict. We recognize that conflicts can have disastrous effects on interpersonal relationships, especially when they lead to escalation and conflict spirals (Pruitt & Rubin, 1986). But conflicts can serve constructive ends, as noted by Deutsch (1973), and as seen in Putnam's (1989) analysis of teacher–school board contract negotiations. The negotiation enabled both sides to exchange information, and it clarified misunderstandings, both of which accounted for a large portion of the variance in predicting satisfaction with the contract. This finding can be extended to the sort of disputes handled by community mediation centers. Disputants who exchange information and reach common understandings in community mediation should be especially satisfied with the outcome of their conflict. Findings on long-term success in mediation support this conclusion (Kressel & Pruitt, 1989).

Acknowledgments

The research reported in this chapter is based in part upon work supported by the National Science Foundation under Grant No. BNS-8809263 to Peter Carnevale. We are grateful to Paul Olczak and Andrea Hollingshead for their helpful comments, and to the Neighborhood Justice of Chicago for allowing the research reported here.

REFERENCES

Carnevale, P. J. (1986). Strategic choice in mediation. *Negotiation Journal, 2,* 41–56.
Carnevale, P. J., & Pegnetter, R. (1985). The selection of mediation tactics in public-sector disputes: A contingency analysis. *Journal of Social Issues, 41,* 65–81.

Deutsch, M. (1973). *The resolution of conflict*. New Haven, CT: Yale University Press.

Donohue, W. A. (in press). *Communication, marital dispute and divorce mediation*. Hillsdale, NJ: Erlbaum.

Donohue, W. A., Weider-Hatfield, D., Hamilton, M., & Diez, M. E. (1985). Relational distance in managing conflict. *Human Communication Research, 11*, 387–406.

Hiltrop, J. M. (1985). Mediator behavior and the settlement of collective bargaining disputes in Britain. *Journal of Social Issues, 41*, 83–99.

Hiltrop, J. M. (1989). Factors associated with successful labor mediation. In K. Kressel, D. G. Pruitt, & Associates (Eds.), *Mediation research: The process and effectiveness of third party intervention* (pp. 241–262). San Francisco: Jossey-Bass.

Jones, T. S. (1988). Phase structures in agreement and no-agreement mediation. *Communication Research, 15*, 470–495.

Jones, T. S. (1989). A taxonomy of effective mediator strategies and tactics for nonlabor–management mediation. In M. A. Rahim (Ed.), *Managing conflict: An interdisciplinary approach* (pp. 221–230). New York: Praeger.

Keltner, J. W. (1987). *Mediation: Toward a civilized system of dispute resolution*. Urbana, IL: ERIC Clearinghouse of Reading and Communication Skills.

Kochan, T. A., & Jick, T. A. (1978). The public sector mediation process: A theory and empirical examination. *Journal of Conflict Resolution, 22*, 209–241.

Kochan, T. A., & Katz, H. C. (1988). *Collective bargaining and industrial relations*. Homewood, IL: Irwin.

Kolb, D. M. (1983). Strategy and tactics of mediation. *Human Relations, 36*, 247–268.

Kolb, D. M., & Rubin, J. Z. (1989, October). Mediation through a disciplinary kaleidoscope: A summary of empirical research. *Dispute Resolution Forum*, pp. 3–8.

Kressel, K. (1972). *Labor mediation: An exploratory survey*. Albany, NY: Association of Labor Mediation Agencies.

Kressel, K. (1985). *The process of divorce*. New York: Basic Books.

Kressel, K., & Pruitt, D. G. (1989). A research perspective on the mediation of social conflict. In K. Kressel, D. G. Pruitt, & Associates (Eds.), *Mediation research: The process and effectiveness of third party intervention* (pp. 394–435). San Francisco: Jossey-Bass.

Lim R. G., & Carnevale, P. J. (1990). Contingencies in the mediation of disputes. *Journal of Personality and Social Psychology, 58*, 259–272.

McGillis, D. (1981). Conflict resolution outside the courts. In L. Bickman (Ed.), *Applied social psychology annual* (Vol. 2, pp. 243–262). Beverly Hills, CA: Sage.

Neighborhood Justice of Chicago. (1987) *Mediator training manual*. Chicago: Author.

Neighborhood Justice of Chicago. (1990). *Eviction court mediation program handbook*. Chicago: Author.

Pruitt, D. G., & Rubin, J. Z. (1986). *Social conflict: Escalation, stalemate, and settlement*. New York: Random House.

Putnam, L. L. (1989, August). *Formal negotiations: The productive side of organiza-*

tional conflict. Paper presented at the annual meeting of the Academy of Mangement, Washington, DC.

Putnam, L. L. (1990). Reframing integrative and distributive bargaining: A process perspective. In B H. Sheppard, M. H. Bazerman, & R. J. Lewicki (Eds.), *Research on negotiation in organizations* (pp. 3–30). Greenwich, CT: JAI Press.

Putnam, L. L., & Poole, M. S. (1987). Conflict and negotiation. In F. M. Jablin, L. L. Putnam, K. H. Roberts, & L. W. Porter (Eds.), *Handbook of organizational communication* (pp. 549–599). Beverly Hills, CA: Sage.

Rubin, J. Z. (1980). Experimental research on third-party intervention in conflict: Toward some generalizations. *Psychological Bulletin. 87*, 379–391.

Rubin, J. Z. (1981). *Dynamics of third party intervention: Kissinger in the Middle East*. New York: Praeger.

Stevens, C. M. (1963). *Strategy and collective bargaining negotiation*. New York: McGraw-Hill.

Thoennes, N. A., & Pearson, J. (1985). Predicting outcomes in divorce mediation: The influence of people and process. *Journal of Social Issues, 41*(2), 115–126.

Wall, J. A., Jr. (1981). Mediation: An analysis, review, and proposed research. *Journal of Conflict Resolution, 25*, 157–180.

Womack, D. F. (1985). The role of argument in mediation styles. *Journal of the American Forensic Association, 21*, 215–225.

Zappa, J., Manusov, V., Cody, M. J., & Donohue, W. A. (1990, April). *The communication and evaluation of accounts during child custody mediations*. Paper presented at the annual convention of the Eastern States Communication Association, Philadelphia.

9

Factors Affecting the Outcome of Mediation: Third-Party and Disputant Behavior

NEIL B. McGILLICUDDY
Research Institute on Alcoholism

DEAN G. PRUITT
State University of New York at Buffalo

GARY L. WELTON
Tabor College

JO M. ZUBEK AND ROBERT S. PEIRCE
State University of New York at Buffalo

The number of community mediation programs in the nation and around the world has increased dramatically in recent years. Research examining these programs has shown an equivalent surge (Kressel & Pruitt, 1989); much energy has been devoted to the examination of the factors involved in successful and unsuccessful mediation. In this chapter, we examine data collected from two large-scale projects conducted by our research team. The data are examined with an eye toward issues relevant to mediators, so that our findings may be implemented into practice. We also discuss areas in which future research may improve mediation services.

The data were collected by the Research Project for the Investigation of the Dynamics of Social Conflict, under the direction of Dean G. Pruitt, at the State University of New York at Buffalo. Both studies involved direct observation of mediation hearings. Study 1, conducted solely at the Dispute Settlement Center (DSC) in Buffalo, New York, provided information about two important issues: (1) the relative strengths and weaknesses of three types of third-party power; and (2) the conditions that lead to caucus sessions (private meetings between the mediator and one disputant), and ways in which these sessions differ from joint sessions in which the two disputants and the mediator are present.

Study 2, conducted at both the DSC and the Neighborhood Justice

Project (NJP) in Elmira, New York, examined the antecedents and characteristics of caucus sessions. Other topics examined in this study were the
antecedents of short-term and long-term success and differences between
complainants (the parties making the original charges) and respondents (the
parties answering the charges).

The typical Buffalo mediation case originates from a judge, district
attorney, or court clerk; the typical Elmira case is self-referred. Hearings
ordinarily involve people who have continuing relationships, such as
spouses, former spouses, relatives, friends, neighbors, or landlords and
tenants. The goal of these hearings is to help disputants reach a mutually
acceptable resolution to their dispute. The mediators are volunteers who
have participated in an extensive training program and typically conduct one
case per month.

A typical hearing begins with an introduction to mediation presented by
the third party, during which assurances of neutrality and confidentiality are
made. The disputants are then provided the opportunity to tell their stories,
with the complainant ordinarily speaking first. Following this, issues are
analyzed, alternatives developed, and an agreement reached. Caucus sessions can be held at any point. If and when agreement is reached, the
mediator writes it and the disputants sign it. These agreements usually enjoy
the status of a contract.

ROLE OF THIRD-PARTY POWER

Study 1 compared three common forms of third-party intervention. These
forms are similar in that the third party first attempts to mediate the dispute,
thereby helping the disputants attain their own agreement. However, the
forms are different with respect to what happens if agreement is not reached.
In "straight mediation," third-party services end, leaving the disputants
without a resolution. In "mediation/arbitration (same)," often abbreviated as
"med/arb(same)," the third party who previously served as mediator becomes the arbitrator and issues a binding decision about the dispute. In
"mediation/arbitration (different)," abbreviated as "med/arb(diff)," a fourth
party, who is not present during the mediation phase, becomes the arbitrator and issues a binding decision about the dispute. We investigated how
these forms of third-party intervention influenced mediator and disputant
behavior *during* the mediation hearing; we did not examine posthearing
phases.

This study is relevant to both practical and theoretical debates in the
field. One debate involves the advisability of using med/arb rather than
straight mediation. Proponents of med/arb argue that it encourages agreement during the mediation phase, because disputants fear loss of control
over their outcomes in the event of arbitration. Hence, the "hammer" of

arbitration should make parties more likely to reach agreement. Opponents of med/arb, however, counter that it is an inferior form of dispute resolution, because if agreement is not reached, responsibility for the settlement is taken away from the disputants, who presumably understand the issues best. These people believe it is better that disputants themselves determine the consequences when agreement is not reached.

Another debate concerns the relative merits of med/arb(same) and med/arb(diff). People who wrestle with this issue believe in the superiority of med/arb over straight mediation, but disagree about the best form of med/arb. Proponents of med/arb(same) argue that having the power to arbitrate gives mediators the prestige necessary to persuade reluctant disputants to make concessions and engage in problem solving. Proponents of med/arb(diff), including many attorneys, argue that mediation is poor preparation for arbitration: Mediators may become partial to one side or to a particular solution, thereby biasing them as they move into the role of arbitrator. The provision of a different arbitrator, they argue, would eradicate that concern. Some critics also worry that mediators who have arbitral powers will become too forceful, making mediation indistinguishable from arbitration. (For a discussion of previous research related to this debate, the reader is referred to Bigoness, 1976; Johnson & Pruitt, 1972; and Kochan & Jick, 1978.)

Method

Study 1 was conducted at the DSC, a branch of the Better Business Bureau Foundation of Western New York, Inc. The cases involved domestic, neighborhood, and minor commercial disagreements. The mediators were trained volunteers whose obligation involved mediating about one case per month. The study was a true field experiment, in that cases originating from Buffalo City Court were randomly assigned (by a clerk who was blind to the hypotheses) to either straight mediation, med/arb(same), or med/arb(diff). Our sample had 36 cases, with 12 cases in each of the three conditions. Disputants were informed of the form of intervention they would experience at least five times prior to the hearing; mediators were provided with this information at least three times. All information was provided by mediation center employees who were blind to our hypotheses.

Immediately before the hearing, the mediator and both disputants were asked whether they would consent to being observed. When all parties agreed (in most cases they did), two observers entered the room. These observers were blind to the form of third-party intervention to be used; they content-analyzed what was said by the parties, recording 28 categories of mediator behavior and 26 categories of disputant behavior by means of an electronic event recorder.

Among the mediator categories were behaviors aimed toward helping the parties reach their own agreement, including statements noting the similarity and interdependence between the parties; behaviors aimed toward helping the mediator and the other party learn each party's priorities, including asking for information; behaviors in which the disputants were criticized for their lack of problem-solving behavior, including negative evaluations of disputants' proposals and threats to end the session; and proposals of possible solutions to end the conflict.

Among the disputant categories were hostile behaviors, including sarcasm and criticism of the other's behavior; competitive behaviors, including favorably comparing the self to the other disputant; and problem-solving behaviors, including giving information about priorities and proposals of possible solutions to end the conflict.

The coding unit was a speaking turn (i.e., everything said from the end of the prior speaker's remarks to the beginning of the next speaker's remarks). When speaking turns lasted more than 30 seconds, a second unit was initiated, and so on for each 30-second interval. A given unit could receive several different codes, but never the same code twice. Only codes that achieved an intercoder reliability of .70 or better were used. The main data consisted of the relative frequency of each content code, calculated as the number of units in which the code was detected divided by the total number of mediator or disputant units. Mediator coding and disputant coding were conducted separately by the two observers.

At the end of the mediation session, the observers rated disputant motivation on three scales, and participants answered questions about their perceptions of the session. All mediators answered the questionnaire, but only 46 of the 72 disputants were willing to do so. For a complete description of the methods employed, see McGillicuddy, Welton, and Pruitt (1987).

Results and Discussion

Our evidence suggests that med/arb(same) produced the most constructive disputant behavior; there were fewer hostile statements and invidious comparisons in this condition than in the other two conditions. There was also more evidence of problem solving in the form of new proposals for resolving the issues. Med/arb(diff) lay intermediate on most of these measures, and straight mediation was least favorable.

A likely explanation for these differences can be derived from the coder ratings of disputant motivation. Disputants in both med/arb conditions seemed more motivated to settle the dispute than those in straight mediation; this suggests that the fear of losing control over one's dispute may foster constructive behavior. Also, disputants in med/arb(same) seemed especially interested in impressing and following the mediator; this suggests that med/arb(same) may elevate the mediator's prestige, encouraging the disputants to take the mediator's instructions for conciliation more seriously.

We also found differences related to mediator behavior. First, pressure tactics (i.e., threats and advocacy of a particular proposal) were used more often in med/arb(same) than in straight mediation, with med/arb(diff) again being in the middle. This might seem to support the criticism that med/arb(same) encourages forceful mediator behavior. However, most of our data suggest that these tactics were employed in the last minutes of mediation, after it became apparent that agreement was unlikely. In addition, disputants in med/arb(same) perceived the mediator as *less* forceful and themselves as *more* involved in the hearing than did disputants in the other two conditions—a finding suggesting that they did not regard the mediator behavior as unduly forceful.

Finally, we found that third parties in med/arb(diff) were less active and involved in the hearing than in either of the other two forms of intervention. These mediators intervened less and broke off the session sooner. Perhaps the mediators in this condition felt less responsible for the case, since they could be replaced by a more powerful individual.

Conclusions

These findings suggest that giving mediators the power to arbitrate encourages disputants' efforts to solve their own problems. We found a little support for the criticism that the power to arbitrate encourages mediators' efforts to dominate, but this did not appear to be a major problem. It could conceivably become a larger problem with mediators who have a constant flow of cases and develop the sense that they know how most cases will turn out. Our data do not speak to the criticism that a prior period of mediation tends to bias an arbitrator. But we did find defects in the standard solution to this problem—having a different person as mediator and arbitrator, or med/arb(diff). Med/arb(diff) did not produce as much disputant problem solving as med/arb(same), probably because the mediator did not have as much prestige under med/arb(diff). Furthermore, having a different person as arbitrator appears to erode the mediator's involvement in the case. A broader implication of our findings, which deserves further research, is that mediator power of any kind serves to strengthen the mediation process.

CAUCUSING

"Caucusing," as mentioned earlier, refers to private meetings between the mediator and one or both parties. We investigated several facets of caucusing. We looked at the events that led a third party to move into caucus. We also examined how behavior by disputants *and* mediators differed between caucus and joint sessions (sessions in which both disputants were present).

We were aware of a debate concerning whether caucusing should be employed in community mediation. Proponents of caucusing recommend it for difficult hearings involving high hostility and low problem solving. They argue that with the other party absent, a disputant will feel freer to provide information about underlying interests and assumptions and will propose more new ideas for possible solutions. Also, proponents argue that mediators can speak more directly in caucus without appearing biased.

Pruitt (1981) presents some arguments against caucusing. These include the notion that joint problem solving—that which occurs *between* disputants—is essential for successful mediation, as it produces better agreements and provides the disputants with practice in solving their own problems. Caucusing involves problem solving between the mediator and *each* disputant. Another argument is that a disputant may make inaccurate statements to the mediator when the other party cannot hear them. This can become especially problematic if the mediator plays a role in forging the settlement by suggesting a solution or acting as an arbitrator.

Method

We employed data on caucusing from both studies (see Welton, Pruitt, & McGillicuddy, 1988; Welton, Pruitt, McGillicuddy, Ippolito, & Zubek, 1990). The second study differed from the first in several ways. First, no variables were manipulated. Second, the two observers transcribed the hearings for later coding rather than conducting the coding on site. Third, a greater number of behavioral categories were coded for both the mediator and the disputants. Fourth, several measures of outcome quality were employed. These included measures of short-term outcome (i.e., whether agreement was reached, whether disputants' goals had been achieved in the hearing, and whether disputants were satisfied with the agreement) and long-term outcome (i.e., the quality of the parties' relationship 4 to 8 months later, whether they had complied with the terms of the agreement, and whether new problems had developed). Fifth, a second research site was utilized for this project; 50 cases were observed at the DSC, while an additional 23 cases were observed at the NJP. The Elmira site was utilized for a number of reasons. First, we wanted to expand the number of cases under study. Second, we wished to have the opportunity to generalize our research findings beyond the Buffalo center. Third, and perhaps most importantly, Elmira stresses joint problem solving over mediator activity, and hence encourages less use of caucusing than Buffalo; consequently, we had the opportunity to study two models of mediation.

Results and Discussion

We present a synthesis of findings from the two studies here, as they were remarkably similar. Nearly 35% of the mediation time was spent in caucus, with the remaining time being spent in joint session. Of the 73 cases, 52 (71%) employed at least one caucus session.

Direct forms of disputant hostility, such as hostile questions, sarcasm, and swearing and angry displays, were more common in joint than in caucus sessions. This suggests that the disputants experienced stronger emotions with their opponents present. A related finding was that third parties made more efforts to control hostility during joint than during caucus sessions.

Though direct hostility was not common during caucus sessions, indirect hostility was. This took the form of character assassination (e.g., "He's an alcoholic") and behavioral criticism (e.g., "He drank too much that day"). Disputants were also more self-complimentary during caucus than during joint sessions. These findings probably result from the fact that a disputant knows that statements in a caucus session cannot be heard and refuted by the opponent. However, if the mediator believes a disputant who disparages the opponent and congratulates himself or herself behind closed doors, mediation outcomes may be seriously affected. Hence, the mediator must listen to such statements cautiously, only believing them if they are confirmed by other evidence (such as statements by the other party).

Problem solving also occurred more frequently in caucus than in joint sessions. Disputants provided more information about underlying feelings, values, and goals, and also offered more new alternatives for settlement of the problem, in caucus than in joint sessions (this latter finding was limited to the Buffalo center). Mediator requests for new proposals tended to produce such proposals; these requests were made more frequently in caucus than in joint sessions. Mediators said more about the other party's perspective and also offered more alternatives of their own in caucus than in joint sessions.

There are at least four possible explanations for the greater prevalence of problem solving in caucus than in joint sessions: (1) Tension is reduced, allowing for creativity in the form of proposal generation. (2) Disputants feel freer to try out new ideas, as each knows the opponent cannot hear what is happening, and hence they cannot be held to statements they make. (3) Because the mediator plays a more dominant role in caucus sessions, his or her broad experience in dispute resolution is more effectively engaged. (4) The mediator feels freer to explain the other party's position and to throw out new ideas, knowing that the other party is not listening.

Our evidence suggests that there was considerable problem solving between disputant and mediator during caucus sessions. Such problem solving may be possible because the mediator feels free to present the perspective of the other party in caucus conversations. Mediators were also more critical of disputants in caucus than joint sessions. Since disputants are not so tense during caucus sessions, such criticism seems likely to open the minds of at least some of them. If this criticism were to occur in joint sessions, the result would probably be destructive, as the mediator would seem to be currying favor with the other party, and consequently would appear biased.

Conclusions

These findings imply that caucus sessions offer an alternative location for problem solving when disputants are hostile and repetitive in joint sessions. Mediators must be cautious about believing the information they hear during caucus sessions, however, as disputants tend to brag a lot and tend to be especially critical of their adversaries in these settings. This confirms another criticism of med/arb(same)—namely, that mediation involving caucusing is especially likely to bias a future arbitrator. There are three possible solutions to this problem. One is to outlaw caucusing in med/arb(same); this is a questionable remedy, since caucusing is a valuable tool in the hands of a mediator. The second is to train mediators to take a constructive role during caucusing but to suspend belief about anything they hear in caucus. A third is to employ two mediators during the mediation phase, one of whom is engaging in caucusing if this procedure seems warranted and the other of whom becomes the arbitrator if mediation fails.[1] The third solution builds on the comediation (two mediators) model, which is fairly common in community mediation.

SHORT-TERM SUCCESS

Another one of our goals was to examine the antecedents of "short-term success" in mediation. Short-term success was defined as whether disputants reached agreement, whether they achieved their goals in the agreement, whether they were satisfied with the agreement, and whether they were satisfied with the way the hearing had been conducted. (For a fuller description of this study, see Zubek, McGillicuddy, Peirce, Pruitt, & Syna, 1990.) Of the 73 hearings at the two centers, 63 resulted in agreement.

Method

The following procedure was employed to measure goal achievement: A list of the issues mentioned by either disputant was made. Each issue was assigned an importance score for each disputant (by coders not present at the hearing) by distributing 100 points among the issues. Each issue was subsequently given a score, ranging from −1 to +1, indicating the extent to which each disputant achieved what he or she wanted. Importance scores were multiplied by these latter scores and summed across the issues to

---

[1]We wish to thank Nicole Sheindlin for this idea.

create a disputant goal achievement score. An overall goal achievement score was calculated for each dyad by summing complainant and respondent goal achievement scores. Satisfaction with the agreement and the hearing was measured by means of 5-point scales in the disputant questionnaires.

Results and Discussion

Hostility, contending, and joint problem solving during the hearing were predictive of short-term success; disputants who were hostile or contentious had lowered goal achievement, whereas disputants who engaged in problem solving achieved elevated goal achievement. These behaviors were, in turn, predicted by two other variables. If conflict had escalated, or if it had centered on principles, there was more hostility and less problem solving, resulting in lower goal achievement.

Several mediator behaviors also encouraged short-term success. These included mentioning issues that needed to be solved, proposing agendas (the order in which issues should be discussed), and challenging the disputants to propose new ideas. Similarly, when mediators played an active role by proposing new ideas or requesting reactions to previously made proposals, agreement was more likely and goal achievement was enhanced. Finally, short-term success was enhanced when mediators displayed a high degree of empathy toward disputants.

Several nonconstructive mediator behaviors were also detected. For instance, our data suggest that criticizing disputants is an ineffective mediator tactic, encouraging lower satisfaction with the conduct of the hearing. Asking embarrassing questions, a form of indirect criticism, had a negative impact on goal achievement. Pressure to reach agreement was also negatively related to all forms of immediate success. These findings held up when initial case difficulty was held constant, but we must nevertheless be careful about drawing conclusions concerning cause and effect. Future research must examine the independent role of mediator criticism in mediation outcome.

Interestingly, assertions of expertise—statements directed toward publicizing one's credentials as an effective mediator—had a negative impact on short-term success. Perhaps stressing one's credentials as a mediator produces *lower* respect, because disputants assume that the third party is qualified, and any protracted discussion becomes overkill. Or perhaps talking about oneself is as damaging for a mediator as for a psychotherapist; the dispute settlement center, not the mediator, should inform disputants about the mediator's credentials.

Mediators also reacted differently according to the disputants' past relationship with each other and their expectation for a future relationship. When a future relationship was anticipated, mediators were more likely to be empathic, to argue for disputant proposals, and to praise disputant behaviors (behaviors all related positively to short-term success). Contrastingly, when disputants were previously hostile, mediators were less empathic, more likely to be critical, and more likely to ask embarrassing questions. Hence, it appears that mediators tailor their behavior to the disputants' behavior and relationship: If the disputants are nonhostile or dependent upon each other, mediators foster problem solving. But if disputants have a past and/or a current history of hostility, achievement of an agreement becomes a mediator's sole objective.

Conclusions

Our data suggest that mediators who want short-term success (perhaps because disputant relationships are expected to continue) should be empathic and should structure the issues and challenge the disputants to think about them. Mediators' proposing ideas on their own is also successful, though efforts to persuade disputants to accept these ideas have no particular value. Criticism and embarrassing questions are somewhat counterproductive, and mediators should not overdo bragging about their credentials.

LONG-TERM SUCCESS

We also examined the hearing conditions related to long-term success, which was measured by means of telephone interviews 4 to 8 months after the mediation. We asked each party about (1) the other party's compliance, (2) the current quality of their relationship, and (3) whether new problems had developed.

Surprisingly, the factors that affected long-term success were not the same as those affecting short-term success. Goal achievement and immediate satisfaction with the agreement were not related to long-term success (Pruitt, Peirce, Zubek, Welton, & Nochajski, 1990). Apparently, a good agreement that speaks to current issues does not produce better relations between the disputants, or even greater compliance. It would appear that the aggrieved relationships of the kind so commonly found in dispute settlement centers are not easily resolved by a simple contract between the parties, even if this contract is of high quality. Similar conclusions have been drawn about the long-term impact of marital contracts (Jacobsen & Follette, 1985).

On the other hand, respondents' immediate satisfaction with the conduct of the hearing and their willingness to endorse the mediation service predicted long-term success. If respondents were happy with how the hearing was conducted, they were likely to report high complainant compliance. Also, if respondents reported the hearing procedure to be fair, complainants reported greater respondent compliance and better long-term relations. Evidently, respondents who thought the hearing was fair had fewer problems with compliance, and this produced greater long-term success. Also, if respondents believed that the true underlying problems had come out in the hearing, complainants reported greater long-term success. Finally, complainants' perceptions that the mediator had understood what they said predicted their reports of long-term success. In short, respondent satisfaction with the conduct of the hearing was crucial for long-term success.

COMPLAINANT–RESPONDENT DIFFERENCES

The results just reviewed suggest differences in complainant and respondent psychology. Our second study revealed a good deal more about these differences. We found attitudinal differences before the hearing, behavioral differences during the hearing, outcome differences immediately after the hearing, and compliance differences months after the hearing. (For a fuller description of this study, see Castrianno, Pruitt, Nochajski, & Zubek, 1988.)

We found complainants to be more competitive than respondents, as they made more demands and posed more issues that needed to be solved. Respondents, on the other hand, were more critical of their own behavior; they took more responsibility for having caused the problem and gave more information prejudicial to their position. In addition, respondents were more yielding than complainants, agreeing more often to the proposals made by the complainants or the mediators. They also engaged in more problem solving: They provided more information about their underlying goals, feelings, and values, and devised more new ideas for solving the problem.

These findings may be related to conditions present prior to the hearing. We found complainants to be more aggrieved than respondents, meaning that they were more bothered about the issues leading to the dispute. This aggravation may help explain why the complainants took their cases to mediation.

With complainants more strident and respondents more meek and yielding, it is not surprising that complainants were more successful than respondents in attaining their goals. Despite this greater objective success, complainants were *not* more satisfied than respondents with the final agreement, and, surprisingly, they were much less satisfied with the conduct of the hearing. This suggests that they expected a good deal more from the hearings than did the respondents.

Finally, we obtained two differences concerning compliance: (1) At the conclusion of the hearing, the complainants thought it likely that the respondents would have difficulty living up to the final agreement. (2) In the follow-up interview, respondents reported having more problems complying with the final agreement. Neither finding is surprising, since complainants achieved more of their goals than did respondents; what is interesting is the complainants' ability to predict respondents' difficulties.

The differences we found between complainants and respondents suggest that these two kinds of disputants should be treated differently by the mediator. Complainants tend to be demanding and hard to satisfy, while respondents are, on the whole, less sure of themselves and more yielding. The result of a typical mediation is an agreement favoring the interests of the complainant and placing larger burdens of compliance on the respondent. Hence, although the complainant is the one who is "making more noise," the respondent is more important for the future of the agreement. This suggests that mediators should make a special effort to be sensitive to the needs of respondents. They must be careful that respondents are not so yielding as to agree to a solution they cannot live with. Furthermore, our findings suggest that a mediator needs to be sure that the respondent is satisfied with the conduct of the hearing—in other words, that he or she sees the procedure as fair and believes that the most important issues were aired. The respondent's perspective seems to be the key to long-term success.

FINAL CONCLUSIONS

Research on the process and outcome of mediation is beginning to be done on a worldwide basis. Our studies have explored the conditions, procedures, and mediator tactics that produce effective results. We hope that our findings will involve policy makers and mediators and will stimulate continued research efforts.

Acknowledgments

Study 1 was supported by National Science Foundation Grant No. BNS83-09167. Study 2 was supported by National Science Foundation Grant No. SES85-20084. We wish to thank the following people: (1) From the Dispute Settlement Center of the Better Business Bureau Foundation of Western New York: Charles Underhill, President; Judith Peter, Director; David Polino, Associate Director; and Barbara Bittner, Mary Beth Cerrone, Mary Beth Goris, Ann Horanburg, James Meloon, and Brenda Ransom. (2) From the Neighborhood Justice Project in Elmira, New York: Joyce Kowalewski, Former Executive Director; David Rynders, Executive Director; and Jill Dorfeld, Eldon K. Hutchinson, and Beverly Stearns. We are also indebted to Lisa Allen, Lynn M. Castrianno, Thomas Christian, Timothy Franz, W. Rick Fry, Bret Grube, Margaret K. Harwood, Angela Iocolano, Carol A. Ippolito, Drew LaStella, Thomas H. Nochajski, Helena Syna, and Michael R. Van Slyck for their contributions to countless aspects of the two projects.

REFERENCES

Bigoness, W. J. (1976). The impact of initial bargaining position and alternative modes of third party intervention in resolving bargaining impasses. *Organizational Behavior and Human Performance, 17,* 185–198.

Castrianno, L. M., Pruitt, D. G., Nochajski, T. H., & Zubek, J. M. (1988). *Complainant–respondent differences in mediation.* Paper presented at the annual meeting of the Eastern Psychological Association, Buffalo, NY.

Jacobsen, N. S., & Follette, W. C. (1985). Clinical significance of improvement resulting from two behavioral, marital therapy components. *Behavior Therapy, 16,* 249–262.

Johnson, D. F., & Pruitt, D. G. (1972). Pre-intervention effects of mediation vs. arbitration. *Journal of Applied Psychology, 56,* 1–10.

Kochan, T. A., & Jick, T. (1978). The public sector mediation process: A theory and empirical examination. *Journal of Conflict Resolution, 22,* 209–240.

Kressel, K., & Pruitt, D. G. (1989). Conclusion: A research perspective on the mediation of social conflict. In K. Kressel, D. G. Pruitt, & Associates (Eds.), *Mediation research: The process and effectiveness of third party intervention.* San Francisco: Jossey-Bass.

McGillicuddy, N. B., Welton, G. L., & Pruitt, D. G. (1987). Third party intervention: A field experiment comparing three different models. *Journal of Personality and Social Psychology, 53,* 104–112.

Pruitt, D. G. (1981). *Negotiation behavior.* New York: Academic Press.

Pruitt, D. G., Peirce, R. S., Zubek, J. M., Welton, G. L., & Nochajski, T. H. (1990). Goal achievement, procedural success, and the success of mediation. *International Journal of Conflict Management, 1,* 33–45.

Welton, G. L., Pruitt, D. G., & McGillicuddy, N. B. (1988). The role of caucusing in community mediation. *Journal of Conflict Resolution, 32,* 181–201.

Welton, G. L., Pruitt, D. G., McGillicuddy, N. B., Ippolito, C. A., & Zubek, J. M. (1990). *Antecedents and characteristics of caucusing in community mediation.* Unpublished manuscript.

Zubek, J. M., McGillicuddy, N. B., Peirce, R. S., Pruitt, D. G., & Syna, H. (1990). *Short-term success in mediation: The effect of prior conditions and mediator and disputant behaviors.* Manuscript submitted for publication.

PART III

ISSUES IN
COMMUNITY MEDIATION

In Part III, we attempt to deal in some depth with a number of critical and timely issues germane to the actual practice of mediation. In the first chapter of this unit, Paul Olczak provides an analysis of the various sources of resistant behavior in mediation by offering a conceptual model of the process, derived from an integration of accumulated knowledge in the domains of social and clinical psychology. The aim of this chapter is to provide the practitioner with some usable clinical skills for handling resistant behavior before, during, and after the hearing, while providing the researcher (and, we hope, the practitioner) with a conceptual model capable of increasing our understanding of the process and generating additional research in this important area of human behavior as well.

In the next chapter, Ellen Cohn and Mae Lynn Neyhart first describe several factors that may affect the public's acceptance of community mediation, and then offer possible solutions. Included in their analysis are such topics as ignorance of the process (e.g., "I never heard of it!" or "How does it work?"); schemas or cognitive biases that may affect a person's ability to perceive the positive aspects of mediation (e.g., a person's beliefs about the purpose of a jury trial); differences in the view of mediation taken by casual observers as opposed to participants; and, finally, researched individual differences that may affect the public's receptivity toward mediation (e.g., legal development level, attributional biases such as "belief in a just world," etc.).

In Chapter 12, Larry Ray offers the reader a comprehensive and provocative view of alternative dispute resolution techniques as seen through the eyes of the legal establishment—that is, members of the American Bar Association. To accomplish his goal, Ray first raises a number of frequently asked questions regarding mediation and then proceeds to answer them from a legal perspective.

In Chapter 13, Albie Davis provides the reader with her incisive and thought-provoking analysis of the issues surrounding the field of mediation today. In particular, she focuses on the issue of credentialing and its effect upon the delivery of high-quality mediation services, as well as future developments in the field such as professionalization and licensure.

Finally, in Chapter 14, Samuel Forlenza presents the reader with an examination of possible parallel processes existing between the areas of mediation and psychotherapy or counseling, from the perspective of a family mediator. Forlenza focuses on areas of common interest between these two approaches (e.g., need for confidentiality), as well as divergences in their orientation (e.g., distinctly separate goals), as they affect the enlistment of various mental health professionals to serve as mediators within the mediation setting.

10

Resistance to Mediation: A Social–Clinical Analysis

PAUL V. OLCZAK
State University of New York at Geneseo
Family Court Psychiatric Clinic, Buffalo, New York

Mediation, defined by Volpe and Bahn (1987) "as a short-term, task-oriented, participatory intervention process in which disputants voluntarily agree to work with a third party to reach a mutually satisfactory and balanced agreement" (p. 297), has blossomed as a dispute resolution technique that has much to offer over traditional adversarial court proceedings for a variety of cases. In keeping with this growth is the fact that preliminary research on a variety of mediation programs has already demonstrated some impressive rates of user satisfaction, greater compliance with the outcome, and reduced likelihood of relitigation for the participants (McGillis, 1986). However, much remains to be learned. Despite these impressive early returns, mediation as an intervention process is not totally devoid of procedural difficulties. Like similar high-stakes interventions into people's lives (e.g., psychotherapy, counseling, etc.), mediation often can produce behavior in the participants that appears "resistant," or seemingly at odds with the process.

This is perhaps surprising, in that mediation is construed as a "win–win" type of situation for both sides in the hearing. The notion of resistance is pervasive in the psychotherapy or mental health fields. Many therapists in various mental health fields find that clients either do not want to change or are at least ambivalent about it. When viewed in this fashion, resistant behavior takes on a strong adversarial quality, often accompanied by a variety of military metaphors (e.g., "attacking the defenses," "strategies to eliminate resistance," etc.) to describe it (O'Hanlon & Weiner-Davis, 1989).

In contrast to the mental health literature, where resistant behavior has long been a topic to be investigated and understood (e.g., Anderson & Stewart, 1983; Strean, 1985), the mediation literature—except for a few recent contributions that have been more impressionistic in nature (e.g.,

Folberg & Taylor, 1984; Volpe & Bahn, 1987)—has been slow to formally address resistant behavior occurring during the mediation process. In fact, much of the discussion on resistance to using alternative dispute resolution mechanisms is based on speculation, for there is a dearth of reliable data (Goldberg, Green, & Sander, 1985). As a result, "practitioners" in the field (i.e., the mediators) have begun to look toward the social sciences, and psychology in particular, for assistance in understanding and dealing with this problematic and counterproductive behavior.

The purpose of this chapter, then, is to help remedy this relative neglect by attempting to achieve two goals. The first of these is to provide a conceptual framework derived from the areas of social and clinical psychology that will provide readers with a better understanding of resistant behavior, and, as a result, of ways to reduce or control it within the mediational setting. It is hoped that this conceptual framework will facilitate research efforts aimed at understanding resistant behavior in this context as well. The second goal is to provide mediators (and other interested or involved professionals) with an increased understanding of resistant behavior by taking a closer look at possible displays of resistance within a mediational context; examples gleaned from the clinical literature are used to provide a greater understanding of this phenomenon.

A recognition that social and clinical psychology have much to offer each other has existed for many years. For example, in his chapter entitled "Social Psychological Approach to Psychotherapy Research," Stanley Strong (1978) credits Kurt Lewin (1948) and some of his students as being the first group to apply social psychology to the field of psychotherapy. For example, former students Leon Festinger's (1957) theory of cognitive dissonance, Darwin Cartwright's (1965) notions of social power, and Harold Kelley's (1967) insights into causal attribution have all generated concepts that have contributed to a better understanding of the psychotherapeutic process. Jerome Frank (1961), who early in his career researched social persuasion in Lewin's lab as well, later published his landmark book *Persuasion and Healing*, in which he viewed varied forms of psychotherapy as resulting from a process of social persuasion and influence.

Since then a number of contributors have continued this link, including Goldstein, Heller, and Sechrest (1966), Carson (1969), Goldstein (1971), Brehm (1976), Weary and Mirels (1982), and Maddux, Stoltenberg, and Rosenwein (1987), to name just a few. To paraphrase Brehm and Smith (1986, p. 70), by 1983 professional interests had come full circle, so that there was sufficient cross-subdiscipline communication to support the creation of a new journalistic merger, the *Journal of Social and Clinical Psychology*. In keeping with this tradition of cross-fertilization between the social and clinical domains, I have specifically chosen the seminal 1966 work of Goldstein et al. to provide a compatible framework for investigating and understanding resistant behavior in mediation.

DEFINITIONS OF RESISTANCE

Let us first examine existing definitions of resistance from the literature in psychotherapy and behavior change. For example, Gottmann and Leiblum (1974) define resistance as "a word used when the client is not meeting the therapist's expectations, or not working in what the therapist considers a goal-directed way" (p. 101). MacKinnon and Michels (1971), operating from a more traditional psychodynamic orientation, define resistance as "any attitude on the part of the patient that opposes the objectives of the treatment" (p. 16).

Similarly, from the mediation literature, Volpe and Bahn (1987) define resistance as "actions by parties, both conscious and unconscious, that forestall, disrupt and/or impede change designed to alter customary behaviors" (p. 298). Although the processes of psychotherapy and mediation vary on a number of dimensions (see Forlenza, Chapter 14, this volume, for a complete discussion), a comparison of the definitions taken from these disparate literatures nevertheless suggests much similarity, especially in how resistance can adversely affect both the process and outcome of psychotherapy as well as mediation. For greater detail on the similarities and differences between psychotherapeutic interventions and mediation, the interested reader can consult recent works by Gold (1985), Grebe (1986), Kelly (1983), and Milne (1985).

In their then innovative attempt at applying existing social-psychological research to psychotherapy, Goldstein et al. (1966) chose to examine resistance using a communicational model proposed independently by Hartley and Hartley (1952) and Cohen (1964). Their choice was motivated by the belief that increases in knowledge regarding resistance would be most adequately advanced by major attention on the part of *both practitioners and researchers* to the nonclinical research findings on behavior change that were available in contemporary general psychology, especially social psychology.

Operating from the same set of beliefs, I believe that this communicational model can be adapted to resistant behavior in the mediation setting. The mediator thus can be conceptualized as a communicator who initiates "therapeutic" or dispute-resolving communiques aimed at achieving a successful outcome for the disputants, who are the communicants or recipients of these communications (see Figure 10.1).

Goldstein et al. (1966) noted that a breakdown in communication, and therefore resistance, can occur at various points in this model. For example, resistance can occur as a function of the characteristics of the communicator (or mediator), of the communicant (disputant or claimant), or even of the message itself. (In mediation, one must remember that it is the claimant who files the complaint, while it is the respondent who responds to the complaint or charges.)

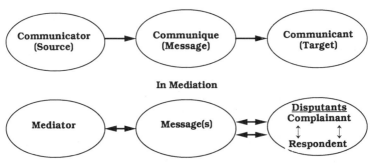

In Communication and Persuasion

FIGURE 10.1.   A communicational model of possible sources of resistance occurring during the mediation hearing. (Adapted from a model proposed independently by Hartley & Hartley, 1952, and Cohen, 1964.)

RESISTANCE AS A FUNCTION OF CHARACTERISTICS OF THE MEDIATOR

First, let us look at possible handling of resistance by the mediator. Everyone seems to agree, both in the psychotherapy literature and in the mediation literature as well, that resistance cannot be ignored, but must be dealt with when it arises. Because of the many forms resistance may take, it is often difficult for a mediator (especially a novice) to be completely prepared for its occurrence. Therefore, as a general strategy, Volpe and Bahn (1987) suggest that the mediator anticipate its occurrence and be prepared to accept resistance as a challenge rather than a threat, which can then be dealt with during the mediation process in a creative manner. For example, a mediator must recognize resistance, but, unlike the therapist, he or she does not need to interpret it. Attempting to achieve a meaningful interpretation not only requires a prohibitive amount of time, but may result in the mediator's being perceived as hostile or aggressive by one of the disputants. For example, if someone is repeatedly late, the mediator should focus on how being late reduces the time spent in working toward a solution, rather than on the "psychodynamic reasons" behind the person's being late. As a general rule of thumb, a mediator does not have to dig deep into every client's psyche, but only to the level required to deal with the mediatable issues. A mediator is not there to "cure" the person, but simply to advance the process (Volpe & Bahn, 1987).

In developing one's skills as a mediator for handling resistance, the first commandment is "Know thyself!" This self-knowledge includes possessing a requisite level of procedural and substantive knowledge regarding the mediation process, as well as an in-depth understanding of one's assets and liabilities as a stimulus object to others.

In regard to the former, Volpe and Bahn (1987) assert that resistant behavior is best handled by a mediator who feels competent, secure, and comfortable with his or her role. According to them, possessing the knowledge that one is sufficiently skilled in the procedural and substantive matters of mediation enables one to think competently and confidently "on one's feet," and therefore to handle most sources of interference with the mediation process as they arise.

In regard to the latter, it is important for the mediator to use his or her feelings and reactions to the clients as valuable data in the encounter. From a clinical perspective, this represents the "transference–countertransference" phenomenon in psychotherapy. I have pointed out earlier that the mediator often invokes or elicits a response to himself or herself from the client "as if" he or she were or represented someone else from the client's past. The mediator is advised to accept this phenomenon as such and not to take its occurrence personally, but to consider it a challenge to be dealt with and mastered.

These transference or "as-if" responses by the client to the mediator may best be handled by legitimizing them and anticipating their occurrence, and announcing them as part of the development of a mediation contract. In this respect, the educational process regarding mediation, whether performed at the intake level or by the mediator himself or herself, can go a long way toward ensuring the success of the enterprise.

For example, the mediator can anticipate and disarm a number of possible transference phenomena and their accompanying resistance by telling both parties beforehand that it is natural to see something like mediation as not working or as being too simplistic, or to see the mediator as being one-sided. Also, the use of a technique borrowed from strategic therapy called "reframing" may prove helpful here, particularly to the practitioner. Changing the way a problem is perceived or classified by the individual has been shown to help circumvent client resistance that poses a barrier to achieving a successful outcome (e.g., see LaClave & Brack, 1989). For example, if one party is focusing on what the other party is "winning" or getting via mediation, the mediator can help that party to refocus on what he or she is also receiving from a successful settlement.

As additional suggestions to mediators for enlisting greater participation in the process, while not becoming defensive themselves, Volpe and Bahn (1987) include the sharing of credentials, experience, and/or neutrality; establishing sufficient structure and ground rules regarding the process; and providing alternatives to the participants. Tactics of this sort, which may be part of setting up the initial mediation contract, may assist in engaging the clients in the process of mediation by reducing subsequent displays of resistance that may be invoked via their ignorance of the process. Thus, the importance of the opening interaction between the mediator and the disputants may be likened to the importance of the initial therapist–patient contact for a successful outcome in psychotherapy. As Rabkin (1977) states, "most of our therapeutic successes can be attributed to the opening phases of psychotherapy. . . . Like chess, the game is either won or lost in the beginning" (p. 11).

From the "countertransference" end of the spectrum, mediators who possess a great deal of self-knowledge regarding their own personalities and the effects they have on other people will have the insight necessary to realize that they may not be able to mediate all types of cases or clients, because of their own personal biases, shortcomings, or "blind spots" (Volpe & Bahn, 1987). For example, a mediator with a history of difficulties interacting with adolescents may find it necessary to exclude himself or herself from cases involving adolescents to remain effective. This suggests that mediators may benefit from training in the human services area prior to their enlistment, with perhaps additional continuing education requirements aimed at sharpening and extending these skills.

In addition, how the communicants (or disputants) perceive the communicator (or mediator) can be influenced by a wide variety of communicator characteristics, such as personality, status, and expertise (Goldstein et al., 1966). In the psychotherapy literature, therapists' credibility and perceived attractiveness have been found to be potent variables in determining their effectiveness and ability to produce change (Strong, 1978). In addition, a wide variety of research in social psychology has demonstrated that communicators with positively valued characteristics (e.g., high credibility, trustworthiness) are more effective than those with negative characteristics (e.g., low credibility & untrustworthiness) (e.g., Hovland & Weiss, 1951; Kelman & Eagly, 1965; Kelman & Hovland, 1953; Weiss & Fine, 1956). Perhaps reflecting the need for additional research in this area is some recent work by Zubek, McGillicuddy, Peirce, Pruitt, and Syna (1990), who found that mediators who "tooted their horn too loudly" by publicizing their own credentials or expertise had a negative effect on such short-term measures of success in mediation as whether the disputants reached an agreement (for a fuller discussion, see McGillicuddy, Pruitt, Welton, Zubek, & Peirce, Chapter 9, this volume).

Several different types of hearing officers have been used to process cases in neighborhood justice and mediation centers, without much research as to how the various types and their effectiveness are perceived by disputants and potential users of these centers. Many experts in mediation (e.g., Bercovitch, 1984; Moore, 1986) suggest that neutral third parties need to establish personal, institutional, and/or procedural credibility as one of their first steps in gaining entrance into others' disputes. Stulberg (1981) has recently defined the functions of a mediator to include many roles; among them are those of a catalyst, an educator, a translator, an expander of resources, a bearer of bad news, an agent of reality, and occasionally a scapegoat.

In regard to carrying out this perhaps difficult role, Murray (1984)—a mediator himself—has postulated a number of characteristics of the mediator, as perceived by the disputants, that he believes contribute to the effectiveness of an intervention. He includes such qualities as knowledge, impartiality, motivation, acceptability, and the timing of the interventions. McGillis (1980), on the other hand, focusing on the qualifications of individuals who can mediate best, states that a variety of mediators from a variety of backgrounds can be used successfully. For instance, he reports that lay citizen mediators' credibility is generally high. However, how does their credibility compare to that of a lawyer or judge handling a dispute via mediation?

A colleague and I (Duffy & Olczak, 1989) recently examined subjects' perceptions of various hypothetical third parties (e.g., a "mediator," a "judge," a "social worker," etc.) as dispute settlers, in a study employing a between-subjects design. Results indicated that college students perceived the "judge" as being somewhat better as a third-party intervenor in disputes than the others, including the target labeled simply as a "mediator." We interpreted this to indicate the potency of the labeling process, as well as the reverence Americans appear to hold for the judiciary. Therefore, it would appear that perceptions of third-party intervenors or mediators are somehow causally related to achieving a successful outcome. Lately this issue is becoming more important because the Academy of Family Mediators, the states of Florida and New Jersey, and others involved in the certification of mediators are beginning to require specific credentials and/or education (e.g., a law degree or a master's degree in behavioral science) prior to certification. (The interested reader can consult Davis, Chapter 13, this volume for more on these issues.)

From the analysis above, it would appear that a great deal more research is needed on the value of existing "relationship enhancement methods" gleaned from the social and clinical literatures (e.g., see Kanfer & Goldstein, 1980) for influencing disputants' perceptions of the mediator and of his or her ability to achieve a successful resolution of their problems.

RESISTANCE AS A FUNCTION OF CHARACTERISTICS OF THE DISPUTANTS

In the psychotherapy literature, resistance is often imputed to qualities or characteristics of a client that make him or her a difficult candidate for treatment. For example, Schofield (1964) surveyed a large number of randomly selected mental health practitioners and found consensus among them for a number of behaviors that rendered a candidate a poor risk for treatment. As deficiencies, an inability to form a close interpersonal relationship, poor verbal ability, and high defensiveness emerged—qualities often found in the same person in the real world. On the other hand, the acronym YAVIS (i.e., "young, attractive, verbal, intelligent, and successful") has been shown to identify the more desirable candidate or the one with a higher potential for a successful outcome in psychotherapy (Schofield, 1964).

Resistance often results from the client's disbelief (either conscious or unconscious) in alternate ways of living. For this individual, holding on to the familiar (i.e., in mediation, the lawsuit or dispute) appears less threatening than any anticipated change resulting from a resolution of the problem. In a sense, then, resistance to mediation may result from a fear of the unknown or of what to expect in a new situation.

Resistance often also results from a disputant's not knowing how to act or what is expected of him or her in the session. In other words, "What am I supposed to do or say in mediation?" Hofrichter (1987) notes that "most parties do not have experience [of] or understand the culture of mediation as they do legal culture. Concepts about judges, due process, rules of evidence, and winning and losing are embedded in the culture. They do not have to be explained" (p. 125). Hofrichter (1987) believes therefore that resistance to mediation emerges, at least in part, "because it is unfamiliar and challenges ordinary assumptions about conflict resolution" (p. 125).

The mediator is cautioned here to remember that it may be absurd to expect a client whose long-standing problem (and perhaps the dispute itself) involves interpersonal relationships or dealing with people to resolve his or her difficulties by building or developing a further relationship with the other party, or even with the mediator. Proficiency in appropriate role-related behavior, perhaps acquired through increased knowledge of the mediation process, may go a long way toward reducing resistance that emanates from a perceived skill deficiency of this type.

Another type of resistance may be shown by an individual who demonstrates a highly dependent personality. Here the disputant or claimant may have difficulty (i.e., show resistance) in learning how to resolve the issue alone in mediation, without the benefit of an advocate (e.g., an attorney) to assist him or her as in a court proceeding.

Progress in our understanding of individual differences has blossomed recently, with social psychologists' new willingness to incorporate a wider variety of personality variables (e.g., authoritarianism and religiosity) into their theories and research strategies (Blass, 1984). In shedding some much-needed light on various dispositional influences on resistant behavior, however, the field of social psychology has overemphasized its study of the conformity process, to the near-exclusion of those who are resistant to influence. One notable exception appears to be in the work of Jack Brehm (1966) and his associates on "psychological reactance," or the tendency of some people to actively resist being influenced by others when they perceive that their freedom has been threatened. Another is the recent work of Robert Cialdini (1985) and his colleagues on social influence and the ability to resist the pressures of compliance.

Traditionally, the "resistant" or perhaps hyperindependent individual has often been labeled and discussed in the psychotherapy literature as a failure in selection or screening, rather than as a challenge to be mastered. Resistance, then, as stated earlier, represents an adversarial approach taken by an individual to the solution of a problem instead of an interactive or conciliatory one. In mediation, except for a few instances in family or divorce mediation, the hearing officer cannot simply label and dismiss resistant disputants as "poor candidates," but must somehow work through these deficiencies in getting the individuals to work toward a satisfactory resolution of their dispute.

Thus, in the area of mediation, cognitive limitations affecting disputants' attention and comprehension of the message, differences in ethnic and/or cultural backgrounds between the participants, and the relationship between motivation and affect must all be investigated as possible sources of resistant behavior that can be altered or controlled. Here, some recent work by Petty and Cacioppo (1986) on their "elaboration likelihood model" of persuasion may prove useful. Stated simply, they argue that there are two routes to persuasion. Under some conditions people are motivated and able to engage in careful, issue-relevant thinking, which Petty and Cacioppo term "central route processing." Under these conditions, attitude arguments are learned and processed carefully before they are accepted. Under other conditions, a type of thinking termed "peripheral route processing" comes into play: Less cognitive effort is exerted, and persuasion is based more on various "rules of thumb" or heuristics, attributions, and moods. Research by Petty and Cacioppo and their colleagues has demonstrated peripheral effects on persuasion for such related variables as perceived credibility of the communicator or source (e.g., Petty, Cacioppo, & Goldman, 1981) and perceived attractiveness or likability of the communicator or source (e.g., Chaiken, 1980). Extrapolation of this model to the persuasion process in counseling and psychotherapy (Stoltenberg & McNeill, 1987) seems to provide an extension of this framework allowing for the integration of a number of variables that may prove useful in mediation, including client or disputant variables, the role of motivation and ability, the role of affect, the nature of cognitive processing, and resistance itself.

RESISTANCE AS A FUNCTION OF THE NATURE OF THE COMMUNICATION OR MESSAGE ITSELF

In the psychotherapy literature, the consensus is that an accurate perception of what will take place in therapy can facilitate the course of treatment and the achievement of a resolution of the problem (e.g., Goldfried & Davison, 1976). Similarly, in the mediation literature, Dan McGillis (1981) has asked, "What types of techniques can be used to improve communication among disputants?" (p. 259). The idea here is that improved communication leads to a better chance for a resolution.

The role of message-related variables in resistance to persuasion has a storied history in the area of social psychology, going back to the Yale Communication Research Program led by Carl Hovland and others and to the publication of their classic *Communication and Persuasion* (Hovland, Janis, & Kelley, 1953) nearly 40 years ago. Since then, research on this component within the communication approach has revealed a number of variables that are related to the acceptance or rejection of a message. For example, discrepancy between the recipient's initial position and the position advocated by the communication, level of threat or fear, personal relevance of the message, the medium used to deliver the message, and repetition have all been shown to affect persuasibility (see Sears, Peplau, Freedman, & Taylor, 1988).

More specific to mediation is the finding that ambiguity of the message or unclear communication is related to perceived increases in threat or anxiety in the target (e.g., Dibner, 1958; Smith, 1957), thus increasing resistance. Again within the elaboration likelihood model, Petty, Ostrom, and Brock (1981) have demonstrated that the personal relevance of the communication affects subsequent cognitive processing; that is, it determines whether the message gets processed in an enhanced or "central" manner, or a more weakened or "peripheral" one. Within the area of mediation, we can probably assume that most messages are high in personal relevance, especially for the complainant. Similarly, Cacioppo and Petty (1985) have demonstrated that the relationship between repetition of a message and persuasibility is a complex one, being dependent on the strength of the target's initial position as well as repeated exposure to the message. Thus, it would appear that more research is also needed on the relationship between these various components of the message and their reception by the disputants within the mediational setting.

Another form of resistance to the message of mediation that must be considered here is resistant behavior originating from the legal community. Recently Salazar (1986) has provided an insightful analysis of the legal profession and its resistance to adopting and utilizing mediation as an alternative form of dispute resolution. Salazar (1986) states that "Much of the problem concerning mediation is a product of ignorance[;] a majority of the legal profession, although familiar with the name, do not really understand the concept or the process" (p. 129). Lawyers in particular need to reduce their fears and apprehension about mediation and learn just what it can do for their clients. In fact, Leonard Riskin (1982) asserts that the future of mediation in the United States rests heavily upon the attitude and future involvement of the legal profession. Salazar (1986)—an attorney herself— goes on to state that attorneys need to develop the understanding that they are dealing with people and not simply isolated acts of behavior. As a result, attorneys must extend their focus from an exclusive concern with winning in court, to satisfying all the needs and feelings of their clients. In certain cases, this may require the utilization of mediation or other alternative dispute resolution techniques.

Salazar (1986) believes that resistance toward mediation from the legal community is often a function of three interrelated areas. First is the socialization process in law school, which indoctrinates developing attorneys with an adversarial, "win–lose" type of mentality for achieving a "true" brand of justice. Included here is a concern by lawyers that only those who cannot afford a lawyer to represent them will submit to mediation; they feel that such people are thus more likely to receive an inferior, "second-class" brand of justice. Second are issues related to perceived economic threats, which seem to result from the belief that an increased use of mediation or other alternative dispute resolution techniques may ultimately lessen any future dependence on lawyers. Third are issues related to the legal community's ignorance of the concept or process of mediation beyond a superficial level. Salazar asserts that the legal community must look beyond its own professional needs, and perhaps those of the justice system, toward better serving *all* of the needs of clients. At times, this may require the utilization of certain alternative dispute resolution forums such as mediation.

As stated earlier, resistance often can be minimized, and the likelihood of a successful outcome enhanced, when greater care is taken to prepare the participants about their roles and any role-related expectations. In addition to the information provided to disputants about mediation at intake or at the onset of the mediation process itself, we must begin to develop a greater awareness of mediation and its capabilities for resolving disputes in all segments of our society. Advertisements in the media, coursework offerings in conflict resolution at the high school and college levels, and other means of disseminating information about mediation and how it works will go a long way toward reducing additional components of resistance toward the process. Finally, it is hoped that the conceptual framework provided will facilitate research efforts aimed at increasing our understanding of resistant behavior in various contexts. Ultimately, all these recommendations may assist mediation in achieving its potential as "an inexpensive method for promptly resolving disputes by allowing the parties themselves to directly communicate, compromise, and negotiate an agreement to their problems" (Salazar, 1986, p. 133).

REFERENCES

Anderson, C., & Stewart, S. (1983). *Mastering resistance: A practical guide to family therapy*. New York: Guilford Press.

Bercovitch, J. (1984). *Social conflicts and third parties*. Boulder, CO: Westview Press.

Blass, T. (1984). Social psychology and personality: Toward a convergence. *Journal of Personality and Social Psychology, 47,* 1013–1027.

Brehm, J. W. (1966). *A theory of psychological reactance.* New York: Academic Press.

Brehm, S. S. (1976). *The applications of social psychology to clinical practice.* Washington, DC: Hemisphere.

Brehm, S. S., & Smith, T. W. (1986). Social psychological approaches to psychotherapy and behavior change. In S. L. Garfield & A. E. Bergin (Eds.), *Handbook of psychotherapy and behavior change* (3rd ed., pp. 69–115). New York: Wiley.

Cacioppo, J. T., & Petty, R. E. (1985). Central and peripheral routes to persuasion: The role of message repetition. In L. F. Alwitt & A. A. Mitchell (Eds.), *Psychological processes and advertising effects: Theory, research, and applications* (pp. 91–111). Hillsdale, NJ: Erlbaum.

Carson, R. C. (1969). *Interaction concepts of personality.* Chicago: Aldine.

Cartwright, D. (1965). Influence, leadership, and control. In J. G. March (Ed.), *Handbook of organizations* (pp. 1–47). Chicago: Rand McNally.

Chaiken, S. (1980). Heuristic versus systematic information processing and the use of source versus message cues in persuasion. *Journal of Personality and Social Psychology, 39,* 752–766.

Cialdini, R. B. (1985). *Influence.* Glenview, IL: Scott, Foresman.

Cohen, A. R. (1964). *Attitude change and social influence.* New York: Basic Books.

Dibner, A. S. (1958). Ambiguity and anxiety. *Journal of Abnormal and Social Psychology, 56,* 165–174.

Duffy, K. G., & Olczak, P. V. (1989). Perceptions of mediated disputes: Some characteristics affecting use. *Journal of Social Behavior and Personality, 4,* 541–554.

Festinger, L. (1957). *A theory of cognitive dissonance.* Stanford, CA: Stanford University Press.

Folberg, J., & Taylor, A. (1984). *Mediation: A comprehensive guide to resolving conflicts without litigation.* San Francisco: Jossey-Bass.

Frank, J. D. (1961). *Persuasion and healing.* Baltimore: Johns Hopkins University Press.

Gold, L. (1985). Reflections on the transition from therapist to mediator. *Mediation Quarterly, 9,* 15–26.

Goldberg, S. B., Green, E. D., & Sander, F. E. (1985). *Dispute resolution.* Boston: Little, Brown.

Goldfried, M. R., & Davison, G. C. (1976). *Clinical behavior therapy.* New York: Holt, Rinehart & Winston.

Goldstein, A. P. (1971). *Psychotherapeutic interaction,* New York: Pergamon Press.

Goldstein, A. P., Heller, K., & Sechrest, L. B. (1966). *Psychotherapy and the psychology of behavior change.* New York: Wiley.

Gottmann, J. M., & Leiblum, S. R. (1974). *How to do psychotherapy and how to evaluate it.* New York: Holt, Rinehart & Winston.

Grebe, S. C. (1986). A comparison of the tasks and definitions of family mediation and those of strategic family therapy. *Mediation Quarterly, 13,* 53–59.

Hartley, E. L., & Hartley, R. E. (1952). *Fundamentals of social psychology.* New York: Knopf.

Hofrichter, R. (1987). *Neighborhood justice in capitalist society*. New York: Greenwood Press.

Hovland, C. I., Janis, I. L., & Kelley, H. H. (1953). *Communication and persuasion*. New Haven, CT: Yale University Press.

Hovland, C. I., & Weiss, W. (1951). The influence of source credibility on communication effectiveness. *Public Opinion Quarterly, 15*, 635–650.

Kanfer, F. H., & Goldstein, A. P. (Eds.). (1980). *Helping people change* (2nd ed.). New York: Pergamon Press.

Kelley, H. H. (1967). Attribution theory in social psychology. In D. Levine (Ed.), *Nebraska Symposium on Motivation* (Vol. 15, pp. 192–238). Lincoln: University of Nebraska Press.

Kelly, J. B. (1983). Mediation and psychotherapy: Distinguishing the differences. *Mediation Quarterly, 1*, 33–44.

Kelman, H. C., & Eagly, A. H. (1965). Attitude toward the communicator, perception of communication content, and attitude change. *Journal of Personality and Social Psychology, 1*, 63–78.

Kelman, H. C., & Hovland, C. I. (1953). "Reinstatement" of the communicator in delayed measurement of opinion change. *Journal of Abnormal and Social Psychology, 48*, 327–335.

LaClave, L. J., & Brack, G. (1989). Reframing to deal with patient resistance: Practical applications. *American Journal of Psychotherapy, 43*, 68–76.

Lewin, K. (1948). *Resolving social conflicts*. New York: Harper.

MacKinnon, R. A., & Michels, R. (1971). *The psychiatric interview in clinical practice*. Philadelphia: W. B. Saunders.

Maddux, J. E., Stoltenberg, C. D., & Rosenwein, R. (Eds.). (1987). *Social processes in clinical and counseling psychology*. New York: Springer-Verlag.

McGillis, D. (1980). Neighborhood justice centers as mechanisms for dispute resolution. In P. D. Lipsett & B. D. Sales (Eds.). *New directions in psycholegal research* (pp. 198–234). New York: Van Nostrand Reinhold.

McGillis, D. (1981). Conflict resolution outside the courts. In L. Bickman (Ed.), *Applied social psychology annual* (Vol. 2, pp. 243–262). Beverly Hills, CA: Sage.

McGillis, D. (1986). *Community dispute resolution programs and public policy*. Washington, DC: National Institute of Justice.

Milne, A. L. (1985). Mediation or therapy—which is it? In S. C. Grebe (Ed.), *Divorce and family mediation* (pp. 1–15). Rockville, MD: Aspen.

Moore, C. W. (1986). *The mediation process: Pretrial strategies for resolving conflict*. San Francisco: Jossey-Bass.

Murray, J. S. (1984). Third-party intervention: Successful entry for the uninvited. *Albany Law Review, 48*, 573–615.

O'Hanlon, W. H., & Weiner-Davis, M. (1989). *In search of solutions: A new direction in psychotherapy*. New York: Norton.

Petty, R. E., & Cacioppo, J. T. (1986). *Communication and persuasion: Central and peripheral routes to attitude change*. New York: Springer-Verlag.

Petty, R. E., Cacioppo, J. T., & Goldman, R. (1981). Personal involvement as a determinant of argument-based persuasion. *Journal of Personality and Social Psychology, 41*, 847–855.

Petty, R. E., Ostrom, T. M., & Brock, T. C. (Eds.). (1981). *Cognitive responses in persuasion*. Hillsdale, NJ: Erlbaum.

Rabkin, R. (1977). *Strategic psychotherapy*. New York: Basic Books.

Riskin, L. L. (1982). Mediation and lawyers. *Ohio State Law Journal, 29*, 41–60.

Salazar, O. M. (1986). Resistance to mediation within the legal profession. In J. Palenski & H. Launer (Eds.), *Mediation: Contexts and challenges* (pp. 125–136). Springfield, IL: Charles C. Thomas.

Schofield, W. (1964). *Psychotherapy: The purchase of friendship*. Englewood Cliffs, NJ: Prentice-Hall.

Sears, D. O., Peplau, L. A., Freedman, J. L., & Taylor, S. E. (1988). *Social psychology* (6th ed.). Englewood Cliffs, NJ: Prentice-Hall.

Smith, E. E. (1957). The effects of clear and unclear role expectations on group productivity and defensiveness. *Journal of Abnormal and Social Psychology, 55*, 213–217.

Stoltenberg, C. D., & McNeill, B. W. (1987). Counseling and persuasion: Extrapolating the elaboration likelihood model. In J. E. Maddux, C. D. Stoltenberg, & R. Rosenwein (Eds.), *Social processes in clinical and counseling psychology* (pp. 55–67). New York: Springer-Verlag.

Strean, H. S. (1985). *Resolving resistances in psychotherapy*. New York: Wiley.

Strong, S. R. (1978). Social psychological approach to psychotherapy research. In S. L. Garfield & A. E. Bergin (Eds.), *Handbook of psychotherapy and behavior change: An empirical analysis* (2nd ed., pp. 101–135). New York: Wiley.

Stulberg, J. (1981). The theory and practice of mediation: A reply to Professor Susskind. *Vermont Law Review, 6*, 85, 91–97.

Volpe, M. R., & Bahn, C. (1987). Resistance to mediation: Understanding and handling it. *Negotiation Journal, 3*, 297–305.

Weary, G., & Mirels, H. L. (Eds.). (1982). *Integration of clinical and social psychology*. New York: Oxford University Press.

Weiss, W., & Fine, B. J. (1956). The effect of induced aggressiveness on opinion change. *Journal of Abnormal and Social Psychology, 52*, 109–114.

Zubek, J. M., McGillicuddy, N. B., Peirce, R. S., Pruitt, D. G., & Syna, H. (1990). *Short-term success in mediation: The effect of prior conditions and mediator and disputant behaviors*. Unpublished manuscript.

11

Factors Affecting Public Acceptance of Mediation

ELLEN S. COHN and MAE LYNN NEYHART
University of New Hampshire

> What we've got here is a failure to communicate.
> —Donn Pearce, *Cool Hand Luke* (1967)

The general public needs to be educated about mediation and its value in order for it to be used widely. Convincing people that mediation is important and should be used is not an easy task. In some of the previous chapters of this volume (e.g., see Folger, Chapter 4, and Olczak, Chapter 10), the authors have discussed the problems of making mediation acceptable to the participants. In this chapter, we focus on factors affecting the public's likelihood of accepting mediation, and corresponding strategies for enhancing the attractiveness of mediation.

There are four aspects of public responses to mediation. First, the public may lack knowledge of mediation. Second, laypeople's view of mediation may be different from that of participants involved in the process. Third, individual differences may affect the public's receptivity toward mediation. Fourth, people may have attributional biases that may affect their ability to perceive the positive aspects of mediation.

What does the public expect to get from mediation? In answering this question, Peachey (1989) maintains that people want different things from mediation, depending on the nature of the crime. Victims of crimes involving property damage and/or loss desire repayment and compensation; victims of personal injury crimes want retribution. Peachey argues that mediation is less acceptable for people who want retribution than for people who want repayment and compensation. He suggests three solutions for these people. First, they can use the courts instead of mediation, so that they have their retribution. Second, they can change their orientation away from retribution, so that they can accept compensation or restitution. Third, they can participate in public educational programs that introduce them to alternatives to retribution. We agree with these solutions, but we suggest others as well.

This chapter extends Peachey's (1989) work to include noncriminal disputes (e.g., divorce) and demonstrates other ways that the public can be convinced to accept mediation. As Peachey does, we invoke social psychological theories to explain some of the problems and limitations in convincing the public about the value of mediation.

LACK OF INFORMATION ABOUT MEDIATION

Often the public's positive response to mediation may be limited by a lack of knowledge. Because mediation is relatively new, people may lack familiarity with the possibility of using it (Christian, 1986). This lack of information may lead to "absent" (Malorzo, Duffy, & Olczak, 1989) attitudes or possibly negative attitudes toward mediation.

There are two different dimensions of lack of information. First, people may be ignorant of mediation. In order to test this assumption, we conducted a study (Cohn, Grosch, Morrison, & Neyhart, 1988) in which we explored several predictors of the likelihood of using mediation, including knowledge about mediation. Second, people may have misconceptions about the process of trial by jury that lead them to ignore the negative aspects of it. Consequently, they may fail to consider the value of mediation as an alternative. People assume that the legal system focuses on truth seeking, not conflict resolution. In reality, the legal system is more concerned with conflict resolution than with truth seeking (Miller & Boster, 1987; Wrightsman, 1991), and in this way it is similar to mediation.

Ignorance of Mediation

Despite the recent interest in mediation and a large number of studies (e.g., Kressel & Pruitt, 1985), few researchers have compared the likelihood of using mediation for an interpersonal conflict versus a property conflict. Roehl and Cook (1985, 1989) do note that mediation does not function well with all kinds of cases. They suggest that cases involving people in an ongoing relationship who have serious, continuing problems are more likely to be mediated, but that the agreements are more likely to break down. In contrast, civil disputes involving conflicts over money and property are difficult to get to mediation, although the agreements arrived at hold over time.

The findings suggest that people may be more likely to say that they would use mediation for interpersonal conflicts than for property and money conflicts, especially if they are unaware of the outcomes of these kinds of mediation. As mentioned above, Peachey (1989) makes different predictions for mediation of cases involving interpersonal crimes and property disputes. He suggests that mediation works better with property disputes, because people are oriented to repayment and compensation in such cases; by contrast, mediation is more difficult with interpersonal crimes, because people in such cases are oriented to retribution, which is incompatible with mediation.

As stated, the literature does not address the factors predicting the likelihood of using *mediation* to resolve interpersonal and property conflicts. To fill this void, we (Cohn et al., 1988) conducted a correlational study in which 75 male and 99 female undergraduates were asked to complete a questionnaire that included several sections. The first part included demographic questions and a short quiz measuring each student's knowledge of facts about mediation. The quiz dealt with some of the basic characteristics of mediation (e.g., "In mediation, an impartial third party assists the disputants in coming to their own resolution"). After completing the quiz, subjects listened to a short oral presentation from a research assistant about the nature of mediation, how it typically works, and how it has been used as a method of conflict resolution.

Next, participants completed the second part of the questionnaire, which contained ratings of general attitudes toward mediation; ratings of how appropriate mediation was for a list of specific conflicts (general disputes, landlord–tenant disputes, and sexual harassment); ratings of how likely they would be to use mediation for each conflict; and estimates of how often they had experienced each conflict.

It was expected that subjects would be more likely to use mediation if they knew more about mediation, had a more positive attitude toward mediation, and had frequently experienced certain conflicts (e.g., landlord–tenant disputes). It was found that subjects were more likely to say they would use mediation in property disputes than in interpersonal conflicts. When the likelihood of using mediation for property disputes was the predicted variable, the two significant predictors were the appropriateness of using mediation for property disputes and general attitudes toward mediation. When the likelihood of using mediation for interpersonal conflicts was the predicted variable, the only significant predictor was the appropriateness of mediation for interpersonal conflicts.

Analyses of variance were conducted to determine the differences between property disputes and interpersonal conflicts in terms of appropriateness, frequency of experiencing the conflicts, and likelihood of using mediation. Property disputes were seen as more appropriate for mediation than interpersonal conflicts. Interestingly, participants reported experiencing significantly more interpersonal conflicts than property disputes, but said that they would be more likely to use mediation for property disputes than for interpersonal conflicts. It seemed that participants were more likely to recommend mediation for more infrequent types of disputes (i.e., property disputes) than for more frequent types of conflicts (i.e., interpersonal conflicts).

The findings in this study suggest that a lack of knowledge about mediation is not an important predictor of people's likelihood of using mediation. Instead, the likelihood of using mediation is more a function of general attitudes toward mediation (in the case of property disputes). It may be that the relation between knowledge and likelihood of mediation is indirect. Moderating variables may include attitudes toward mediation or other variables not measured in the study.

In an experimental study, the information provided was manipulated between the different conditions; this may be a better test of the relation between information and mediation attitudes. Malorzo et al. (1989) extended our findings (Cohn et al., 1988). They were interested in the effects of information and the source of information on changes in factual knowledge, behaviors, and attitudes regarding mediation. Christian (1986) suggested that the public is unaware of mediation, whereas both we (Cohn et al., 1988) and Duffy and Olczak (1989) found negative attitudes about the appropriateness of mediation for certain disputes (e.g., roommate disagreements).

Participants in the Malorzo et al. (1989) study were 63 male and 67 female college subjects. Subjects were given a pretest, in which their mediation knowledge and attitudes and behaviors toward mediation were measured by revisions of the scales we used (Cohn et al., 1988). After this pretest, subjects read information about mediation. The experimenters had a control condition in which information irrelevant to mediation was presented; in the experimental conditions, they varied the source of the mediation information (nonexpert similar peer, nonexpert dissimilar peer, expert similar peer, expert dissimilar peer, expert judge from a local court, and no specific communicator). After the mediation information was read, subjects completed a questionnaire that used the same measures of mediation knowledge, attitudes, and behaviors as the pretest.

It was found that the source of the mediation information had no effect on knowledge, attitudes, or behavior regarding mediation in the posttest. Instead, the strongest difference in the posttest was found between people who received information about mediation and those who received no information. People who received written communication about mediation scored higher on the knowledge scale. They also reported more positive mediation attitudes and behavior than those who did not receive the written communication.

The findings in this study demonstrate that information per se can affect not only people's knowledge about mediation, but also their attitudes and behaviors. We (Cohn et al., 1988) measured people's knowledge of mediation before giving *all* subjects information about mediation. Then we measured the subjects' mediation attitudes, behaviors, and likelihood of using mediation after they received information about mediation. If information is as important as Malorzo et al. (1989) suggest, then our subjects were responding to the attitude and behavior scales in the same way as subjects completing the posttest in the information condition in Malorzo et al. (1989). This would lead to less variability in subjects' scores on these scales. Therefore, no relation was found between the pretest of knowledge of mediation and later measures of attitudes, behaviors, and likelihood of use of mediation.

Taken together, these studies are important for understanding two problems with lack of information. First, our findings (Cohn et al., 1988) do support the suggestions of Peachey (1989) that people are more likely to use mediation for property disputes than for personal issues (personal injury for Peachey and personal conflicts for Cohn et al.), possibly because they seek repayment and compensation for property problems but retribution for personal issues. Second, Malorzo et al. (1989) found that information improves people's knowledge and attitudes toward mediation.

Misconceptions about the Jury Trial

Another problem in educating the public about mediation may be that they have a misconception about the purpose of a jury trial. Miller and Boster (1987) identify three different images of the jury trial: the trial as a rational, rule-governed event; the trial as a test of credibility; and the trial as a conflict-resolving ritual. The first image, that of the trial as a rational event, assumes that all parties are involved in a collective search for truth. It assumes that attorneys, jurors, and judges can lay aside personal prejudices and biases in this search. The second image, that of the trial as a test of credibility, assumes that jurors and judges can evaluate the truth of each piece of evidence. The third image, that of the trial as a conflict resolution mechanism, is very different from the first two images. It assumes that the truth can never be known; instead, the trial serves to solve the dispute between the two parties.

The first two images of the trial are similar to Wrightsman's (1991) notion of discovering the truth, and the third image is almost identical to his notion of resolving conflicts. Wrightsman argues that there is a dilemma in the legal system between discovering the truth and resolving conflicts. The public would like to believe that the legal process can result in finding the truth behind each case. It is difficult and perhaps impossible to know the truth, however, because jurors and judges have biases both before the trial begins and as they process the information being presented. Even the information about the case is presented in a biased way by the prosecuting and defense attorneys. In reality, the jury trial simply results in conflict resolution between the two parties involved in the case.

If members of the public were to recognize that conflict resolution is the true outcome of most trials, they might be more responsive to mediation. No one pretends that finding the truth is the major goal of the mediation process; the entire process is oriented to getting an agreement between the two parties. Unlike the process of a jury trial, the process of mediation is private and open only to the two parties and the mediator. The parties represent themselves and try to work together on a solution that is acceptable to both parties. The mediator is only there as a facilitator, but not as a decision maker (such as a judge). Participants actually have *more* to say than in the jury trial; therefore, mediation may be more satisfying.

A Solution to the Lack-of-Information Problem: Mediation as an Alternative within the Legal System

Some mediation programs are run separately from the legal system. This may make the programs less well known to members of the public, who are more oriented to the traditional legal process. In Boston's Middlesex Superior Court, a pilot program called the "multi-door courthouse" has been established to offer mediation as one of a series of alternatives to the jury trial (Kennedy, 1990; Sander, 1976; see also Ostermeyer, Chapter 6, and Ray, Chapter 12, this volume, for further discussion of the multi-door concept).

The program is the brainchild of Harvard law professor Frank E. A. Sander (1976), who developed the idea as a way of offering options to disputants in place of conventional litigation. Sander said, "I was really struck with the fact that we're trying to do too much with the court system. We're sort of dumping everything that can't be handled anywhere else and wondering why it's become swamped" (quoted in Kennedy, 1990, p. 102). Sander sees the value of such a program in reducing people's dissatisfaction with the legal system. Under the pilot program, any lawsuit that has been in the legal system for 7 months is eligible to pass through one of the "doors." The doors include mediation, as well as arbitration and case evaluation. Sander argues that such a program will benefit the entire legal system by leading to faster, less expensive, and more satisfying results for litigants.

This solution may expose to mediation those individuals who come in contact with the legal system and were previously unfamiliar with it. It also may lead to a system that is perceived as more procedurally fair by disputants. Now people have an opportunity for mediation within the structure of the legal system.

The next section explores the problem of lay versus role reasoning about mediation. Those intimately involved in the mediation system may have a very different orientation to the mediation process from that of laypeople who have not been involved in mediation.

LAY REASONING VERSUS ROLE REASONING
ABOUT MEDIATION

In order to decide how best to make mediation acceptable to the public, it is important to understand first how the public actually thinks about mediation. Recently, Furnham (1988) and Antaki (1981) have suggested that we can no longer assume, as Heider (1958) did, that people want to be "naive scientists" and use the same rules governing social behavior as experts do. Instead, they argue that laypeople may reason very differently from experts about a number of areas, including health, law, and business.

This suggests that the public may think about mediation differently than the participants in the process do. In fact, Cohn and White (1989) argue that the law is one sphere in which the public reasons very differently from the experts, including jurors, judges, and attorneys. Laypeople are free from the constraints that bind actors in the legal system, such as "reasonable doubt" or a "preponderance of evidence." It may be that mediation is an aspect of the law where the same kind of phenomenon can be observed.

Cohn and White (1989) suggest that there are four kinds of lay legal reasoning. First, the public frequently makes claims about legal rights. These claims are made in the context of conflict. This kind of legal reasoning may prevent the public from accepting mediation, because they do not want to give up their rights claim. Second, lay legal reasoning involves judging the conduct of others. Unlike mediation, which places certain constraints on the conduct of mediators and participants, the public is free to make any judgments about the case. The third kind of lay legal reasoning involves decisions about personal conduct (e.g., whether or not to obey a speed limit law). One does not need to consider the other party, as in mediation. The last kind of lay legal reasoning is public evaluation of the legal process (e.g., when a person on the street is interviewed about the Oliver North case). The whole process of mediation is private between the disputing parties and not open to public scrutiny.

These four examples suggest that lay legal reasoning is a pervasive human activity. It may lead the public to think about mediation in a different way from that of participants in the process.

Tyler (1987) argues that disputants are more concerned about procedural fairness or the fairness of the process, than they are about distributive fairness, or the fairness of the outcome. It may be that the public is focusing more on distributive justice, or the outcome of the case. They believe that people will only have satisfaction if they win their cases. In a series of studies involving litigants in both civil and criminal cases, Tyler and his associates (Lind & Tyler, 1988; Tyler, 1987; Tyler & Folger, 1980) have found that procedural fairness is a better predictor of satisfaction with the legal system than is distributive fairness. It may be that the public needs to be told this. If more people were aware of the importance of procedural fairness, they might be convinced that disputants have a larger voice in a mediation session than they do in a court session.

INDIVIDUAL DIFFERENCES

In addition to lack of information and lay reasoning about mediation, particular individuals may be more or less receptive to mediation because of individual difference factors. In this section, we explore two of these factors: legal development level and belief in a just world. Legal development level (Cohn & White, 1990; Levine & Tapp, 1977; Tapp & Kohlberg, 1977) refers to the three ways people reason about legal issues: law deference, law maintenance, and law creation. The three levels of legal development are distinct, but parallel Kohlberg's (1958, 1984) levels of moral development. Belief in a just world (Lerner, 1970, 1980; Lerner & Miller, 1980; Rubin & Peplau, 1975) is the belief that the world is a fair and just place where people get what they deserve. For example, people may believe that victims deserve what happened to them, even if the victims are not actually responsible.

Legal Development Level

One possible factor affecting people's receptivity to mediation may be their individual level of reasoning about the law generally and mediation specifically. Tapp and her associates (Levine, 1979; Levine & Tapp, 1977; Tapp, 1970; Tapp & Kohlberg, 1977) have developed the Tapp–Levine Rule-Law Inventory (TLRLI), a scale to measure how people reason about the law. Based on Kohlberg's (1958, 1984) scale to measure moral reasoning, the TLRLI divides respondents into three different levels of legal reasoning. People at the lowest or preconventional level are concerned with avoiding punishment and obeying authority. People at the middle or conventional level are concerned with social desirability and conformity. Finally, those at the highest or postconventional level focus on principled reasons (e.g., quality of life is more important than length of life) and are willing to accept or reject rules on the same basis. This suggests that people who reason differently about the law may reason differently about mediation. Preconventional reasoners should be least likely to accept mediation, because there are no arbitrary rules to guide the mediation; instead, the two parties or disputants decide on what is a rule. Mediation should be much more compatible with the way both conventional and postconventional reasoners operate. Because much of conventional reasoning is based on social conformity, the two parties can work together to arrive at a solution to the conflict. Postconventional reasoners can adapt to mediation, because they are used to accepting or rejecting rules based on principles.

Cohn and White (1990) have reported results from a longitudinal study conducted with college students living in one of three residential settings: a peer authority hall, where students ran their own judicial system and decided on their own rules; an external authority hall, where the students had little control and the hall staff strictly enforced all rule infractions; and two control residence halls, where the usual university procedures were followed. The legal development level of these students was measured both at the beginning of the fall semester and at the end of the spring semester. Legal development level was a better predictor of legal attitudes than was residential setting: The higher one's legal development level, the more one approved of enforcing rules against rule-violating behaviors, and the less one approved of these rule-violating behaviors. It will be interesting to learn whether legal development level can similarly predict attitudes toward mediation.

If legal development level does predict attitudes toward mediation, it will be important to determine whether any situational variables can affect legal development level. Cohn and White (1990) did find that the interaction between legal development level and residence situation predicted attitudes toward the law. From fall to spring, the only residence hall that showed an increase in legal development level was the peer authority hall, where students were encouraged to decide about rule enforcement in their own dorms. In both of the other residential environments, legal development level decreased from fall to spring. The peer authority hall was the only residence to demonstrate increases in approval of rule enforcement and decreases in approval of rule-violating behaviors. In the other halls, approval of rule enforcement decreased and approval of rule-violating behaviors increased.

Cohn and White's (1990) data suggest that giving students an opportunity to have their own judicial system and to decide on rule enforcement increases legal development level and approval of rule enforcement, while decreasing approval of rule-violating behaviors. Perhaps this kind of experiment needs to be undertaken in local communities to convince the public about the usefulness of mediation. A community example is Sander's (1976) "multi-door" approach in Boston, where mediation is an alternative to a jury trial. This approach does have the limitation that the public does not need to take the mediation option. A more radical solution would be for the legal system to require that certain kinds of cases *must* go through mediation. For example, the state of Maine requires that any couple filing for divorce must go through a mediation process. An interesting research question will be whether the public is more receptive when given a choice to participate in mediation or when participation is mandatory.

Belief in a Just World

Lerner (1970, 1980; Lerner & Miller, 1980; Lerner & Simmons, 1966) developed the belief in a just world concept as a style that characterizes people's need to have predictability and control in their lives. Rubin and Peplau (1975) extended Lerner's concept by developing a scale to measure the extent to which people believe in a just world. They argued that belief in a just world was not just a style, but an individual difference factor that could differentiate between people who scored high versus low on the scale. Zuckerman, Gerbasi, Kravitz, and Wheeler (1975) found that subjects having a low belief in a just world rated the victim of a crime more favorably than subjects having a high belief in a just world.

Lerner (1980) described both rational and nonrational strategies people use to eliminate threats to the belief in the just world. The rational tactics, which are not problematic in mediation, include (1) prevention and restitution and (2) acceptance of one's limitations. People engage in prevention and restitution by their individual contributions to charitable organizations that work to prevent or reduce suffering. They show their acceptance of their limitations by making a cost–benefit analysis of which organizations to support. None of these strategies seems particularly detrimental to mediation.

More problematic for mediation are the nonrational strategies that people use to deal with belief in a just world, including (1) denial–withdrawal and (2) reinterpretation of the event (Lerner, 1980). People who deny and withdraw are those who avoid situations where they would have to see suffering by others. These people may be particularly reluctant to engage in mediation, because there they would have to confront their problems directly.

Those who reinterpret a negative event can do so by reinterpreting the outcome, the cause, or the character of the victim. The outcome of the event can be reinterpreted by concluding that the person is a better person because of suffering. For example, people may say that an AIDS patient is a better person because he or she has had to endure the disease. The cause of the event can be reinterpreted by blaming something the person did for the misfortune. For example, a rape victim can be (and often is) said to be responsible for the rape because she walked down a dark alley alone. Finally, the character of the victim can be reinterpreted by saying that poor people or members of certain ethnic and racial groups deserve to suffer. All of these nonrational approaches to the belief in a just world are problematic, because they place a great deal of distance between the two parties and may reduce the likelihood of mediation's being acceptable.

ATTRIBUTIONAL BIASES AND MEDIATION

We have discussed nonrational cognitive approaches that reduce the likelihood that an individual will be amenable to mediation. Systematic biases in causal attribution can affect a person's orientation toward mediation as well. According to Peachey (1989), victims' views about the cause of offenders' behavior have profound effects on their approach to justice, and hence on the mediation process. An important psychological concept that Peachey discusses is known as the fundamental attribution error. The fundamental attribution error is the tendency for people to ignore situational causes for the behavior of others and to attribute the behavior of others to internal, dispositional causes (Heider, 1958; Jones & Davis, 1965; Ross, 1977). The actor–observer effect (Jones & Harris, 1967; Jones & Nisbett, 1972) is a related phenomenon; the term refers to the tendency for actors to see their own behavior as constrained by the situation and to see the behavior of others as dispositionally caused. As well as providing the basis for many psychological experiments, the fundamental attribution error and the actor–observer effect have implications for conflict resolution. Peachey points out that crime victims will not want to deal with the offenders in a mediational setting as long as they make dispositional attributions about the behavior of the offenders. Rather, they will want to see "justice done" and see the "bad persons" put away.

Experimental social psychologists have been able to reverse the actor–observer effect in the laboratory (e.g., Storms, 1973). In other words, actors come to see the behavior of others as more situationally caused, and their own behavior as more dispositionally caused. This suggests that people's attributions can be changed so that they will see mediation as more acceptable and appropriate. A consequence of the actor–observer effect may be that victims want more stringent punishment for the offender, and therefore they will be less likely to want to enter into mediation. The mediation process generally leads to compromise, and often to less stringent punishment for the offenders. Peachey contends that a person who attributes the other person's wrongdoing to temporary internal or external causes will prefer restitution or compensation—outcomes that are common to mediation. The critical question, and the one that Peachey (1989) asks, is how it may be possible to change people's attributions to more external, situational factors so that mediation will be seen as more acceptable.

The approach that we take to answer Peachey's question is to consider the explanations that have been suggested for the actor–observer effect (Fiske & Taylor, 1984). These include an informational explanation and a perceptual explanation.

One reason for the tendency to attribute another's behavior to dispositional factors may be that the person making an attribution simply lacks any information about the other person's background or immediate situation that may serve as the cause for the behavior. Thus, a person may have no choice but to make inferences about disposition based on the act itself. In fact, some psychologists have asked whether subjects commit the fundamental attribution error in the laboratory because they lack any other information about the stimulus person other than the person's behavior (Funder, 1987; Kahneman & Tversky, 1982; Miller & Larson, 1989). For example, the public viewing the people involved in a conflict may have had no prior experience with or information about the disputants; therefore, they attribute the disputants' behavior to dispositional factors. The work of Jones and Nisbett (1972) also supports this conclusion. They argue that the actor–observer effect occurs because the actor and the observer have different information available to them. The actor possesses information about the variability of his or her own behavior, but lacks any such information about the other person. Therefore, he or she can only compare the person's behavior to the behavior of others and evaluate it in a dispositional way.

Storms (1973) demonstrated that an observer's attributions about the cause of another person's behavior can be changed from dispositional to situational by reversing the person's physical point of view. When subjects must literally take the perspective of another person (by viewing their own behavior on tape), their attributions about the other person's behavior became more situational. Peachey (1989) discusses the importance of helping each disputing party understand the reasons for the other disputant's behavior, because it leads the disputants to make external (or situational) attributions about the behavior in question.

Several other investigators have shown that the fundamental attribution error can be reduced in a number of ways. As we have suggested, one way is to provide the subjects with more information about the stimulus person. A laboratory study by Miller and Larson (1989) demonstrated that, if given the option of having more information about another person, subjects were less likely to commit the fundamental attribution error. In addition, Doob and Roberts (1983) found that as subjects were given more facts about a particular case, their judgment became less severe. Only 14.8% of respondents who read a 500-word summary of a case thought the sentence was too lenient; in contrast, 80% of the participants who were not provided with a summary thought the sentence was too lenient.

It has also been found that the actor–observer effect can be reversed by providing subjects with what have been called empathy set instructions (Gould & Segal, 1977; Regan & Totten, 1975; Wegner & Finstruen, 1977). Subjects in these studies are told to put themselves in the place of the individual who performs the action. It has been shown that when told to do this, observers actually become more like actors and begin to make more situational attributions about behavior. In other words, if a subject empathizes with another person, the subject is less likely to make a dispositional attribution (Wolfson & Salancik, 1977).

Other research has shown that discussing the behavior about which an attribution is to be made can often help to avoid the fundamental attribution error. Wells, Petty, Harkins, Kagehiro, and Harvey (1977) found that subjects who expected to discuss their attributions about an actor's behavior made fewer dispositionally based attributions than subjects who did not expect to discuss their attributions. In addition, it seems that simply taking time to think about an actor's behavior helps observers to see the behavior as more situationally caused. In a typical courtroom situation, all the thinking is done by the lawyer, judge, and jury. The disputants are assigned the role of passive observers. It is not surprising that a dispositional perspective would prevail in such a situation. In mediation, the persons involved do the thinking on their own. With regard to attributional style, this change in perspective could make all the difference. For example, Bierbauer (1979) found that observers who had to think about an actor's behavior for an extended period of time explained the behavior much more situationally than subjects who rated the behavior after a shorter interval.

Jones, Riggs, and Quattrone (1979) showed that when their subjects were asked to make attributions first immediately, and then 1 week later, attributions were more situational at the latter time. Data from a British crime survey (Wright, 1989) indicate that more victims express punitive feelings about burglars in general than about their own offenders. They may feel differently about their own offenders because of empathy or more information. They know *something* about their offenders as opposed to criminals in general.

It seems that people's tendency toward dispositional attributions could be reduced by a mandatory waiting period before individuals begin the legal process (filing charges, hiring an attorney, etc.). It is possible that during that time a disputant may be better able to take the other disputant's point of view. As we have seen, that person may then be more willing to enter into mediation. If that same person had gone out and invested effort in hiring a lawyer immediately, while still holding a dispositional attribution, the individual would probably feel unable to change his or her mind later on.

After a person is freed from the tendency to place blame on such stable factors as the other disputant's personality or demeanor, that person may be in a more receptive frame of mind for mediation. Once the parties are in mediation, it is almost a certainty that the act of discussion can only continue to alleviate the dispositional bias. Wright and Wells (1985) demonstrated that groups discussing questions of attribution were less likely to commit the fundamental attribution error than individuals making decisions on their own without a discussion.

SUMMARY

We have argued that four factors affect the public acceptance of mediation: lack of information, lay conceptions of the legal system, individual differences (legal development level, belief in a just world), and attributional biases. Each of these factors leads to different solutions to the problem of acceptance.

The first factor explored, lack of information, includes both ignorance and misconceptions about mediation. In addition to ignorance, people mistakenly assume that jury trials lead to truth instead of conflict resolution (Miller & Boster, 1987; Wrightsman, 1987). In practice, the outcome of mediation may be more similar to that of jury trials than the public perceives. A solution offered for this lack of information problem is Sander's (1976; Kennedy, 1990) "multi-door courthouse," where mediation is one of the alternatives offered in place of jury trials. This ties mediation directly to the traditional criminal justice system.

A second factor is the orientation of laypeople versus participants in the legal system. Tyler (1987) suggests that disputants are more concerned with procedural fairness (the fairness of the process) than with distributive fairness (the justice of the outcome). In contrast, laypeople may focus more on distributive fairness than on procedural fairness. The solution to this problem is to convince laypeople about the importance of fair procedures, instead of focusing on the outcome.

A third factor involves two individual difference factors, legal development level (Levine, 1979; Levine & Tapp, 1977; Tapp, 1970; Tapp & Kohlberg, 1977) and belief in a just world (Lerner, 1970, 1980; Lerner & Miller, 1980; Lerner & Simmons, 1966). Research by Cohn and White (1990) suggests that people who reason at the preconventional level may be more resistant to using mediation than others. A solution is to raise the legal development level of preconventional reasoners by giving them the opportunity to be part of the mediation process. People high in the belief in a just world are less sympathetic to victims than those low in this belief (Lerner, 1980; Lerner & Miller, 1980; Zuckerman et al., 1975). They may also be less sympathetic to mediation between victims and defendants. The nonrational strategies used to eliminate threats to belief in a just world are especially problematic to mediation, because they involve avoiding direct confrontation with problems. A solution is to get people who are high in the belief in a just world to change to more rational strategies that would not eliminate the possibility of direct confrontation in mediation.

The last factor involves attributional biases, including the fundamental attributional error (Heider, 1958; Jones & Davis, 1965; Ross, 1977) and actor–observer differences (Jones & Harris, 1967; Jones & Nisbett, 1972). One solution is to give disputants more situational information about each other; another solution is to force a waiting period before mediation begins, so that disputants have more of an opportunity to understand situational factors that may explain the source of the conflict.

REFERENCES

Antaki, C. (Ed.). (1981). *The psychology of ordinary explanations of social behaviour*. London: Academic Press.

Bierbauer, G. (1979). Why did he do it? Attributions of obedience and the phenomenon of dispositional bias. *European Journal of Social Psychology, 9,* 67–84.

Christian, T. (1986). A resource for all seasons: A state-wide network of community dispute resolution centers. In J. Palenski & H. Launier (Eds.), *Mediation: Contexts and challenges* (pp. 85–94). Springfield, IL: Charles C Thomas.

Cohn, E. S., Grosch, J. W., Morrison, M., & Neyhart, M. L. (1988, April). *Predicting likelihood of using mediation for property and interpersonal conflicts.* Paper presented at the annual meeting of the Eastern Psychological Association, Buffalo, NY.

Cohn, E. S., & White, S. O. (1989, June). *What do we mean by legal reasoning?* Paper presented at the annual meeting of the Law and Society Association, Madison, WI.

Cohn, E. S., & White, S. O. (1990). *Legal socialization: A study of norms and rules.* New York: Springer-Verlag.

Doob, A. N., & Roberts, J. V. (1983). *Sentencing: An analysis of the public's view of sentencing.* Ottawa: Department of Justice.

Duffy, K. G., & Olczak, P. V. (1989). Perceptions of mediated disputes: Some characteristics affecting use. *Journal of Social Behavior and Personality, 4,* 541–554.

Fiske, S. E., & Taylor, S. E. (1984). *Social cognition.* Reading, MA: Addison-Wesley.

Funder, D. C. (1987). Errors and mistakes: Evaluating the accuracy of personality judgements. *Psychological Bulletin, 101,* 75–90.

Furnham, A. (1988). *Lay theories.* Oxford, England: Pergamon Press.

Gould, R., & Segal, H. (1977). The effects of empathy and outcome on attribution: An examination of the divergent perspectives hypothesis. *Journal of Experimental Social Psychology, 13,* 480–491.

Heider, F. (1958). *The psychology of interpersonal relations.* New York: Wiley.

Jones, E. E., & Davis, K. E. (1965). From acts to dispositions: The attribution process in person perception. In L. Berkowitz (Ed.), *Advances in experimental social psychology* (Vol. 2, pp. 219–266). New York: Academic Press.

Jones, E. E., & Harris, V. A. (1967). The attribution of attitudes. *Journal of Experimental Social Psychology, 3,* 1–24.

Jones, E. E., & Nisbett, R. E. (1972). The actor and the observer: Divergent perceptions of the causes of behavior. In E. E. Jones, D. E. Kanouse, H. H. Kelley, R. E. Nisbett, S. Valins, & B. Weiner (Eds.), *Attribution: Perceiving the cause of behavior* (pp. 79–94). Morristown, NJ: General Learning Press.

Jones, E. E., Riggs, J. M., & Quattrone, G. (1979). Observer bias in the attitude attribution paradigm: Effect of time and information order. *Journal of Personality and Social Psychology, 37,* 1230–1238.

Kahneman, D., & Tversky, A. (1982). Subjective probability: A judgement of representativeness. *Cognitive Psychology, 3,* 430–454.

Kennedy, J. H. (1990, March 11). Law professor's idea of broader legal options to get its day in court. *Boston Globe,* p. 102.

Kohlberg, L. (1958). *The development of modes of moral thinking and choice in the years ten to sixteen.* Unpublished doctoral dissertation, University of Chicago.

Kohlberg, L. (1984). *The psychology of moral development: The nature and validity of moral stages.* New York: Harper & Row.

Kressel, K., & Pruitt, D. G. (1985). Themes in the mediation of social conflict. *Journal of Social Issues, 41*, 179–198.

Lerner, M. J. (1970). The desire for justice and reactions to victims. In J. Macauley & L. Berkowitz (Eds.), *Altruism and helping behavior* (pp. 205–229). New York: Academic Press.

Lerner, M. J. (1980). *The belief in a just world: A fundamental delusion*. New York: Plenum.

Lerner, M. J., & Miller, D. T. (1980). Just world research and the attribution process: Looking back and ahead. *Psychological Bulletin, 85*, 1030–1051.

Lerner, M. J., & Simmons, C. H. (1966). The observer's reaction to the "innocent victim": Compassion or rejection? *Journal of Personality and Social Psychology, 4*, 203–210.

Levine, F. J. (1979). *The legal reasoning of youth: Dimensions and correlates*. Unpublished doctoral dissertation, University of Chicago.

Levine, F. J., & Tapp, J. L. (1977). The dialectic of legal socialization in community and school. In J. L. Tapp & F. J. Levine (Eds.), *Law, justice, and the individual in society* (pp. 163–182). New York: Holt, Rinehart & Winston.

Lind, E. A., & Tyler, T. R. (1988). *The social psychology of procedural justice*. New York: Plenum Press.

Malorzo, L., Duffy, K. G., & Olczak, P. V. (1989, March). *Communicator characteristics and attitudes toward mediation*. Paper presented at the annual meeting of the Eastern Psychological Association, Boston.

Miller, A. G., & Larson, T. (1989). The effect of an informational option on the fundamental attribution error. *Personality and Social Psychology Bulletin, 15*, 194–204.

Miller, G. R., & Boster, F. J. (1987). Three images of the trial: Their implications for psychological research. In B. D. Sales (Ed.), *Psychology in the legal process* (pp. 19–38). New York: Spectrum.

Peachey, D. E. (1989). What people want from mediation. In K. Kressel, D. G. Pruitt, & Associates (Eds.), *Mediation research: The process and effectiveness of third party interventions* (pp. 300–321). San Francisco: Jossey-Bass.

Regan, D. T., & Totten, J. (1975). Empathy and attribution: Turning observers into actors. *Journal of Personality and Social Psychology, 32*, 850–856.

Roehl, J. A., & Cook, R. F. (1985). Issues in mediation: Rhetoric and reality revisited. *Journal of Social Issues, 41*, 161–178.

Roehl, J. A., & Cook, R. F. (1989). Mediation in interpersonal disputes: Effectiveness and limitations. In K. Kressel, D. G. Pruitt, & Associates (Eds.), *Mediation research: The process and effectiveness of third party interventions* (pp. 31–52). San Francisco: Jossey-Bass.

Ross, L. (1977). The intuitive psychologist and his shortcomings: Distortions in the attribution process. In L. Berkowitz (Ed.), *Advances in experimental social psychology* (Vol. 10, pp. 337–387). New York: Academic Press.

Rubin, Z., & Peplau, A. (1975). Who believes in a just world: *Journal of Social Issues, 31*, 65–89.

Sander, F. (1976). The multi-door courthouse: Settling disputes in the year 2000. *The Barrister, 3*, 18–21, 40–42.

Storms, M. D. (1973). Videotape and the attribution process: Reversing actors' and observers' points of view. *Journal of Personality and Social Psychology, 27*, 165–175.

Tapp, J. L. (1970). What rule? What role? Reacting to Polier's rule of law and role of psychiatry. *UCLA Law Review, 17*, 1333–1344.

Tapp, J. L., & Kohlberg, L. (1977). Developing senses of law and legal justice. In J. L. Tapp & F. J. Levine (Eds.), *Law, justice and the individual in society* (pp. 89–105). New York: Holt, Rinehart & Winston.

Tyler, T. R. (1987). The psychology of disputant concerns in mediation. *Negotiation Journal, 3*, 367–374.

Tyler, T. R., & Folger, R. (1980). Distributional and procedural aspects of satisfaction with citizen–police encounters. *Basic and Applied Social Psychology, 1*, 281–292.

Wegner, D. M., & Finstruen, K. (1977). Observers' focus of attention in the simulation of self-perception. *Journal of Personality and Social Psychology, 35*, 56–62.

Wells, G. L., Petty, R. E., Harkins, S. G., Kagehiro, D. & Harvey, J. H. (1977). Anticipated discussion of interpretation eliminates actor–observer differences in attribution of causality. *Sociometry, 40*, 247–253.

Wolfson, M. R., & Salancik, G. R. (1977). Observer orientation and actor–observer differences in attributions for failure. *Journal of Experimental Social Psychology, 5*, 441–451.

Wright, E. F., & Wells, G. L. (1985). Does group discussion attenuate the dispositional bias? *Journal of Applied Social Psychology, 15*, 531–546.

Wright, M. (1989). What the public wants. In M. Wright & B. Galaway (Eds.), *Mediation and criminal justice: Victims, offenders and community* (pp. 264–269). Newbury Park, CA: Sage.

Wrightsman, L. S. (1991). *Psychology and the legal system*. Monterey, CA: Brooks/Cole.

Zuckerman, M., Gerbasi, K. C., Kravitz, R. I., & Wheeler, L. (1975). The belief in a just world and reactions to innocent victims. *JSAS: Catalog of Selected Documents in Psychology, 5*, 326.

12

The Legal System Discovers New Tools: Dispute Resolution Techniques

LARRY RAY
Standing Committee on Dispute Resolution,
American Bar Association

Much of the legal system reflects society's general belief that "through a conflict of views, truth emerges." This long-standing belief has led to the adversarial approach usually used in courthouses and in negotiations. During the past 10 years, however, lawyers have begun to realize that the adversarial mode leaves them with only one tool; this may remind them of the saying, "If your only tool is a hammer, everything looks like a nail." Their clients' problems all begin to look like nails, with the adversarial hammer being the only approach.

But each client case is unique, and a toolbox full of diverse dispute resolution tools has become a necessity for "good lawyering." Diagnosing the case and matching it to the most appropriate dispute resolution process have become valued skills in best meeting the needs of the clients. Associate Supreme Court Justice Sandra Day O'Connor described the essence of a good legal system when she stated,

> The courts of this country should not be the place where the resolution of disputes begin. They should be the places where disputes end—after alternative methods of resolving disputes have been considered and tried. The courts of our various jurisdictions should be considered "the courts of last resort." (O'Connor, 1983, p. 2)

An increasing number of lawyers are discovering that they themselves enjoy being neutral third parties (i.e., mediators, arbitrators, private judges). Some perform this service as a profession; others serve on a volunteer, pro bono basis. This new perception of dispute resolution is leading the legal system closer to former Chief Justice Warren Burger's hope "that someday all lawyers will be viewed as healers of human conflict" (American Bar Association, Standing Committee on Dispute Resolution, 1985). The

185

burgeoning movement toward alternative dispute resolution (ADR) used to be viewed only as a method for unclogging court dockets of irritating minor disputes. But today ADR is viewed as a vital tool for lawyers and the courts.

USE OF ALTERNATIVE DISPUTE RESOLUTION TOOLS NATIONWIDE

When criminal filing fees were ruled unconstitutional by a local Columbus, Ohio court in 1971, legal system leaders thought that the floodgates had been opened; it seemed that every case showed up on the docket. In response, the city prosecutor and Capital University Law School spawned the Columbus Night Prosecutor's Mediation Program as a joint venture. The program, one of the first to be developed, has proven to be a successful model. During the first year, 120 spats involving barking dogs and noise were referred to mediation. Today, the program mediates more than 14,000 interpersonal disputes each year. One-third of all potential criminal charges, including assaults, threats, and thefts, are scheduled for mediation as a first step. It is said that a defense lawyer cannot practice effectively in Columbus today without in-depth awareness of mediation.

The Columbus program is symbolic of the national dispute resolution landscape. A quick look at national statistics demonstrates the growth of ADR.

The Vital Role of the Bar Associations

Bar associations have played pivotal roles in promoting dispute resolution. For example, the Houston Bar Association formed a committee in 1979 to study ADR programs throughout the country. Panel members, led by Chief Justice Frank G. Evans of the Court of Appeals, First Supreme Judicial District of Texas, visited model programs in San Francisco, Columbus, Chicago, New York City, and Fort Lauderdale. Each model demonstrated excellent attributes: in San Francisco, community orientation; in Columbus, high rates of utilization; in Chicago, bar association involvement; in New York, institutionalization throughout the justice system; and in Fort Lauderdale, emphasis on juveniles.

Synthesizing these characteristics, the Houston Bar Association created the Neighborhood Justice Center, Inc. In only 3 years, the center became one of the best mediation programs in the nation. The program is bar-sponsored, has satellite community centers, has built up an impressive caseload, involves hundreds of attorneys and community mediators, enjoys a close association with the legal system, and has a juvenile component.

The excellence of the Houston program led the American Bar Association (ABA) Standing Committee on Dispute Resolution to select Houston, along with Tulsa, Oklahoma, and the District of Columbia, as a site for its Multi-Door Courthouse (Dispute Resolution) Centers Project. Harvard law professor Frank E. A. Sander, chair (1986–1989) of the ABA Standing Committee on Dispute Resolution, created the concept of the multi-door courthouse. The phrase "fitting the forum to the fuss" captures the essence of his idea. At all three sites, disputes and complaints are analyzed, diagnosed, and then referred on a voluntary basis to the most appropriate ADR "door": mediation, conciliation, arbitration, minitrial, summary jury trial, moderated settlement conference, or another alternative.

The results of the multi-door experiment have been impressive. More than 90% of citizen users have expressed great satisfaction with the help they received from intake specialists, according to a 1986 study by the National Institute of Justice (Roehl, 1986). In most communities, citizens seek assistance from a hodgepodge of services with no identifiable pattern of access. Residents in the pilot communities indicated that multi-door personnel guided them through this administrative maze and that they learned new tools for managing conflicts, communicating, and resolving disputes. Roughly 95% of those who tried mediation said they would use it again (Roehl, 1986). The State Justice Institute is now financing a series of workshops to promote multi-door centers.

Nationally, more than 90% of those who have used mediation express high satisfaction with the services. A National Institute of Justice study (Cook, Roehl, & Sheppard, 1980) found that if both parties appeared for the mediation session, 85–90% said that they left with a mutually acceptable agreement.

State and local bar associations also sponsor a variety of other projects. An annual Settlement Week has interested and encouraged the involvement of many bars, such as those in West Virginia; Ohio; St. Louis; Indianapolis; Orange County, California; and the District of Columbia. Often in conjunction with Law Week, the courts and the bar set aside a week to provide negotiation, mediation, and arbitration to clear case backlog. Hundreds of trained attorneys serve as dispute resolvers, especially in cases that have been pending on court calendars for a long time.

In encouraging bar association activity, the professional education of lawyers in using dispute resolution tools is essential. The state bar of Texas devoted a special issue of its journal to this topic (see *Texas Bar Journal*, Volume 51, No. 1, January 1988). Both the Colorado and the District of Columbia bars have produced handbooks that describe and make referrals to dispute resolution options. The Ohio State Bar Association has included an insert on dispute resolution services in the *Ohio Lawyer* (Volume 1, No. 3, May–June 1987). The bar associations of Minnesota; Michigan; Washington; Virginia; Boston; and Wichita, Kansas have sponsored regional or statewide conferences and seminars on ADR.

Many bar associations have created study groups in conjunction with state supreme courts. Minnesota, California, Arizona, New Jersey, and Massachusetts are identifying and forming recommendations on the appropriate role of the bar. In June of 1985 the North Carolina Bar Association's 1-year study committee issued a series of recommendations that included promotion of community justice centers, experimentation with mandatory court arbitration, and institution of a publication series, one of which was a statewide directory of dispute resolution services.

In the last few years, the Chicago and Los Angeles County Bar Associations have invested a great deal of time and money in their neighborhood justice centers. These centers provide mediation for a wide variety of complaints. Lawyers and laypeople serve as volunteers on mediation panels.

Several programs are exploring the use of mediation in new areas of conflict. A few AIDS cases have been mediated by the Atlanta Bar Association, with the support of the Atlanta Neighborhood Justice Center and the New York City Institute for Mediation and Conflict Resolution.

Emphasis on older Americans, both as mediators and disputants, is evidenced by a joint project of the American Association of Retired Persons and the ADA in Washington.

The Richmond Dispute Resolution Center, sponsored by the Virginia State Bar and the Better Business Bureau, is taking a fresh look at arbitration. Emphasis is on a structured, step-by-step approach to arbitration, including improved communication and increased negotiation opportunities. "Possibly, if arbitration is viewed as a distinct dispute resolution process with special advantages instead of a second-class adjudication, more attorneys will use it voluntarily," said the center's executive director, Karen Donegan (personal communication, 1987).

LEGISLATIVE TOOLS

Professionalism, certification, and licensing in mediation are on most bar associations' agendas. The Society for Professionals in Dispute Resolution has set up a special commission on these topics. Generally, the controversy is between professionals such as lawyers, psychologists, and social workers on the one hand, who wish to increase professionalism in the field, and volunteer mediators on the other, who claim that requirements such as professional degrees do not translate into higher-quality mediation service. Until now, bar associations have played observers' roles. The only standards the ABA recommends are those for attorneys acting as family mediators (see Davis, Chapter 13, this volume, for a discussion of credentialing).

Closely aligned with the issue of standards is that of institutionalization. Supporters feel that institutionalizing dispute resolution increases access to and sustains the life of ADR programs. Others, recalling the origins of the movement, oppose an institutional flavor. Recent Florida legislation alarms some and delights others. A new law there permits use of almost any dispute resolution tool and links professional degrees with high-quality mediators. But legislation in Texas may have captured the careful balance between reform and institutionalization. The so-called "multi-door bill" establishes as public policy the encouragement of dispute resolution options. In so doing, the bill gives all judges authority to refer appropriate cases to alternative processes.

Statewide dispute resolution initiatives seem to be a wave of the future. The supreme courts of Virginia, Arizona, and Ohio are among those in 18 states that have set up groups to study the states' dispute resolution roles. Their recommendations will wield substantial influence with legislators on the progress and methods of ADR.

QUESTIONS FREQUENTLY ASKED BY JUDGES

Generally, the judiciary has embraced the idea of dispute resolution. Reviewing some of judges' most frequently asked questions and the responses provides insight into the philosophies and reasons for endorsement.

1. What is the relationship between ADR programs and the courts?

Courts and ADR processes and programs have a close and beneficial relationship. Thomas F. Christian, director of the Community Dispute Resolution Centers Program, State of New York Unified Court Systems, Office of Management Support, has divided ADR programs and processes into three categories (Rosenblatt & Christian, 1989):

> *Court-annexed programs*—programs that are sponsored, funded, and often staffed and administered directly by the courts
> *Court-linked programs*—programs that have contracted with the courts or public agencies to provide dispute resolution services
> *Independent programs*—profit or nonprofit agencies available to the community for a variety of referral sources

The Superior Court of the District of Columbia's Multi-Door Dispute Resolution Center falls into the first category, that of court-annexed programs. The center offers mediation and arbitration along with other ADR services, such as summary jury trials. Federal courts also sponsor programs. Approximately 16 federal courts offer arbitration. U.S. District Court Judges Thomas A Lambros (Northern District of Illinois) and Richard A. Enslen (Western District of Michigan) have implemented the summary jury trial process in their districts. U.S. District Court Judge A. Joseph Fish (Northern District of Texas) often uses mediation to assist parties in resolving problems.

The Asheville, North Carolina, Mediation Center represents the second category, that of court-linked programs. Volunteers from this program sit in the courtroom, and judges refer appropriate cases to them.

In the third category is the San Francisco Community Boards, an independent community-based dispute resolution program. Citizens are encouraged to bring their disputes directly to the boards before contacting the courts.

Independent not-for-profit and for-profit entities also offer dispute resolution services. The American Arbitration Association, the Center for Public Resources, and the U.S. Arbitration Services are examples.

Generally, courts have been receptive to ADR for a variety of reasons:

- Reduction in court caseload
- Savings of time and money
- Improved methods for resolving disputes

Many judges and courts feel it is best to institute comprehensive ADR programs gradually. They have experimented with particular types of cases or processes. Many believe that testing an ADR procedure is beneficial before parties use trial court docket time.

2. Under what authority do judges or courts refer cases to ADR?

"The role of the judiciary . . . is more complex than simply adjudicating disputes. The judiciary takes on executive functions to the extent that the judges are involved with the administration of the litigation system" (National Center for State Courts, 1978, pp. 144–145).

Some federal judges state that specific authority for using an ADR program can be found under the Federal Rules of Civil Procedure's broad pretrial management provisions (Fed. R. Civ. P. 16(a)(1), (a)(5), (c)(7), and (c)(11)). For judges who feel a need for additional authority, legislation and court rules exist in some jurisdictions.

For example, the 1987 Texas Alternative Dispute Resolution Procedures Act (Tex. Civ. Prac. & Rem. Code Ann. tit. 7, § 154) states that all trial and appellate courts and their court administrators have responsibility for carrying out policies to encourage the peaceable resolution of disputes and to facilitate early settlement of pending litigation through voluntary settlement procedures. The Texas law further provides that upon the motion of any party, or upon the court's own motion, the court may mandatorily refer a matter to an ADR process.

Florida law (Fla. Stat. §§ 44.301–306, 1988) gives circuit and county judges the power to refer contested civil actions to mediation or nonbinding arbitration and give disputants the right to request binding arbitration. In addition, the law allows judges to create such programs where they do not exist.

For federal courts, the Court-Annexed Arbitration Act (H.R. 2127, 28

USC § 651–658, 1988; passed as part of the 1988 Judicial Improvements & Access to Justice Act) amended Title 28 of the United States Code to encourage prompt, informal, and inexpensive resolution of civil cases in U.S. district courts by the use of arbitration.

3. How are ADR techniques distinguishable from traditional pretrial conferences or from attorneys negotiating "on the courthouse steps"?

Much of the emphasis in ADR is on the process. The way in which cases are settled may be as important as the final result. Traditional pretrial conferences or attorneys negotiating "on the courthouse steps" focus only on the final result or settlement and are usually of an ad hoc nature.

ADR provides a logical step-by-step procedure that increases communication and participation by the parties and facilitates agreement or settlement. Research demonstrates that when parties have a significant role in the dispute resolution process, they are more satisfied with the outcome and compliance is higher (Rosenblatt & Christian, 1988). ADR can be initiated soon after filing; therefore, settlements usually are achieved earlier, conserving court time and resources. ADR is sometimes viewed as an excellent docket management tool. With ADR's structural framework available, more litigants and lawyers are likely to use ADR to reach a settlement than would, by chance, settle at pretrial conferences or on the courthouse steps.

4. How is the appropriate process selected?

Deciding which cases go to which dispute resolution process is a complex and developing field of study, called "dispute taxonomy" or "dispute typology." Understanding this taxonomy is at the heart of the ABA's Multi-Door Courthouse (Dispute Resolution) Centers Project.

Presently, the following discernible operational practices exist: Cases are referred to mediation (1) when disputants know each other (e.g., neighbors, families); (2) when disputes involve ongoing relationships (e.g., landlord–tenant, consumer); (3) in criminal cases where no violence has occurred; and (4) in commercial cases when the court or the parties think settlement is possible. Monetary amounts generally determine when arbitration is applied. Small claims are not often referred to arbitration. In Colorado, cases of less than $50,000, but more than $5,000, are submitted to mandatory arbitration. Conciliation is the most frequently used dispute resolution process for consumer and landlord–tenant disputes. Minitrials and summary jury trials are applied to complex or highly technical cases. Often the selected third party is an expert in the particular area of the case.

Most of the operational guides above have evolved from informal beliefs or personal theories. They may be implemented for political or pragmatic reasons rather than through evaluation of the effectiveness of the chosen process.

Research is planned to study placement aspects further. If an evaluation were to incorporate a completely random referral method, mediation might prove as successful in stranger-to-stranger cases as in disputes between neighbors. Monetary amounts may not be an appropriate guide for deciding when to apply arbitration. However, it is certain that whatever the guidelines are, proper screening and thorough intake procedures are necessary. In fact, a key element of the Multi-Door Courthouse Centers Project is placing well-trained intake specialists "up front" to conduct sophisticated interviews with the disputants. These specialists assist in diagnosing the situation and selecting the most appropriate first step in the dispute resolution process.

5. Which criminal cases can be referred to mediation?

Although mediation is viewed as a method for settling civil cases, in actual practice thousands of potential or filed criminal cases are mediated each year. Most of the more than 350 neighborhood justice centers or community dispute centers in the United States mediate minor criminal matters. New York and Ohio lead in the use of mediation for criminal cases.

New York has experimented successfully with mediation in various criminal matters. In 1981, then Chief Judge Lawrence H. Cooke (Supreme Court of the State of New York) led the effort to pass the Community Dispute Resolution Centers Program (N.Y. Jud. Law § 21-A, ch. 847, McKinney 1981). The purpose was "to provide: an alternative to courts for resolution of minor criminal disputes involving neighbors or other persons with a continuing relationship" (p. 2). Cases included harassment, criminal mischief, vandalism, larceny, criminal trespass, assault, bad checks, forgery, menacing, restitution for damages, theft of services, uncontrolled pets, and excessive noise.

Some cases were excluded. Mediation was not available in cases where the defendant had been indicted for a felony or had been charged with a violent felony or a serious drug offense. It also was not available to a defendant who, if convicted, would be a second-felony offender. Other inappropriate cases for mediation were those in which violence had occurred or in which there appeared to have been a high potential for violence. The legislation creating this experimental program also amended the New York Criminal Procedure Law (N.Y. Crim. Proc. Law § 170.55, McKinney 1981) to provide that a court might grant an adjournment in contemplation of dismissal, on the condition that the defendant would participate in mediation and comply with any settlement from such a process.

This experiment was declared a success 3 years later. As a result, funding for dispute resolution centers was institutionalized into the state court budget. Now New York State has programs in all 62 counties (Rosenblatt & Christian, 1988). Research from this program indicates that 87% of the cases that reached mediation resulted in successful resolution. In fact, 97% of the parties involved in mediations stated that they would participate in the process again. Chief Justice Frank G. Evans of the First District Court of Appeals of Texas represents many court leaders who believe that mediation has the potential of preventing future criminal behavior: "Mediation is future oriented and attempts to teach citizens how to more effectively deal with everyday frustrations and problems" (Evans & Kovach, 1987, p. 7).

New York has broadened the scope of appropriate cases for mediation as a result of these promising statistics. For example, the New York City Police Department (1986) has stated in an operations order, "Dispute Resolution personnel also resolve conflicts involving strangers, particularly in those instances where a form of restitution can be awarded" (p. 1). Also, Chapter 837 Laws of 1986 permits courts to refer "select felonies" to mediation "upon or after arraignment" (N.Y. Crim. Pro. Law § 170.55, ch. 837). Violent felonies, drug offenses, and serious felonies are still excluded. Cases involving large amounts of money, criminal mischief, and people who know each other are considered potentially suitable for mediation.

Although New York is unique in institutionalizing the mediation of criminal disputes, more than 47 programs throughout the country mediate between victims and offenders, sometimes after conviction (Gehm & Umbreit, 1986; see also Woolpert, Chapter 17, this volume, for a discussion of these issues). Oklahoma has a statewide program through the Department of Corrections. A model program in Elkhart County, Indiana reports a victim satisfaction rate of 70% (Gehm & Umbreit, 1986).

6. What kind of ADR program or processes will help reduce court backlog?

Measuring the impact of ADR on court overload has been problematic. Research is increasing in the dispute resolution field, but the actual reduction of backlog because of ADR is still being evaluated. Many programs and processes have been implemented in reaction to the high number of cases. Those who are closely involved in such programs state that there is a definite impact. Administrators of Tulsa, Oklahoma's Early Settlement Program noted a 4% decrease in filings during 1986. They attributed this decrease to the newly instituted mediation program (Terry Simonson, Director, personal communication, May, 1988).

One small Ohio town reduced the mayor's court time by one-third after implementing a mediation program that handled neighborhood and other minor disputes. The Night Prosecutor's Mediation Program in Columbus, Ohio, mediates over 10,000 criminal misdemeanor cases a year. Program coordinators note that although misdemeanor criminal filings have held steady, felonies and civil filings, for which mediation is not available, have increased.

Court-annexed arbitration has also been implemented in an attempt to manage the burgeoning caseloads. Today, over 100 trial courts in at least 12 states have adopted such programs, and experimental programs have been implemented in three federal courts (National Institute for Dispute Resolution, 1985). Pennsylvania instituted the first court-ordered arbitration program in 1952. A 1983 study indicated that the backlog of cases in Pennsylvania was reduced from 48 months to 21 months (Levin, 1983).

A 1982 study of the Michigan programs indicated that 36% of federal and 63% of state cases set for arbitration were removed from the trial calendar either by acceptance of the panel's award, removal of cases abandoned or determined to be below the jurisdictional amount for the court, or settlement (Goldberg, Green, & Sander, 1985).

Although both mediation and arbitration hold great promise for reducing courts' caseloads, most proponents emphasize that improved quality of justice should be the primary reason for implementing dispute resolution programs and processes.

7. What has the ABA learned during the formative stages of the Multi-Door Courthouse (Dispute Resolution) Centers Project?

The most important lessons learned from the Multi-Door Courthouse (Dispute Resolution) Centers Project thus far are as follows: (1) the need to be more cautious about assumptions that underlie case analysis; (2) the value of a sophisticated initial and ongoing case analysis process; and (3) an appreciation of the complexity of developing a dispute taxonomy.

Professor Frank E. A. Sander of the Harvard University Law School first developed the concept of a multifaceted ADR courthouse in 1976 at the National Conference on the Popular Dissatisfaction with the Administration of Justice, St. Paul, Minnesota (see Sander, 1976). The ABA Standing Committee on Dispute Resolution piloted his idea in 1984 at three sites: Tulsa, Houston, and the District of Columbia.

Phase I focused on the development of an intake analysis unit. Lawyers and counselors were hired as intake officers at each site and were stationed at the courthouse and bar association to help disputants. Phase II emphasized the creation of ADR processes within the courthouse. Phase III, which began in January 1988 and is still in progress, involves disseminating the knowledge obtained from the project to judges and bar association executives in both local and state jurisdictions.

The Multi-Door Courthouse Centers Project has demonstrated conclusively that the court is an appropriate and valuable location for ADR processes and programs.

QUESTIONS FREQUENTLY ASKED BY LAWYERS

1. What is the lawyer's role in ADR?

Lawyers now play a variety of roles in dispute resolution. One of their most valuable roles occurs during the initial client interview and diagnosis stage, when a client is being asked questions to determine whether a case can be prosecuted or litigated. With increased awareness of dispute resolution, attorneys are now trying to discern how they can best assist their clients in using all the available tools.

In addition, the traditional adversarial negotiations that often take place during initial stages of a case are giving way to the *Getting to Yes* (Fisher & Ury, 1981) style of negotiation. Instead of focusing exclusively on financial or other awards for the client, the attorney considers the desires of all involved parties, while keeping the client's interests at the forefront.

This nonadversarial style of negotiation may evidence itself during another role that the attorney can play in dispute resolution. That role is one of an advocate during the process. For example, when a mediation is scheduled, the attorney may research the mediation deliverer and the process. Then the attorney, if the client desires, attends the mediation itself. Sometimes the attorney is merely an onlooker; at other times, the attorney may actively participate. The attorney's presence or participation may promote the success of the process by balancing the power of sides or protecting information or rights of the client.

Beyond these two roles, the attorney may play a role outside of or after the mediation process. An agreement secured during the process may then be taken to the parties' respective attorneys for checking and approval. The fourth role that attorneys can play is that of a neutral third party. Hundreds of attorneys have taken mediation or arbitration training and are volunteering or receiving pay for their services to ADR programs, such as the Multi-Door Dispute Resolution Program of the Superior Court of the District of Columbia or the Maryland Attorney General Office Arbitration Program.

2. What types of cases use attorney involvement?

Presently, attorneys are involved in all types of cases. In neighborhood and small-claims cases, attorneys often chat with their clients before and after the session. In family and divorce questions, attorneys often are with their clients during the session. In actuality, 95% of all cases, including commercial and business cases, are settled without a trial (Goldberg, Green, & Sander, 1985, p. 5). Increasingly, dispute resolution techiques such as the summary jury trial, the moderated settlement conference, and the minitrial are being used in public disputes as well as tort cases (including medical malpractice).

3. Does dispute resolution add to the bureaucracy?

At present, dispute resolution does not appear to be adding to the bureaucracy; however, attorneys and other professionals must ensure that it does not, or there will be a search for alternatives to the alternatives. Ten years ago, "dispute resolution" referred to those processes being used outside the courthouse and as alternatives to traditional litigation and prosecution. Paperwork and procedures in such programs as the Night Prosecutor's Mediation Program in Columbus, Ohio, were minimal. Even the agreements were oral, not written. Despite this, or maybe because of it, a high compliance rate existed. Results of these calls in the annual report of 1979 showed that approximately 90% of the participants substantially fulfilled their agreements. During follow-up, each party was called to verify compliance.

Today, dispute resolution programs are much more widespread, and many more disputes are being referred to them. Many professionals, including attorneys, are expressing concerns about quality control and a desire to validate the professional, private, neutral third party. The result seems to be an increasing complexity of dispute resolution. This complexity involves standards and guidelines, now more than ever, mandated by court rules and legislation. Although rules and legislation often help clarify ADR's role, practitioners must retain their goal of keeping ADR a true alternative.

4. Isn't dispute resolution part and parcel of an attorney's job? Is there a real need to call upon outside resources?

Progressive lawyers do use many ADR tools and skills in their everyday delivery of service. These skills include the art of effective questioning, listening and communicating, conflict prevention, conflict management, and interest negotiation. Dispute resolution does not supplant those skills, but instead supplements them. In many cases, no matter how skillful an attorney is, no settlement can be reached. In these cases, dispute resolution offers more tools for resolving and overcoming obstacles.

5. What are the ethical problems of lawyers' operating in dispute resolution?

The role of the lawyer in representing a client in one of the dispute resolution procedures is similar to his or her role in any other process: The lawyer looks out for the best interests of the client as well as the interests of the other parties. If the lawyer is the mediator, then the lawyer does not represent either party.

The ABA standards of practice for family lawyer mediators (American Bar Association, Standing Committee on Dispute Resolution, 1985) gives excellent advice to the lawyer/mediator. The lawyer/mediator must stay neutral, should not give legal advice to any parties, should make clear to all involved that he or she is not involved in a lawyer–client relationship, and should not mediate disputes that involve previous clients.

The ethical situation of a lawyer/mediator needs increased attention from lawyers. The ABA Standing Committee on Dispute Resolution is at work presently on a model rule that should prove helpful (see, e.g., McKay, 1990).

6. What about the legal rights and due process of the client?

Most dispute resolution procedures are voluntary and include the basic characteristics of due process. Sometimes, in the interest of privacy or efficiency, citizens may voluntarily decide to waive their rights to a jury trial or appeal, especially in arbitrated cases.

When dispute resolution processes are mandated, as is increasingly the case, attorneys become more concerned about due process protections. Due process rights are protected if parties are free to reject the results of the ADR procedure and are not thereafter prejudiced in obtaining the full panoply of legal rights available in the justice system. Nonetheless, some courts have found that the mandated ADR process violates due process or other significant rights if the required process is unduly burdensome, although this same criticism is made about pretrial hearings. At least one court has found due process violations if mandatory mediation results in a report to the trier of fact without an opportunity to cross-examine the mediator (*McLaughlin v. Superior Court,* 1983).

7. Are dispute resolution processes confidential?

Confidentiality concerns many attorneys. Some proponents of dispute resolution have alleged that attorneys attend mediation hearings in order to perform informal discovery. Nevertheless, most attorneys agree that confidentiality is important, especially in family cases or cases that contain underlying personal issues. Confidentiality can be ensured in a variety of ways. One way is through a voluntary agreement of all parties, ideally in writing. A protective order against discovery of confidential proceedings where litigation is pending can also ensure confidentiality. Obtaining such an order involves showing the court that the need to protect confidentiality outweighs the merits of disclosure (see Fed. R. Civ. P. 26(c) and its state counterparts).

If a subpoena for confidential information is received, the mediator can seek to quash the subpoena on the basis of any of the following grounds: (1) Evidentiary exclusions preclude the admission of this evidence in court;

(2) common law favors protection of compromise and settlement negotiations (Fed. R. Evid. 408 and its state counterparts extend this protection); (3) a mediation privilege, where enacted by statute or rule, provides the clearest protection (see, e.g., N.Y. Jud. Law § 849-B(6), McKinney 1983–1984); or (4) public policy favors voluntary settlement of disputes, and confidentiality is essential to dispute settlement negotiations.

8. How are agreements enforced?

Enforcement issues arise in two contexts: (1) whether an agreement to submit a future dispute to some form of ADR is enforceable, and (2) whether an agreement reached as a result of ADR is enforceable in court. The answer to these questions will depend in part on the type of ADR utilized. For example, in most states, agreements to arbitrate are enforceable by statute, as are arbitration awards. The law governing mediation is far less clear. In court-connected mediation programs, whether the original agreement to resolve a dispute by mediation can be enforced in court depends on the philosophy of the mediation program, its affiliation with local court agencies, and the status of current state legislation. When a mediated agreement is breached, programs attempt to contact the accused party and to inform him or her of the alleged breach. If possible, the problem is re-mediated for a more workable solution. If the accused party will not cooperate, or ignores the "breach" or "warning" letter concerning the agreement, various steps may be taken.

In general, three models of enforcement are used. In the first model, the mediation program does not participate on an active level, but informs the complainant of possible channels through which to pursue the dispute further. Civil complainants are advised that assistance may be found through small-claims courts, private attorneys, landlord–tenant courts, or other appropriate channels.

In the second model, the program may have drafted the agreement as a potentially enforceable contract on the basis of which the client may sue. A variation of this is the arbitration model, in which the mediated agreement is incorporated into an arbitration award that may be enforced civilly.

In the third model, the original complaint may have been referred from a court, where an arrested individual is given a chance to avoid charges by participating in mediation. The criminal charge is "put on hold" for a specified time, after which the case is re-evaluated. If mediation is unsuccessful, prosecution is continued. If mediation is successful, the charge is dismissed. During mediation hearings, both parties are told that their agreement can be upheld by a court of law and that it can be viewed as a valid contract. Programs refer to this method as the "adjourn in contemplation of dismissal" process.

Some agreements are fully self-executing. They can be completely carried out at the time of acceptance (e.g., a single sum of money paid after the agreement is signed, an apology, or an exchange of property). Self-executing strategies encourage compliance but do not ensure it (e.g., disputants may make private oral exchanges or promises in the presence of the mediator or an authority figure). Parties may publicly exchange promises (e.g., at a press conference) or may draft informal written agreements such as memoranda of understanding, which also work effectively to encourage compliance.

Other agreements require continued performance over a period of time (e.g., child support payments or environmental standards performance). Disputants often develop their own standards and scheduling for performance and review of compliance. Parties may monitor their own agreement or, in multiparty disputes, may select a joint committee composed of party representatives. Finally, disputants may select a third party (other than the mediator) whom they trust and respect to be their monitor. Monitors' roles are clearly defined in the agreement. These roles vary from merely reviewing progress and reporting on compliance, to overseeing agreement implementation, to generating grievance procedures in instances of noncompliance.

Traditional methods of enforcement are also available. Agreements may be written into a legally binding contract. Parties may agree to have the settlement incorporated into the court order. Economic incentives are sometimes used to encourage compliance. In cases where the violations can be tracked and measured, disputants may agree to an indemnification procedure in which the party who breaches the contract will compensate the nonbreaching party. Performance bonds are another measure used to ensure that assets are available if noncompliance occurs.

Implementation of agreements and compliance occur more readily with an ADR case when certain initial precautionary measures are followed scrupulously, in order to lessen the need for enforcement procedures. First, proper screening and intake procedures are needed to determine the appropriateness of a case for ADR. Parties to an ADR proceeding must understand their rights and obligations and should be given a full explanation, both written and oral, of the process. Finally, any agreement reached by the parties should be written in clear language, stating dates, places, times, and the like, to allow for ease of implementation.

LOOKING TO THE FUTURE: A CAREFUL BALANCING ACT FOR THE LEGAL SYSTEM

In the beginning of the current dispute resolution movement, "alternative dispute resolution" (ADR) was the term used to describe the process. Today, in Canada, the term "better dispute resolution" is being used; New Jersey uses "complementary dispute resolution"; Florida calls it "effective dispute resolution"; the Association of Trial Lawyers Association refers to it as "flexible dispute resolution"; Los Angeles County calls it "improved dispute resolution"; Ohio Governor Richard Celeste has called it "peaceful dispute resolution"; and, making the full circle, Massachusetts uses the term "appropriate dispute resolution." Although this search for the right adjective is somewhat amusing, it is also evidence of the search to describe the role of dispute resolution within society and its relationship to the legal system.

Descriptions of the evolution of dispute resolution vary, according to the perspective of the describers. If the story is told from the American Arbitration Association (AAA) perspective, the movement began when AAA was founded in 1912. If it is related by some community programs, dispute resolution was discovered by community activists in the mid-1970s. If the tale is told by someone associated with the Columbus Night Prosecutor's Mediation Program, the movement began about 1971, when that program was instituted.

Regardless of when dispute resolution was "discovered," attorneys and the legal system have been in the front of the bandwagon during the past 15 years. A majority of the mediation programs were founded by legal system participants. As noted earlier, Chief Justice Frank Evans of the Texas First District Court of Appeals began the successful Houston Neighborhood Justice Center. The Chicago Bar Association created the solid Neighborhood Justice of Chicago Center. Law professor John Palmer established the Columbus Night Prosecutor's Mediation Program. Even some of the most widely known community dispute resolution activists, such as Paul Wahrhaftig of Pittsburg and Ray Schonholtz of San Francisco, are attorneys.

The future looks bright for the growth of dispute resolution. The rate of past growth—from 100 mediation programs in 1976 to more than 400 in 1989—suggests that fairly soon every jurisdiction in the United States will contain such a program. Assisted by legislation, the states of New York and Texas now claim that all of their citizens have access to mediation. Attorneys and the legal system will continue to play a major role in creating and volunteering in such programs.

A major concern with ADR programs will be institutionalization. Even the term conjures up negative bureaucratic characteristics of delay, costs, insensitivity, excess paperwork, and so on. Signs of institutionalization are already evident in some older programs. Often, in the zest for increasing access and reducing caseload, court rules and legislation that promote negative bureaucratic system characteristics are hastily passed. Ideally, lawyers and the legal system will be in the forefront of recognizing and correcting these problems. Ideally, people will remember that many of these programs were created to provide alternatives to these system characteristics. Dispute resolution has evidenced great success in terms of citizen satisfaction and decreases in costs and delays, without a lot of rules, regulations, standards, and guidelines. Mediation is being listed as one of "the hot new professions."

In the future, many more lawyers will begin to incorporate dispute resolution tools into their private practices. Progressive attorneys will view their roles as almost "mini-multi-door services."

Increasingly, lawyer referral services will have dispute resolution referral panels. Attorney general offices will begin to operate in a multi-door dispute resolution fashion. Bar associations will expand their attorney–client fee arbitration programs into multi-door dispute resolution services for all types of attorney and client disputes.

Careful balancing away from institutionalization and toward integration may be the key. Fortunately, such organizations as the State Justice Institute, the Society for Professionals in Dispute Resolution, the National Institute for Dispute Resolution, and of course the ABA Standing Committee on Dispute Resolution seem to have already captured the idea of careful balancing and will continue their vital guidance to the developing dispute resolution field. With the lessons of the past and the promise of the future, lawyers and bar associations have the potential to guide this reform, increasing citizens' access to prompt, appropriate, and affordable justice.

REFERENCES

American Bar Association, Standing Committee on Dispute Resolution. (1985). Standards of practice for lawyer mediators in family disputes. In American Bar Association Family Law Section (Ed.), *Divorce mediation: Readings* (pp. 597–605). Washington, DC: American Bar Association.

Cook, R., Roehl, J., & Sheppard, D. (1980). *Neighborhood justice centers field test: Final evaluation report*. Washington, DC: U.S. Government Printing Office.

Evans, F. G., & Kovach, K. K. (1987). An overview of dispute resolution in Texas [Special Issue, 1986 Dispute Resolution annual report]. *The Houston Lawyer*, 7–8.

Fed. R. Civ. P. 16(a)(1), (a)(5), (c)(7), (c)(11).

Fed. R. Civ. P. 26(a).

Fed. R. Evid. 408.

Fisher, R., & Ury, W. (1981). *Getting to yes*. Boston: Houghton Mifflin.

Fla. Stat. §§ 44.301–.306 (1988).

Gehm, J., & Umbreit, M. (1986). *Victim–offender reconciliation and mediation program directory*. Valparaiso, IN: Prisoner and Community Together Institute of Justice.

Goldberg, S. B., Green, E. D., & Sander, F. E. (1985). *Dispute resolution*. Boston: Little, Brown.

H.R. 2127, 100th Cong., 1st Sess. (1987).

H.R. 3152, 100th Cong., 1st Sess. (1987).

Keilitz, Susan (1990, Fall). A court manager's guide to the ADR database. *State Court Journal, 14*(4).

Levin, A. L. (1983). Court-annexed arbitration. *University of Michigan Journal of Law Reform, 16*, 537–548.

McKay, R. B. (1990). Ethical considerations in alternative dispute resolution. *Arbitration Journal, 45,* 16–28.

McLaughlin v. Superior Court, 140 Cal. 3d 473, 189 Cal. Rptr. 479 (1983).

National Center for State Courts. (1978). *State Courts: A blueprint for the future.* Second National Conference on the Judiciary. Williamsburg, VA: Author.

National Institute for Dispute Resolution. (1985, August). Court-ordered arbitration issue: A report of the First National Conference on Court-Ordered Arbitration, *Dispute Resolution Forum,* N.D.R.

N.Y. Crim. Proc. Law § 170.55 (McKinney 1981).

N.Y. Crim. Proc. Law § 170.55, ch. 837 (McKinney 1981).

New York City Police Department. (1986, May 19). *Referral of certain misdemeanor and violation offenses to conflict resolution dispute centers* (Operations Order No. 53). New York: Author.

N.Y. Jud. Law § 21-A, ch. 847 (McKinney 1981).

N.Y. Jud. Law § 849-B(6) (McKinney 1983–1984).

O'Connor, S. D. (1983, January). *Consumer dispute resolution: Exploring the alternatives.* Keynote address presented at the American Bar Association National Conference, Washington, DC.

Roch, J. A. (July, 1986). *Toward the multi-door courthouse: Dispute resolution intake and referral.* (NIJ Reports 2–7, U.S. Department of Justice). Washington, DC: National Institute of Justice.

Roehl, J. A. (1986). *The Multi-Door Courthouse Project of the American Bar Association Special Committee on Dispute Resolution: Phase I. Intake and referral assessment* (National Institute of Justice Grant Executive Summary). Washington, DC: National Institute of Justice.

Rosenblatt, A. M., & Christian, T. F. (1988). *The Community Dispute Resolution Centers Program annual report.* Albany, NY: Office of Court Administration.

Rosenblatt, A. M., & Christian, T. F. (1989). *The Community Dispute Resolution Centers Program annual report.* Albany, NY: Unified Court System Office of Management Support.

Sander, F. (1976). The multi-door courthouse: Settling disputes in the year 2000. *The Barrister, 3,* 18–21, 40–42.

Tex. Civ. Prac. & Rem. Code Ann. tit. 7, § 154 (Vernon 1987).

13

How to Ensure High-Quality Mediation Services: The Issue of Credentialing

ALBIE M. DAVIS
District Court Department,
Commonwealth of Massachusetts

How can community mediation programs ensure the quality of their services? The answer to this question can be found by examining two interrelated perspectives: internal (i.e., those actions local programs can take on their own accord) and external (e.g., credentialing imposed by others). I do not claim to be neutral on the subject and therefore feel it proper to explain my own background and biases.

I first became exposed to community mediation in the late 1970s. In 1980 I was trained as a mediator with the Urban Court Program in Dorchester, one of Boston's most diverse neighborhoods, and I have been mediating for my community since that time. The attraction was, and remains, the fundamentally respectful nature of the process—when it is done well. The history of mediation in Dorchester has been both impressive and tumultuous, especially in regard to the issues of quality of services and treatment of volunteers. As a consequence, I have a personal, and sometimes painful, involvement in the question. Since 1983, I have been director of mediation for the District Court Department in Massachusetts. From that vantage point I have been able to chart the growth of the field in one state. Because I act as a clearinghouse for information about mediation, I am particularly conscious of the growing numbers of people who are attracted to the field for reasons quite different from my own. My associations with national organizations—for example, the committee that drafted standards of practice for the Society of Professionals in Dispute Resolution (SPIDR) and the Community Justice Task Force of the National Institute for Dispute Resolution (NIDR)—have allowed me to develop a broader national and even international perspective.

Mention the word "credentialing" and hear community mediation advocates (myself included) cry, "Ouch!" For many, the attraction to mediation is its ability to draw conflicts away from the *so-called* experts (e.g., attorneys and judges) and return them to the *real* experts (people embroiled in differences). Although mediators care greatly about the quality of service delivered by local programs and do not like to see the mediation process taken lightly, they fear two negative outcomes from credentialing. First, it may distance them from those they serve; that is, it may establish mediators as the new caste of experts. Second, credentialing may represent the first step on the slippery slope toward a new profession—one that digs moats around its members and pours hot oil on those who dare to scale the ramparts.

Mediators are caught in a dilemma: how to ensure the quality and integrity of the services provided, without creating a new mystique—a cult of mediation. This dilemma, no matter how distressing, is not going away. As the field of mediation expands at a geometric rate, the applications for mediation appear endless, and hybrid processes proliferate. Of economic necessity, community mediation programs are shedding their grassroots image and assuming a more entrepreneurial posture. In addition, each day new practitioners hang out their shingles. Some are competent, caring, and ethical. Others are not. It is extremely difficult for the initiated to understand these alternatives and their implications, let alone to ensure their quality. The uninitiated are at a severe disadvantage. "Buyer beware" is the best advice one can give to the average consumer who needs to sort out his or her options. In sum, mediation is so far down the slope toward professionalism, there is no turning back. The best strategy for community mediation is to sharpen its vision, ski skillfully, and aim for a positive outcome.

THE INEVITABLE STAGES OF PROFESSIONALIZATION

One way to improve vision is temporarily to draw back from the fray and look at the big picture. For over a decade, mediation practitioners and theorists have been alert to the trend toward professionalization and wary of its pitfalls. Unusual insights into this issue are found in a surprisingly humorous article, "The Social Organization in Alternative Dispute Resolution: Implications for Professionalization of Mediation" (Pipkin & Rifkin, 1984). As a prelude to discussing their findings about the staff and mediator composition of mediation programs, the authors describe the classic stages of the rise of any new profession, as charted 20 years earlier by Harold L. Wilensky (1964, p. 137). I quote Pipkin and Rifkin at some length because their analysis helped me cut through my denial that professionalism is already a fact, forced me to drop my self-righteous attitude about its consequences, and allowed me to view such developments with a sense of history *and* a sense of humor.

> [The process] starts by people "doing full time the thing that needs doing." Next, practitioners, clients, or [members of] a professional association press for the establishment of training schools. The first teachers are the

"enthusiastic leaders of the movement," "protagonists of some new technique," or both. If training schools do not begin in universities, they always try to end up there. "A corps of people who teach rather than practice is an inevitable accomplishment." The third stage is to form a professional association. "Activists in the association engage in much soul-searching—on whether the occupation is a profession, what the professional tasks are, how to raise the quality of recruits, and so on."

During the third stage, a number of subdevelopments occur. One is a self-conscious effort to define and redefine the core tasks of the occupation. Typically, an order of delegation emerges through these redefinitions which internally stratifies the group. Conflict is likely between those who win and those who lose under hierarchical rearrangements. Conflicts also arise between those who are committed to the old locations and organizations that helped launch the enterprise and the new cohorts of practitioners who lack these attachments. In addition to the internecine struggles, externally directed conflict with other occupations [that] claim the same territory or expertise is likely at this stage.

In the fourth stage, professional associations seek the support of law to impose certification requirements on the practice. Licensure is sought to protect the territory and exclude the unqualified and unscrupulous. Finally, the fifth and last stage is for the profession to codify its rules of ethics as the bases for self-regulation. (Pipkin & Rifkin, 1984, p. 205)

Most readers will recognize that, to some degree or another, the field of mediation has experienced all five stages. Signals that stage five is here, or near, are "grandfathering" clauses in legislation or standards that allow one last cohort of "underqualified" practitioners to join the ranks before the doors to the profession are closed. Pipkin and Rifkin see two primary issues at stake in the move toward professionalization: (1) Will mediation be a new and autonomous profession or a subset of existing professions, such as law, mental health, or social work, and thus regulated by them? (2) Will the goal of "community building" through lay dispute resolution, which implies interest in one's community, be threatened by attempts to define mediation as an intervention based upon "individual expertise and professional disinterest rather than community engagement"? They conclude that resolution of these questions "may depend on which groups are best able to stake out first territorial claims and command the allegiance of participants" (Pipkin & Rifkin, 1984, p. 207).

Can community mediation meet this territorial challenge and quest for allegiance? How often do mediators remind others that the Chinese word for crisis is composed of the two characters "danger" and "opportunity"? Now is the time for the community mediation field to heed its own advice—to face the crisis and untangle the opportunity from the danger. This exercise requires mediators to reflect upon the usual stages of the rise of a new profession and to ask tough but fundamental questions. What trends are occurring in the field and why? What developments appear positive, and which ones may contain the seeds of eventual destruction? What is essential about the nature of community mediation? What, on the other hand, is habit? History? Self-serving rhetoric? And, given the rapid pace of change and limited resources, where are the critical junctures where well-timed and well-conceived interventions might produce positive results?

THE ROOTS OF COMMUNITY MEDIATION

The focus of this chapter is upon those mediation programs that embrace community building as part of their mission—in other words, those that recruit, train, and use volunteers and consider the parties' ability to shape their own agreements as integral to their definition of mediation. Many programs, even those that place primary emphasis on reducing court backlog or costs, fall within this definition. In general, community mediation programs are run by private, nonprofit organizations; however, many times they are housed in courts, government agencies, or colleges and universities (McGillis, 1986, pp. 19–30). No doubt the growing numbers of programs that train elementary and secondary students and teachers to mediate conflicts deserve to be included in the count.

Three distinguishing features of community mediation programs are (1) their use of volunteers (2) who come from all types of backgrounds and (3) who begin providing service after a relatively brief period of training. As a starting point in staking its claim to this new profession, the community mediation field must first re-examine and then put in perspective these three characteristics, which run counter to those of most traditional professions.

How did these features emerge? And what is the rationale for each? In answering these questions, it is useful to recall the history of community mediation—in particular, our labor mediation and community empowerment roots. Our labor ancestors saw mediation as more an art than a science. The authors of a Canadian labor mediation manual note that to those who believe mediation is an art form, the question of choosing and preparing mediators is simple—"select only 'great men' and expose them to 'trial by combat.' After a reasonable apprenticeship period with a seasoned mediator, and a subsequent term of direct 'hands-on experience,' a labor relations agency simply retains those who survive and replaces those who did not" (Education Relations Commission, 1983, p. 1).

George Nicolau, labor arbitrator and mediator and former president of the SPIDR, was highly instrumental in adapting the skills of labor mediation to the community setting. He took something that had been passed along anecdotally or through "war stories," but was not generally accessible, and put his thoughts and experiences into a written curriculum that has influenced practice throughout the nation. He did not fall into the trap of the "great man" theory, however, for along with his labor arbitration and mediation background, he brought the insights he had gained as a Peace Corps staff member, as regional director of the Office of Economic Opportunity, and as the first commissioner of community development for New York City. He saw mediation as an art that could be learned by people from all backgrounds in a relatively short period of time (Nicolau, 1975).

In a 1986 talk to a statewide gathering of community mediators in Massachusetts, Nicolau reminisced about the founding days of the field as he experienced it from his vantage point. In 1973, at the urging of two staff members from the New York City Department of Corrections, Ann Weisbrod and Sandy Feinberg, the Institute for Mediation and Conflict Resolution (IMRC) agreed to recruit and train volunteers to mediate community conflicts. "There was virtually nothing out there," Nicolau noted. "Community mediation, alternative dispute resolution, ADR, did not exist—not as a considered concept, as a trend, as a movement, or even as an acronym" (Nicolau, 1986, p. 3). IMCR had trained people from the Federal Department of Justice and the New York City Police Department, as well as various community leaders from diverse ethnic backgrounds and levels of leadership, in general conflict resolution skills. This successful experience influenced their approach.

> We set no formal educational standards or requirements. We didn't really care whether this person had a college degree or a high school diploma or was a dropout, because we didn't believe that education was a relevant measure of what we were looking for. We were looking for people who could postpone judgment, who did not try to impose their values on participants in the process, who were not upset by, but sensitive to and able to deal with cultural differences, people who could listen with understanding. We knew that if we could find such individuals, we could give them the skills to bring people together. We recruited our first class (of volunteers) and put them through a rigorous training program. Fifty-five hours of training—building, shaping, and honing conflict resolution skills. (Nicolau, 1986, pp. 3–4)

VOLUNTARISM, BRIEF TRAINING, AND OPEN ADMISSIONS

The precedent was established early—in New York City; Philadelphia; Columbus, Ohio; San Francisco; Rochester, New York; and Boston—that community mediation skills could be taught to volunteers from all backgrounds in a short, experiential manner (McGillis, 1986, p. 5). Elements of that tradition are still holding. Across the nation, thousands of volunteers are providing mediation services. New York State gives its count as 1,500 (Rogers, Kanrich, & Steinhauser, 1989, p. 1), and Massachusetts has over 1,000 (Davis, 1986, p. 31). The average hours requirement for mediation training in Massachusetts is 30 hours (Davis, 1986); New York's and North Carolina's volunteers must complete 25 hours of training (Freedman, 1984, pp. 109, 117); 25 hours of classroom instruction and a 10-hour practicum are required for Californians (Division of Consumer Services, 1987, p. 5). An Illinois law requires 30 hours of mediation training plus peer review and further states that "mediators shall perform their duties as volunteers, and shall not receive any compensation for their services" (Brodigan, Sideris, Price, Murtagh, & Steele, 1988, Appendix C).

However, given the evolution of other professions, one has to wonder what the future holds. As long as community mediation programs focused upon cases involving persons of little means, who were entangled in difficult-to-resolve and often highly charged conflicts, competition for territory was infrequent. Critics of the emerging field might bemoan mediation as second-class justice, noting that "diversion of disputes to alternative forums might indeed lighten the judicial burden; but it would do so at the risk of 'transforming powerless people into victims who can secure relief neither in the courts nor anywhere else' " (Auerbauch, 1983, p. 125). But few fought for the right to provide these same clients with either legal or mediation services.

Now several forces are working together in a circular and reinforcing fashion to make the boundaries between voluntarism and paid work highly permeable and to put the traditions of voluntarism, short training, and open admissions at risk. As a starting point, zealous community mediators, all carriers of a new way of resolving conflict, have trained thousands of other people in the process. The supply of mediators available for community work far exceeds the demand. At the same time, for every trainee who responds to the community-empowering potential of the process, another two see in mediation an exciting new career possibility. Originally, academics were merely curious about this new development, but soon they offered lectures, then units, classes, courses of study, clinical experience at nearby community mediation centers, and eventually degrees in conflict resolution. Their activities further raised expectations about career opportunities and "upped the ante" for the amount of preparation necessary for dispute resolvers. With a minuscule number of careers to select from, those eager to earn their living through practice sought ways to stimulate demand. The smallest successes on the demand side were all that were needed to nurture the supply side. And so on.

Finally, the staffs of community-based programs, weary from long years in the vineyards, began to question their own wisdom. Why should they, the experienced trainers and mediators, continue to work at sacrificial wages when their neophytes were moving off into the world of free enterprise with dollar signs in their eyes? One solution was to leave community work and set up their own businesses. Another was to become more entrepreneurial in the management of their community programs, take on new initiatives, and raise their own salaries. Many did both. Often the results were internal confusion and strife within their programs because of the blurring of lines between activities that should be carried on by their agencies and matters that were suitable for private consulting. With so many community mediation programs and their staff members or graduates reaching into new territories where others (attorneys and therapists, for example) were already earning a living—divorce, insurance claims, major civil cases, and environmental disputes—the question of who should be eligible to mediate became more intense. For better or worse, local programs had always assumed responsibility for "credentialing" their own mediators. The cavalier way in which these program-based credentials were used by the newly trained to leverage careers caused even the most hard-nosed anticredentialists to rethink their philosophy on this issue. Credentialing began to look attractive to many people for vastly different reasons. Now community mediation programs, those interested in developing new careers, and those who were already paid professionals sought ways to define who could mediate.

CREDENTIALING THROUGH LEGISLATION

"Creeping legislation is beginning to define what it is to be a mediator," notes Jay Folberg, president of the Academy of Family Mediators (quoted in Bureau of National Affairs, 1989b, p. 303). Indeed, while professional societies debate the issue, de facto and de jure qualifications are evolving, usually on a state-by-state basis. The way in which legislation or regulations answer three questions— (1) Who is eligible to mediate? (2) Who certifies the eligible? and (3) Who can mediate what kind of cases?—has profound implications for the future of the field. Through legislation, the fates of the volunteer and the paid mediator become intimately entwined.

In the area of divorce mediation, the tendency toward using other degrees as entry requirements to the "profession" was set rather early. Folberg expressed this phenomenon in a 1983 address to the American Bar Association (ABA) Section on Family Law, noting that divorce is a "family process within a legal context" and as such has traditionally involved lawyers and mental health professionals. These two professions "may not eagerly cooperate in creating joint roles nor in relinquishing their traditional domain. They may, however, become strange bedfellows in checking the emergence of a new 'profession' of family mediators" (quoted in Goldberg, Green, & Sander, 1985, pp. 315–316). When California passed its Family Conciliation Court Law in 1979, requiring mediation of child custody or visitation rights, it set out minimum qualifications including "a master's degree in psychology, social work, marriage, family and child counseling, or other behavioral sciences substantially related to marriage and family interpersonal relationships" (Freedman, 1984, p. 25).

Other states show the influence of California's approach, but also have added a law degree as a ticket for admission. In Alaska, 1983 legislation allows the presiding judge to maintain a list of persons "who certify that they meet the following minimum requirements: A law degree or a master's degree in psychology, social work, marriage, family and child counseling, or *other behavioral science substantially related to marriage and family interpersonal relationships*" (Freedman, 1984, p. 25, italics mine). The 1982 Michigan "friend of the court act" stipulates that domestic relations mediators must meet one of several qualifications—for example, "licensed psychologist; or five years experience in family counseling; or a graduate degree in behavioral science, plus mediation training; or, membership in the bar, plus mediation training" (Freedman, 1984, p. 81).

Interestingly, in New Hampshire, where the use of volunteers to mediate divorces gained an early foothold, the hegemony of the legal and mental health professions (so prevalent in other states) was avoided. A 1989 act "established a board of marital mediator certification with members to include one superior court judge, one full-time marital master, one attorney, two public members, one mental health professional, and three marital mediators" (Bureau of National Affairs, 1989d, p. 324). Mediators must complete 48 hours of training, complete an internship with a certified marital mediator, and submit three recommendations. Certification must be renewed every 3 years. No mention is made of qualifying degrees. On the west coast, the state of Oregon forbids the use of "formal education in any particular field" as a prerequisite to serving as a mediator (Oregon Revised Statutes, 1989).

Most typically, legislation identifies the judiciary as the one certifying agency. In Florida, "no person may be appointed to serve as a mediator or arbitrator unless he has been certified by the chief judge of a circuit in accordance with the standards established by the Supreme Court" (Brodigan et al., 1988, Appendix C). The standards finally approved by the Florida Supreme Court call for three types of mediators with three sets of qualifications to handle three categories of cases. County court mediators, who handle cases "involving non-complex issues," can come from any walk of life, as long as they successfully complete 20 hours of training and an apprenticeship. Family mediators must either (1) have a master's degree in social work, mental health, or other behavioral or social sciences; or (2) be a certified psychiatrist; or (3) be an attorney or a certified public accountant. They must have 4 years of practical experience in one of these fields. In addition, they must complete a minimum of 40 hours of training. Civil mediators, who mediate cases where attorneys usually negotiate on behalf of their clients, must be former judges or members of the Florida bar for 5 years. They too must complete 40 hours of mediation training (Bureau of National Affairs, 1988b, pp. 434–435). By contrast, a Massachusetts civil mediation program, which pays its mediators $150 an hour, intentionally recruits both attorney and nonattorney mediators (Massachusetts Mediation Service, 1988).

In Texas, courts also appoint mediators, according to set standards, but may waive these requirements "if the court bases its appointment on legal or other professional training or experience in particular dispute resolution processes" (Brodigan et al., 1988, Appendix C).

Some states are moving toward statewide advisories, with representation from other branches of government and outside agencies. The Oklahoma Dispute Resolution Act allows for mediator certification by local mediation agencies, which in turn must be certified by a statewide Dispute Resolution Advisory Board appointed by the Oklahoma Supreme Court. The 15-member board must be composed of representatives from "state and local governments, business organizations, the academic community, the law enforcement field, the legal profession, the judiciary, the field of corrections, retired citizen organizations, the district attorney profession, consumer organizations, social service agencies, and three members at large" (Brodigan et al., 1988, Appendix C).

Appointments to the legislatively created 12-member Ohio Commission on Dispute Resolution and Conflict Management are made by the governor (four), the chief justice of the Ohio Supreme Court (four), the president of the state senate (two), and the speaker of the state house (two). Although the act does not specifically grant the Ohio commission the right to certify mediators, the legislature has appropriated over $1 million to support local programs and has given the commission the right to evaluate those programs. Oregon recently established a five-member commission to develop standards for mediators and the community programs, with appointments made by the governor (Bureau of National Affairs, 1989a, p. 285).

In some instances, certification has "sneaked in through the back door," so to speak. Massachusetts offers an interesting example. When mediation advocates sought a free-standing confidentiality statute in 1985, without any accompanying legislation to provide a context, legislators quite naturally wanted to know to whom they were granting such broad coverage. They inquired about mediator training, and, having just done a survey on the topic, I told them that the average training requirement for community programs was 30 hours. When the actual bill emerged from the legislative process, I was surprised by the "compromise" definition of a mediator that was appended to the brief bill:

> For the purposes of this section a "mediator" shall mean a person not a party to a dispute who enters into a written agreement with the parties to assist them in resolving their disputes and has completed at least thirty hours of training in mediation and who either has four years of professional experience as a mediator or is accountable to a dispute resolution organization which has been in existence for a least three years or one who has been appointed to mediate by a judicial or a governmental body. (Davis, 1986, p. 31)

By the stroke of a pen, the former *average* of 30 hours for community volunteers was thereby established as the new *minimum standard* for everyone. (Labor mediation, which already had confidentiality statutes, was exempted from this act.)

Clearly, state legislatures, which are usually dominated by attorneys, are playing a pivotal role in shaping the nature of the field. Some states place the certification of mediators in the hands of the judiciary; others have established commissions to answer such questions; some leave discretion at the local level; and still others are silent on the matter. It can be argued that many of these laws only regulate those programs funded by the government and do not regulate the free marketplace. Nevertheless, the trends are being set.

There has been relatively less legislative activity on the federal level, especially in relation to qualifications of mediators. For a time, expectations for federal support for the field were high when, after a major organized campaign, the Dispute Resolution Act was signed into law by President Carter in 1980. Although the act authorized the expenditure of $11 million annually for dispute resolution programs, Congress never appropriated the funds. The energy of the ADR field was redirected toward passage of the State Justice Institute Act. Since 1987, the State Justice Institute (SJI) has awarded $15 million to support programs affecting state judiciaries, with some of the funds going to ADR (State Justice Institute, 1989). In 1990, the SJI awarded a grant to the Institute for Judicial Administration to develop national standards for court affiliated mediation programs.

One intriguing piece of federal legislation is the Farmer–Lender Act, which provides that the federal government shall make loans to farmers and ranchers only in states that have procedures for mediating defaults of such loans. Each state must establish a commission responsible for appointing mediators. In its fiscal year 1989 report, the U.S. Department of Agriculture, which administers the program, has recommended that Congress consider requiring participation in farm credit mediation by other federal creditors, including the Internal Revenue Service and the U.S. Attorney's offices (Bureau of National Affairs, 1989c, pp. 435–437). Federal farmer–lender mediation is worth watching, for much of the impetus for the program came from the successful experience of the Iowa Farmer Creditor Mediation Service. To this day, Iowa's statewide service does not require academic degrees of its mediators, many of whom are farmers or community mediators. However, the issue of credentialing has become controversial, and there is a move toward using a 4-year academic degree as entry to a standardized mediation training program (G. Boothginna, personal communication, April 18, 1990).

PROFESSIONAL ASSOCIATIONS' VIEWS ON QUALIFICATIONS

Ray Shonholtz, founder of the San Francisco Community Boards and a long-time advocate for the separation of mediation from the judiciary, asserts that the certification debate "forces to the forefront perhaps that most critical issue facing the maturing field of conflict resolution: whether conflict resolution processes are consumer–disputant options or only alternatives to litigation, controlled by judges and attorneys" (quoted in Bureau of National Affairs, 1988a, p. 349). Margaret Shaw, a member of the SPIDR Commission on Qualifications, sees the issue through a slightly different lens, which she calls the "windshield wiper" approach to qualifications. Shaw proposes that private and public dispute resolution can coexist, with the key variable being the degree of choice a consumer exercises over the nature of the dispute resolution process, the program, and the neutral third party.

> On one side of the windshield, there's complete free choice; in that situation, SPIDR takes the position that there ought to be a complete free market. On the other side of the windshield, when a disputant has no choice . . . there ought to be mandatory qualifications standards. (Shaw, quoted in Bureau of National Affairs, 1989b, p. 303)

Although one might expect an organization called the "Society of Professionals in Dispute Resolution" to take an exclusionary stance, in its 1989 report the SPIDR Commission on Qualifications kept the doors to the profession wide open. It acknowledged that knowledge gained while acquiring degrees could be useful, but concluded:

> At this time and for the foreseeable future, no such degree in itself ensures competence as a neutral [third party]. Furthermore, requiring a degree would foreclose alternative avenues of demonstrating dispute resolution competence. Consequently, no degree should be considered a prerequisite for service as a neutral. (SPIDR, 1989, p. 4)

In drafting its 1989 report, "Principles Concerning Qualifications," the commission stayed within SPIDR's tradition of using experience as a criterion for membership, and at the same time was extremely sensitive to the diversity of SPIDR's membership, which by then included many community mediators philosophically committed to open admissions. The Academy of Family Mediators followed suit. In the spring of 1990, the board of this 9-year-old group decided to change membership requirements. Greater diversity of membership will be encouraged, the Academy determined, by giving weight to "integrated, [high-]quality mediation training as an alternative to the previously required academic degrees or academy-approved training. Voluntary certification will be explored" (Bureau of National Affairs, 1990, p. 166).

STATEWIDE ASSOCIATIONS OF MEDIATION PROGRAMS

Since credentialing is occurring, whether one is an activist for a point of view or merely a silent observer, how can community mediation programs make their influence felt? Through their involvement in such associations as

SPIDR, they already have. Moreover, some statewide associations are being formed—New York, Massachusetts, North Carolina, Colorado, Pennsylvania, and California offer early examples. In 1982, the Colorado Council of Mediation Organizations pre-empted the legislature by developing standards of its own prior to the legislature's intervention (Colorado Council of Mediation Organizations, 1982). In New York, the state association and the court system, which is the primary funder of community mediation, worked collaboratively to develop standards relative to domestic violence and mediation (State of New York Unified Court System, 1983).

Organization at the statewide level is critical. Depending upon the degree and complexity of ADR activity in a particular state, it may become necessary for community mediation programs to define minimal community mediation certification collaboratively, before it is done by others, or the doors to practice are closed altogether. Although the thought of establishing credentials may be frightening, the reality may be less so. I like to use the analogy of the Red Cross lifesaving certificate, which has national validity, but is granted at the local level. As members of society, we want our lifesavers trained in a most practical sense. When a person is drowning, we want the lifesaver to demonstrate the ability to jump in the water, swim to the person in distress, rescue and bring the person ashore, and (if necessary) clear the lungs of water and administer cardiopulmonary resuscitation. It matters not if the rescuer has earned a PhD in aquatic science, marine history, or medicine. So it is with our community mediators. Over the years, experience has proven that volunteers from all walks of life can participate in relatively brief training and then demonstrate the ability to offer practical assistance to those drowning in conflict. This concept is in keeping with that urged by the SPIDR Commission on Qualifications, which recommends that "any requirements concerning who can practice as a neutral should be based upon performance . . . not the education or other method by which an individual acquired the knowledge or skills" (SPIDR, 1989, p. 4).

Statewide or regional organizations provide additional benefits that can reinforce community mediation's reputation for good service as well as its actual quality. First of all, these formal or informal networks allow mediators to pool information, perceptions, and ideas. As the preceding section suggests, staying on top of legislative developments is essential. Second, once networks are established, collaborative activities can be undertaken for mutual gain. For example, most statewide associations hold annual or periodic conferences for purposes of skill building, issue discussion, and public education. The Massachusetts Association of Mediation Programs, in cooperation with the state's District Court Department, has held two trainers' institutes designed to enhance the ability of local programs to conduct their own training and to encourage cross-fertilization. The North Carolina Mediation Network acts as a subgrantor to local programs for Interest on Lawyers Trust Accounts (IOLTA) funds. In New York, the state association, capitalizing upon its network of over 40 local centers, sought and obtained a contract from a state agency to mediate conflicts relating to mobile homes. Another contract was awarded to the association by the New York City Department of Education to provide conflict resolution training on a system-wide basis. In some geographic areas, statewide groups work together to sponsor regional events. For example, in 1990, the newly formed Arizona Coalition on Dispute Resolution, the Colorado Council of Mediation Organizations, and the New Mexico Mediation Association pooled their expertise to present the Southwest Conference on Peacemaking and Dispute Resolution with a focus on multiculturalism.

IS A NATIONAL APPROACH NEEDED?

Should community mediation programs form a national alliance? That is a pregnant question. An early attempt to unite the community field, spearheaded by the San Francisco Community Boards, resulted in the formation of the National Association for Community Justice. Although this association grappled with start-up activities for a few years, it was never able to capture the attention or loyalty of local programs. In 1989, it died a quiet death (P. Wahrhaftig, personal communication, September 1, 1989).

Without its own organization, national leadership for community mediation falls by default to other groups, such as the ABA Standing Committee on Dispute Resolution (which for many years has provided technical assistance to new programs and served as the primary clearinghouse for information about mediation) or subcommittees of professional associations, such as SPIDR or the Academy of Family Mediators. The biennial gatherings sponsored by the National Conference for Peacemaking and Conflict Resolution certainly attract many community mediators; however, this conference not only has limited resources, but has a broader constituency and a more global mission than community justice.

In 1989, the National Institute for Dispute Resolution (NIDR), which in the past had called together "focus groups" of community mediators, instituted a 3-year community justice program. During 1989 and 1990, NIDR convened a meeting of a dozen or more community mediation leaders from all over the United States to address the question of the quality of services at the local level. The task force will publish a self-evaluation handbook for mediation programs, and plans are being made to provide technical assistance to community mediation programs on a regional basis (NIDR, 1988). Will the NIDR effort spur the development of a second national approach? Even in the best of times, it will be difficult for community programs to organize on a national basis. Their minimal budgets and small staffs make extensive travel, or even long-distance phone calls, prohibitive. However, the growing number of state associations, the severity of the issues facing the field, and the interest of foundations such as NIDR may signal that the time is ripe for the formation of a new national community mediation network.

A CALL FOR ADAPTATION TO CHANGING TIMES

"Trends are bottom up, fads top down," notes John Naisbitt, author of *Megatrends* (Naisbitt, 1982, p. 3). The grassroots appeal of community mediation has allowed it to survive, defying those who early on tagged it a fad and predicted its demise. Programs have been in operation long enough to have demonstrated many points—primarily that the mediation process works; that people from all backgrounds can be trained to mediate; and that when they are, they love it. But the grassroots nature of mediation is deceptive. The attraction to mediation still remains strongest among the providers of the service rather than the users. It is also important to remember that community mediation arose at a time when activism flourished in areas such as reform of the justice system, civil rights, feminism, community empowerment, self-help, voluntarism (Peace Corps, VISTA), and consensual problem solving. Many threads were woven together to form a new fabric. The federal government was willing to play a major role in supporting the growth of such efforts through grants backed by guidelines calling for community involvement and equitable representation.

In the 1990s the conditions and priorities have changed. The general population no longer looks to the federal government for support or innovation. Both the public and politicians are more conscious of fiscal limitations. Activism centers around such issues as AIDS, drugs, homelessness, the balance of trade, and threats to the environment. If community mediation is to flourish, it must find its place in this new era. In a fiscally austere period where every expenditure must be justified on the basis of cost-effectiveness—a measure not known for its subtlety or ability to incorporate long-range savings—community mediation must prove both the quality of its service and its reason for being. It is not enough to say, "Support us because we love doing this!" The field must re-examine, reshape, and then market itself so that funders and referral sources understand its value and users can make intelligent choices about their options.

THE POTENTIAL OF COMMUNITY MEDIATION

What is the potential of community mediation? A thoughtfully designed program can meet many needs. First and foremost, it can build a flexible, responsive, community-based problem-solving capacity. The component skills of mediation have infinite applications, as most local programs have discovered. Programs that started with a single focus—perhaps mediating small claims or handling criminal cases in court—may use their skills to develop curricula for elementary or secondary students, to handle conflicts between the elderly and nursing homes, or to facilitate public policy disputes. For a relatively small investment, a community can enjoy a service that can accommodate itself to ever-changing needs.

Second, if a program takes conscious steps to reflect the population it serves, it can capitalize upon its diversity, which is an invaluable resource. Regardless of one's background, mediation training provides a level playing field where the significance of age, race, gender, ethnicity, academic and professional background, or economic means fades while other qualities emerge. When people from various backgrounds participate in the same training experience, some powerful outcomes occur. The quality of the training is enhanced, for the sum is greater than its parts when each participant can contribute to and learn from the collective wisdom. Many of the barriers that traditionally separate people from one another are lessened, and a unique form of bridge building and bonding takes place. Each mediator can be a link with other resources—schools, churches, social clubs, social service agencies, and so on. This remarkable collective capacity can be used to address garden-variety disputes as well as those difficult community conflicts that center around differing values.

Community mediation programs can be the standard-bearers for the entire field of mediation. Local centers, provided that they enjoy adequate support, are in a position to monitor and improve the quality of their services in a way that is difficult for solo practitioners, small firms, or even government agencies employing full-time mediators. Opportunities for supervision of the mediators by staff and evaluation by clients are readily available. Co-mediation, which is used in many programs, provides mediators with the chance to learn from one another and to reflect upon their own and others' skills. Burnout, the inevitable "I've seen this case a thousand times" syndrome, which often develops for full-time practitioners, is usually not an issue for volunteers, who may mediate once or twice a month. (It is an issue for some high-volume community programs that use the same "volunteers" day after day.) Education committees can conduct ongoing analysis of the needs of clients and volunteers, and can use that knowledge to reshape basic training and design continuing education programs for the experienced. Because so many community mediation programs serve as the training ground for colleges and universities, the expertise of each institution can be tapped to the benefit of all.

Finally, the vast majority of referrals to community mediation programs come from the courts (State of New York Unified Court System, 1989, pp. 60–61). If mediators are well trained, and the process they use honors the disputing parties' rights and competence, the infusion of laypeople into the justice system can soften its harsh edges, in much the same way that a jury of one's peers softens the application of the law to the individual. This concept is controversial, for an argument can be made that the closer community mediation gets to the courts, the more it will become like them—bureaucratic, rule-bound, and rigid. Although eternal vigilance is required to avoid the natural tendency of an organization to take on the goals and qualities of its referring or funding agencies, the potential of community mediation to improve the administration of justice still holds promise.

ENSURING QUALITY AT THE LOCAL LEVEL

If the community mediation movement is to flourish, each program must take responsibility for ensuring the quality of its own services. Several activities are essential.

Programs must be structured in a way that encourages continuous re-evaluation of the philosophy, assumptions, goals, models, applications, and outcomes of the service. This dialogue should involve all the key players—users, mediators, staff members, board members, agencies making referrals to mediation, agencies to which referrals for service are made, funders, evaluators, legislators, and so on. Periodically, fundamental questions should be asked, such as the following: What is our philosophy? Are the conditions that led us to develop a particular goal, approach, or model still in place? What new factors have arisen that may test the limits of our current ways? What are the short- and long-range outcomes of the services we provide? This whole-system approach toward mediation allows a program to fine-tune or even overhaul itself, in order to address critical issues. As mentioned earlier, contemporary mediation grew out of the labor field, where repeat players came to the table with a list of demands and usually knew the rules of the game. The ethical considerations of a labor case are not identical to those faced in a parent–child mediation, where parties are new to the process and unsure of the stakes, and where power issues abound. Many troubling issues are facing local programs: How should domestic violence cases be treated? Should fee-for-service options be explored? Can a program use both volunteers and paid mediators? Each time a new issue or a new application for mediation is encountered, fresh thinking must occur.

Program diversity is an asset that must be nurtured. Unfortunately, many programs do not make diversity a priority. Research has shown that mediator panels tend "to reflect the personal characteristics of agency administrators" who "have held the doors open slightly wider for people like themselves" (Pipkin & Rifkin, 1984, p. 221). (It is important to note here that all the forces in society that lead to gender, race, ethnic, and class stratification of our institutions are at play in the field of mediation. This negative trend should be of major concern to leaders at the local, state, national, and international levels.) Programs that do articulate diversity as a priority often fail to compose themselves initially in a way that supports that goal. As a consequence, a primarily white, middle-class "we" tries in vain to attract "the other"—a hopeless dynamic. Ideally, a program committed to diversity would begin with an integrated organizing core and prepare itself for continous growth and change. If such is not the case, an existing program will have to make diversity a top priority and do considerable soul searching to see why it has evolved so narrowly. A series of actions will be needed to bring about the desired change. The board or controlling group must be integrated. Recruitment of volunteers must follow affirmative action practices. Outreach to the appropriate communities must be tireless. All procedures and qualifications must be examined to make sure that they are inclusive rather than artificially restrictive. In the end, such a program must be prepared to re-examine and reshape everything about itself, including its basic philosophy.

A sound relationship with volunteer mediators is central to the success of a program. Roles, relationships, and responsibilities must be clarified from the beginning. At the recruitment stage, a program should clearly explain its methods and procedures for selection, and should express its commitment to help each trainee successfully complete the training. At the same time, it should also clarify that not everyone is suited for the role. When I train mediators, I use the analogy of a person eager to become an emergency medical technician, who may come to all classes, do all required homework, show growth in skill development, but nevertheless faint at the sight of blood. If the response cannot be modified, the person, no matter how sincere his or her intentions, will not be useful in the technician's role. In the case of mediation, fainting at the sight of blood will (we hope) not be the issue, but an inability to suspend one's own judgment or a tendency to panic at strong emotions may be.

Program directors should also provide realistic assessments of the opportunities for new volunteers to mediate. A study of volunteers in New York State confirmed that the biggest reason why mediators leave programs is that they feel underutilized (Rogers et al., 1989, p. 5). The authors of the study made several recommendations for improving mediator morale and commitment to the parent agency (Rogers et al., 1989, pp. 7–8), which are summarized here:

• Alert new and old mediators to the potential for underutilization, fluctuations in caseload, and the "no-show" problem (parties failing to show up for a scheduled mediation). Engage volunteers in joint problem-solving around these issues.

• Be more creative about using volunteers. For example, volunteers may conduct intake, do follow-up, confront "no-show" rates, conduct outreach, or write newsletters.

• Give volunteers recognition for mediation *and* other forms of service.

• Design methods for periodic feedback about volunteers' performance and skill development. Do not solve a problem of poor performance by merely not requesting a particular volunteer's services again!

• Keep an updated roster of volunteers indicating who is active, who is on leave, and who is eligible for or interested in particular kinds of cases.

• Provide an environment that encourages communication among mediators. For example, make sure the space where mediation occurs is comfortable, and schedule mediations so that several mediators can have contact with one another at the same time.

I would add that volunteers need to know what is expected of them after they complete their initial basic training. Many programs require an apprenticeship period, during which time a trainee will mediate with a more experienced mediator. Several program directors in Massachusetts have reported to me that their more experienced mediators can "go stale" and teach new mediators bad habits. Or a more experienced mediator who is not committed to the growth of a novice can dominate a session to such an extent that the novice's confidence is actually lowered rather than raised. If this apprenticeship model is used, programs must prepare experienced mediators for the role.

Ongoing education is essential for all mediators, and I believe it should be viewed as a requirement for continued membership as an active mediator. The number of issues to be addressed is endless, from the basics (e.g., confidentiality, listening skills, and writing agreements) to new applications (e.g., landlord–tenant problems, small claims, and parent–child difficulties). Programs would be wise to create a variety of ways to meet continuing education requirements. Certainly, credit should be given for classes taken at local educational institutions. On a more informal basis, several volunteers can conduct a role play in one of their homes. A volunteer who helps with intake can receive credit for teaching another volunteer the required skills. If programs network on a regional basis, some of the responsibility for organizing continuing education can be shared with other organizations. Such cross-program activities can be highly energizing. The idea of continuing education is not to ensure that everyone has an identical experience, but to keep each volunteer in a growth trajectory.

A mediation program's introductory training is the building block upon which all other features of program quality rest. It is at this time that the philosophy of the program is conveyed, a mediator's attitude about his or her role in relation to the parties is shaped, and the requisite skills and knowledge of process are developed. My strong bias is toward the "thinking mediator"; that is, I like to emphasize the philosophy behind mediation, the assumptions it embodies, the ethics it requires, and the reasoning behind each aspect of the process. Tactics flow from the application of these principles to the actual situation at hand. I find that this approach encourages trainees to question my assumptions, analyze and even challenge my interventions, and invent their own, rather than mimic what I do. They can also decide whether mediation is an appropriate forum in a particular case.

I have other biases as well, and I put them forward to spark discussion. The initial training must be well thought out. I suggest the use of a culturally diverse training team, which tailors the training to the goals of the program and the needs, talents, and expertise of those being trained. Learning styles vary, and so should the methods of presenting information and honing skills. A good training program should include a balance of presentations by trainers, full-group and small-group discussions, opportunities to experiment, one-on-one critiques, and complementary video or print materials.

Time on task is important. The simulated mediation is the central focus of most mediation training, for good reason. An effective mediator must integrate numerous skills simultaneously in response to an ever-changing set of dynamics. Exercising a skill out of context is not the same as calling upon it during mediation. The role play is the best substitute for the real thing. In fact, because the trainer may interrupt a simulation in order to make a timely point or re-enact various options, the role play may be superior to the real thing for entry-level training. The experience of playing a disputant or being an active observer is as valuable as playing the role of mediator. There is nothing as informative to a trainee as playing a disputant and sensing personally how a mediator may open a party up with an appropriate word, or shut a person down with a subtle glance. In the observer role, a trainee can watch the interaction of all parties with a certain analytical distance. The trainer should spend time at the beginning of a training program to explain the roles of mediator, parties, observer, and coach. It is worth the investment.

From experience, I have concluded that 30 hours of training is not enough; 40 to 50 hours makes more sense. I recommend that each trainee mediate at least three times (and participate in nine simulations). The first time is needed to overcome the tension of learning a new skill and displaying it before others. The second time provides an opportunity to spot strengths and areas where improvement is needed. By the third time, the training team should be able to make a judgment about the participant's ability to enter an apprenticeship or supervised phase. Four or more opportunities to mediate might be even better, but at a certain point the law of diminishing returns applies and the best course of action is to begin actual mediations under supervision.

The evaluation process leading to judgments about mediator readiness should be spelled out in advance. Early on, it is useful to provide trainees with a list of the skills by which they will be judged. At the same time, a mutual commitment between the trainers and participants should be developed. Trainers should promise to speak to individuals if they have particular concerns about their performance to date and to make remedial suggestions for improvement. Similarly, a participant who is experiencing difficulty is responsible for notifying a trainer, so that special assistance can be provided if necessary.

The ideal ratio of trainers to trainees is 1:6. This allows for highly individualized critiquing of each participant and ample opportunity for all questions to be addressed. Toward the end of the course, the members of the training team should pool their perceptions to make an assessment of each trainee. Individualized written evaluations with suggestions for follow-up learning are highly desirable. Usually, most persons will be moving nicely in the right direction. Some may need additional guidance but show enough promise to warrant a further investment of program time. Not infrequently, however, one or two persons will not show promise. It is vital at this juncture that programs deal with this observation straightforwardly. It is unfair, unkind, and (I believe) unethical to ignore this judgment, graduate such persons, and either never use their services or use them in the awareness that they are not suitable for the task. As painful as it may be, trainers should meet with these trainees, explain the reasons behind their analysis, indicate the ways in which they have already tried to address the shortcomings, and spell out the consequences. Other roles with the program may be available. Opportunities to observe mediation could be offered, along with a chance to try out for a future training program. Or the relationship may simply need to be ended. I am not downplaying the difficulty of these discussions. During the first and second trainers' institutes held by the Massachusetts Association of Mediation Programs and the District Court Department, mock "terminal interviews" were held. The decision was unanimous that program directors and trainers need much more practice in this delicate art form.

A special set of problems arises for new programs, especially when everyone is a novice and there is no internal training capacity. If an outside trainer is hired, several factors should be taken into consideration. The ratio of trainers to trainees should be thought through and agreed upon in advance, as should the trainer's role in evaluation. If the trainer does not offer evaluation services, the program should postpone credentialing until it can develop a sound method for doing so. If possible, the contract should include follow-up consulting and a method for continuing education. In states where mediation is established, assistance is often available from neighboring programs.

AN EDUCATED CONSTITUENCY:
THE BEST GUARANTEE OF QUALITY

It is easy to become overenthusiastic about mediation and promote it as the answer to all conflict. This is a mistake. It has led to what I consider some of the excesses of the field—mandatory mediation, penalties for those who do not mediate in good faith, the promotion of quantity at the cost of quality, and failure to acknowledge the need for advocacy. The appropriateness of mediation for certain conflicts is still a matter of open debate. As eager as mediators are to expand the field, they should exercise some restraint. Public education about mediation must be approached as a dialogue in which users, referral sources, funders, sponsoring agencies, the community at large, special-interest groups, the media, and legislative bodies all have a voice. The actual long-range outcomes of mediation must become part of this dialogue.

CONCLUSION

The debate about credentialing is a lively one. I have expressed my own views on the issue as candidly as possible, but I would be remiss if I did not confess that my thoughts are in flux, for "the times they are a-changing." As I have mentioned at the beginning of this chapter, my own attraction to mediation has to do with its respectful nature. It assumes that people are competent. By that, I mean that mediation encourages people to be the experts in the resolution of their own disputes. Mary Parker Follett, a pioneer in the field of creative conflict resolution, wrote about the dynamic tension between "the expert" and "the people":

> I wish we could understand the word expert as expressing an attitude of mind which we can all acquire, rather than the collecting of information by a special caste. . . . The training of the citizen must include both how to form opinion on expert testimony and how to watch one's own experience and draw conclusions from it. (Follett, 1924, p. 29)

Although I applaud the efforts of those who mediate to become "expert" at their craft, and I fully understand the excitement that mediation holds as a career, I feel obliged to offer some cautions. As the profession of mediation grows, what will happen to community mediation? Teachers, practitioners, and advocates of ADR must not lose sight of community mediation's contributions to the field and its empowering potential. Those of us who are genuinely concerned about the quality of mediation services must avoid the easy route of exclusivity, lest we become that special caste Follett warned us against. Instead, let us use our considerable problem-solving skills to promote quality creatively, while leaving the doors open for diversity.

REFERENCES

Auerbauch, J. S. (1983). *Justice without laws: Resolving disputes without lawyers*. New York: Oxford University Press.

Brodigan, B., Sideris, N., Price, J., Murtagh, L., & Steele, J. (Eds.). (1988). *State legislation on dispute resolution.* Washington, DC: American Bar Association, Standing Committee on Dispute Resolution.

Bureau of National Affairs. (1988a). Professional qualification: Consumers should qualify dispute resolvers, Community Boards chief response to Nicolau. *Alternative Dispute Resolution Report, 2*(20), 349–351.

Bureau of National Affairs. (1988b). Professional qualifications: Florida explains court rules, in face of continuing controversy. *Alternative Dispute Resolution Report, 2*(25), 434–435.

Bureau of National Affairs. (1989a). Court-adjunct ADR: Alternative dispute resolution bill signed by Oregon governor. *Alternative Dispute Resolution Report, 3*(17), 285.

Bureau of National Affairs. (1989b). Family disputes: Family mediators' academy considers qualifications, new directions. *Alternative Dispute Resolution Report, 3*(1), 303–305.

Bureau of National Affairs. (1989c). Farmer–lender mediation: FMHA tells Congress loan mediation in state programs is cost effective. *Alternative Dispute Resolution Report, 3*(26), 436–438.

Bureau of National Affairs. (1989d). New laws and bills. *Alternative Dispute Resolution Report, 3*(19), 324.

Bureau of National Affairs. (1990). Family mediators' academy moves toward skill based certification. *Alternative Dispute Resolution Report, 4*, 166.

Colorado Council of Mediation Organizations. (1982). *Code of professional conduct for mediators.* Denver: Author.

Davis, A. M. (1986). *Community mediation in Massachusetts: A decade of development, 1975–1985.* Salem: District Court Department, Commonwealth of Massachusetts.

Division of Consumer Services, Legal Services Unit, State of California. (1987). *Proposed guidelines for local dispute resolution programs.* Sacramento: Author.

Education Relations Commission. (1983). *The bargaining process and mediation.* Toronto: Author.

Follett, M. P. (1924). *Creative experience.* New York: Peter Smith.

Freedman, L. (Ed.). (1984). *Legislation on dispute resolution.* Washington, DC: American Bar Association, Special Committee on Dispute Resolution.

Goldberg, S. B., Green, E. D., & Sander, F. E. (1985). *Dispute resolution.* Boston: Little, Brown.

Massachusetts Mediation Service. (1988). *Massachusetts Mediation Service: Annual report, July 1987–June 1988.* Boston: Commonwealth of Massachusetts.

McGillis, D. (1986). *Community dispute resolution programs and public policy.* Washington, DC: National Institute of Justice.

Naisbitt, J. (1982). *Megatrends: Ten new directions transforming our lives.* New York: Warner Books.

National Institute for Dispute Resolution (NIDR). (1988). The status of community justice. *Dispute Resolution Forum,* p. 2.

Nicolau, G. (1975). *Community mediator training manual for the mediation unit of the Dorchester District Court.* Dorchester, MA: Urban Court Program.

Nicolau, G. (1986). Community mediation: Progress and problems. *Viewpoint on Mediation, 1*(3), 3.

Oregon Revised Statutes (1989). Sec. 36.155(1)(b).

Pipkin, R. M., & Rifkin, J. (1984). The social organization in alternative dispute resolution: Implications for professionalization of mediation. *Justice System Journal, 2*, 204–227.

Rogers, S. J., Kanrich, S., & Steinhauser, I. (1989). *Understanding our criminal justice volunteers: A study of community mediators in New York State*. New York: Brooklyn Mediation Center.

Society for Professionals in Dispute Resolution (SPIDR). (1989) *Principles concerning qualifications*. Washington, DC: Author.

State Justice Institute. (1989). Information about SJI grant programs to improve the administration of justice in the state courts. *SJI News, 1*(1), 1–8.

State of New York Unified Court System. (1983). *The Community Dispute Resolution Centers Program: Annual report, April 1, 1982 to March 31, 1983*. New York: Author.

State of New York Unified Court System. (1989). *The Community Dispute Resolution Centers Program: Annual report, April 1, 1988 to March 31, 1989*. Albany, New York: Author.

Wilensky, H. L. (1964). The professionalization of everyone? *American Journal of Sociology, 70*, 137.

14

Mediation and Psychotherapy: Parallel Processes

SAMUEL G. FORLENZA
Family Mediation Program,
Superior Court of New Jersey, Newark

Mediation as an alternative to the traditional adversarial system of conflict resolution continues to grow and gain national acceptance (Folberg & Taylor, 1984). Mediators, both volunteer and nonvolunteer, have come from diverse backgrounds. Professional family mediators have come predominantly from the legal or mental health fields (Girdner, 1986). Increasingly, mental health professionals, including psychologists, marriage and family therapists, social workers, and counselors, are working in the interdisciplinary field of mediation in either a paid or a voluntary capacity. They are frequently part of community mediation programs.

This chapter examines the parallel processes of mediation and psychotherapy or counseling. It looks at the convergence and divergence of these two parallel processes. For the present purposes, no distinction is made among "psychotherapy," "counseling," and "therapy," the three terms are used interchangeably. It is useful to note that the current discussion is written from the perspective of a family mediator. Although the material presented reflects this framework, it can easily be seen to have wider application beyond family disputes.

Mediation and psychotherapy have been compared by a number of authors (Brown, 1988; Folberg & Taylor, 1984; Gold, 1985; Grebe, 1986; Kelly, 1983; Milne, 1985) and have been found to be parallel processes in several dimensions. Although mediation is often found to be therapeutic, it is not to be confused with therapy. A clear distinction between the two interventions is essential for effective service delivery. This is particularly true for mediators with a mental health orientation or for therapists who have expanded their practice to include mediation. Without a clear understanding of each process, already blurred boundaries may dissolve. This is probably most apparent with such interpersonal conflicts as parent–child,

The views expressed in this chapter are my own and do not necessarily reflect those of the New Jersey judiciary.

227

custody, and divorce disputes. At times, the two processes may seem indistinguishable.

The task for the mental health professional is to integrate his or her background, skills, and training as a therapist into the process of mediation without losing sight of the separate goal of mediation. Once mediation becomes just another form of therapeutic treatment, the clinician/mediator is defeated. When the clinically trained mediator focuses primarily on the therapeutic elements and on offering therapeutic services at the expense of the issues in conflict, then the therapist/mediator is no longer acting as a mediator.

Mediation and therapy can be compared at different points on several distinct continuums (Brown, 1988; Folberg & Taylor, 1984; Gold, 1985; Kelly, Zlatchin, & Shawn, 1985; Kelly, 1983; Milne, 1985). Before I proceed any further I must briefly define the two interventions as discussed here. "Mediation" can be defined as the process of intervening between conflicting parties to resolve their dispute. The process utilizes a neutral third party (sometimes more than one) to facilitate communication between the disputants, to assist them in defining the issues in dispute, to help them develop options and alternatives, and to reach a consensual resolution that is satisfactory and agreeable to all involved (Folberg & Taylor, 1984; Kelly, 1983; Milne, 1985). Mediation as a problem-solving intervention is both goal-directed and issue-oriented. The goals of mediation are the resolution of a dispute and the development of an agreement, frequently in the form of a written document. According to the setting, this document may be referred to as a "consent order," a "consent agreement," or a "memorandum of understanding."

"Psychotherapy" is a specialized interpersonal helping relationship characterized by psychological interventions designed to modify personality and behavior. It is concerned with improved human functioning, psychological health, and general well-being. Therapy focuses on the person or persons and has as its goal cognitive, behavioral, and/or affective change (Strupp, 1978, 1986).

Since there are numerous models or approaches to mediation, and even more therapeutic paradigms, it is impossible to demonstrate all the various distinguishing characteristics. The present comparison addresses major distinctions, although I realize that there may be exceptions with differing approaches to either mediation or therapy. Guided by a table of comparison (see Table 14.1), this chapter systematically examines each element as utilized in each intervention. This examination is followed by several sections that address issues of role conflict and client expectations; role stress; and cautions and ethical considerations. The entire discussion closes with a summary of the parallel processes of therapy and mediation.

TABLE 14.1. Points of Comparison in Mediation and Psychotherapy

Element	Mediation	Psychotherapy
Primary focus	Problem/issue	Person/relationship
Time frame	Short-term	Short- or long-term
Structure	Mediator-led process	Client-led process
Role of the interventionist	Active role	Active or passive role
Role of the emotions	Contained/directed	Explored/encouraged
Client–interventionist relationship	Secondary	Primary
Time orientation	Present and future (nonhistorical)	Past and present (historical)
Therapeutic focus	Secondary to process	Primary to process
Background data	Less availability	Greater availability
Process constraints	Greater	Lesser
Therapeutic techniques	Utilized secondarily	Utilized primarily
Nature of the process	Legal or quasi-legal event	Psychological/personal event
Confidentiality	Critical to process	Critical to process

GENERAL COMPARISON OF MEDIATION AND PSYCHOTHERAPY

Primary Focus

There is an essential distinction in the primary focus of mediation and psychotherapy. Although they are both human, helping relationships, psychotherapy, as noted above, is a specialized interpersonal helping relationship designed to facilitate cognitive, affective, and/or behavioral changes (Strupp, 1978, 1986); mediation is a problem- or issue-oriented intervention whose goal is the resolution of a dispute and the development of an agreement (Kelly, 1983; Milne, 1985). Unlike therapy, mediation is not a treatment modality. Certainly, both focus on the participants, whether they are called "clients" or "patients," or if they are individuals, couples, or families, but the primary focus of each intervention is quite distinct.

Time Frame

On a time frame continuum, consisting of very brief interventions at one end and indefinite or unlimited time at the other, mediation is found at the time-limited end. Therapy may be located at almost any point on the continuum. It may be of very short duration, as in some behavioral approaches, or may extend indefinitely, as in psychoanalysis.

Mediation is generally a short-term process that may be limited to as few as one to three sessions. Its time frame more closely resembles that of brief term psychotherapy. The length of time permitted for the therapeutic process may vary according to the approach taken and the problem addressed. In mediation it may vary, but generally only within this brief framework. In both processes, the parties may return in the future to resolve any new conflicts that develop.

Structure

There are critical distinctions in the structure of the two processes. Therapy is primarily a client-led process, whereas the mediator leads and directs (sometimes quite forcefully) the process of mediation.

Typically, therapy is a more open, loosely structured, and fluid process. When compared to mediation, it allows for much greater flexibility on the part of all the participants. In treatment, issues or feelings may be addressed repeatedly and at any time the client desires. Mediation, as a contained, step-by-step process (Folberg & Taylor, 1984), attempts to control the discussion of feelings and is more likely to take the participants through stages. Issues may be addressed systematically, beginning with the most easily resolved matters and proceeding to the most strongly contested issues (Fisher & Ury, 1981). Mediation is a structured, task-focused process of dispute resolution. Therapy, as an interpersonal investigation, may explore and proceed with considerable freedom and may simply be guided by the patient's unconscious.

Role of the Interventionist

The role of the interventionist or facilitator may vary according to the model of mediation or the therapeutic modality. Most often, however, mediators will be more active, directive, and involved in attending to the task, while therapists will be less active and will attend more to feelings. The mediator's role most closely resembles that of the therapist in certain behavioral (Milner, 1985) or strategic therapies (Grebe, 1986), which are more directive interventions (Haley, 1976; Hansen & L'Abate, 1982). The mediator is a conflict manager and resolution facilitator. The psychotherapist and the mediator both encourage the parties to be in control of the process.

Role of Emotions

The affective domain is critical to both processes but is viewed quite differently in each. Most, if not all, counseling paradigms consider the therapeutic release of emotions ("catharsis") as a significant component of the curative process. Clinicians encourage the exploration of emotions and emotional issues as a method for understanding and resolving psychological conflicts. This in-depth examination of feelings is thought to facilitate emotional growth (Gilliland, James, Roberts, & Bowman, 1984). This is not the task or the desire of mediation.

Feelings are controlled and directed in mediation. The criterion is the furthering of the dispute resolution. If the expression of emotions can be channeled to facilitate this process, such expression is then considered useful and productive. Effective mediation views ventilation to have a significant but more limited role. In contrast to psychotherapy, conflict management does not and cannot permit this free and unrestricted exploration. Although feelings cannot be ignored, their containment and redirection seem to be most useful in promoting agreement (Folberg & Taylor, 1984; Forlenza, 1988), which of course is the goal of mediation.

Client–Interventionist Relationship

The relationship between the client and the interventionist is an essential ingredient in both mediation and therapy, but in each it is approached from a different perspective. Traditional psychotherapeutic paradigms—that is, psychodynamic or psychoanalytically oriented therapies—consider the patient–therapist relationship ("transference") to be at the core of the process (Prochaska, 1984).

Mediation, as a more task-oriented intervention, does not focus on the client–mediator relationship in the same manner. Maintaining a positive relationship; remaining acceptable to all parties; listening empathically; demonstrating warmth, caring, and genuineness; and showing a sincere interest are all vital to the process of mediation. Mediation differs from therapy in that the relationship between the mediator and the parties is not exhaustively studied and analyzed. It is more important for the mediator to secure the faith and confidence of the disputants—for the disputants to perceive the mediator as a competent helper who can assist them in resolving their conflict.

Time Orientation

There is a major distinction in the time orientations of these two interventions. Mediation is a present- and future-oriented process, unlike psychotherapy, which is primarily a past- and present-oriented modality.

Mediation is a nonhistorical approach. The dispute resolution process does not dwell on the history of the conflict, but rather looks to see what may be done in the present to change future events. Mediation is concerned with the past to the extent that such a focus may aid the parties to develop a workable solution. A detailed examination of the past, although considered desirable and beneficial in therapy, is discouraged in mediation (Kelly, 1983). Rather, clients are urged to build on the present and work toward a more productive future.

Typically, therapy takes a historical approach; it examines past events to determine how they are related to and have affected the present. The belief is that all ongoing psychological problems have their basis in the past. It is thought that unless the past is understood, current symptoms will reappear later (Milne, 1985). By contrast, mediators maintain a future orientation (Kelly, 1983), which discourages the parties from dwelling on the background and history of their conflict. This approach is designed to minimize fault finding, blaming, and any tangential recounting of the events that have led to the current dispute.

Therapeutic Focus

Although both mediation and psychotherapy may be therapeutic to the participants, only psychotherapy has that as its explicit goal. Psychotherapy by its very nature is intended to be therapeutic; mediation is not (Folberg & Taylor, 1984; Kelly et al., 1985). According to the model of mediation, varying degrees of emphasis may be placed on therapeutic benefits (Brown, 1985; Kressel, 1985). However, any therapeutic advantages are clearly secondary to the process. It is useful to remember that a conflict may be successfully mediated without any concomitant significant therapeutic change.

The goal of psychotherapy is to achieve a therapeutic effect. For therapy to be considered successful, it must achieve some level of therapeutic change. It must produce improved mental, emotional, and/or psychological functioning in the client. Usually there will be some change in cognition, affect, or behavior (or possibly some combination).

The clinically trained mediator will want to maintain a realistic view of mediation and to recognize that as a short-term intervention it is not designed to offer the potential benefits that long-term psychotherapy may achieve. As noted earlier, mediation, in several respects resembles certain short-term behavioral approaches. Both are often time- and goal-limited; both maintain a sharp focus; and both involve a highly active and directive interventionist.

Background Data

Background data, or information regarding the parties and a history of their problems, are addressed from a different perspective in each intervention.

In counseling or therapy, the clinician generally has background information on the client (Saposnek, 1983). The therapist may have access to psychological test scores or may administer such tests to obtain further data about the client and the client's problem. These data may provide the psychotherapist with certain insights and clues regarding the client and his or her problem. The clinician has information from which to formulate tentative hypotheses, strategies, and treatment plans.

Mediators typically work with a minimum of information about the disputants and their conflict. Little more than the parties' names may be known until the disputants are seen. This lack of knowledge may force the mediator to attempt quickly to gather pertinent data about the parties, as well as about their conflict. The mediator lacks a context for the dispute. In a relatively brief period, the mediator must collect the data, develop a hypothesis, and formulate strategies without alienating the disputants or losing neutrality. It seems that therapists have an advantage over mediators in this regard. They do not have the pressures to accomplish so much in so little time.

It may be argued that this lack of information ensures mediator neutrality (Haynes, 1981). Familiarity with the case background or intake information may result in mediator bias. However, it seems to be of greater benefit to have sufficient background data with which to formulate a basic hypothesis and an initial framework for the dispute. These data provide structure and direction to the mediation, which can be modified and adapted as the process continues (Kressel, Forlenza, Butler, & Wilcox, 1988).

Process Constraints

Mediation and psychotherapy are both challenging tasks, but there appear to be greater constraints and pressures in the alternative dispute resolution process. Mediators have a more expanded role and are expected to attend to more disparate elements. They are concerned about staying within time limitations, monitoring emotions, identifying issues, and developing a resolution, all while still trying to maintain their acceptability to the parties. No small task!

Although therapy may be more constrained by internal or intrapsychic pressures, mediation seems to be subject to greater external pressures. Such constraints may derive from the pressure to obtain a settlement, also known as "settlement mania" (Kressel et al., 1988). In an attempt to justify their work, to improve statistics, or to assure funding or the future of their programs, mediators may feel driven to produce settlements that clearly demonstrate the efficacy of their intervention.

Therapeutic Techniques

Whether in the context of mediation or of psychotherapy, therapeutic techniques and strategies are useful tools for conflict resolution. This is another element that the two processes share.

The mental health professional has a repertoire of interventions that can be utilized in mediation (Gold, 1985). With the wide range of therapeutic modalities come a number of different techniques and strategies that can be transferred from psychotherapy to mediation. The clinician's theoretical orientation (e.g., psychodynamic, behavioral, humanistic) and treatment modality (individual, group, family, marital) will influence which interventions he or she favors. The therapist/mediator will want to determine which clinical techniques work most productively with his or her style of mediation.

Some therapeutic techniques that can be utilized in the conflict resolution setting include clarification, validation and normalization of feelings, and reflective listening (Saposnek, 1983); relabeling and reframing (Grebe, 1986; Lam, Rifkin, & Townley, 1989); paradoxical techniques and the use of metaphors (Yale, 1988); and directives, both paradoxical and straightforward (Grebe, 1986).

The written agreement developed in mediation, sometimes referred to as a "memorandum of understanding," is similar to contracts used in behaviorally oriented therapies.

For effective mediation, it is essential to determine which therapeutic strategies lend themselves best to the mediation process.

Nature of the Processes

There is a significant distinction between the nature of therapy and that of mediation. Mediation may be viewed as a legal or quasi-legal event, particularly in court-connected or court-sponsored programs. It is a blend of both legal and personal concerns. Mediators may be accountable to judges or other outside authorities. Although mediation is frequently voluntarily entered into, it may be court-ordered or court-recommended. Often attorneys are or have been involved with the dispute. A lawyer may draw up the agreement document or may be consulted regarding it. The agreement may be included in a court order, which will then require a judge's signature. Successful mediation concludes with an agreement or memorandum of understanding between the parties, which is the objective of the process. This consensual agreement may be converted into a binding, written document sometimes known as a "consent agreement."

Therapy is primarily a psychological or personal event that is self-initiated (Herron & Rouslin, 1982). There may be instances when therapy is mandated by a court order, but more usually it is a psychological evaluation or assessment that is ordered. Therapists do not require the support of judges or attorneys and in their therapeutic work are seldom accountable to them (Saposnek, 1983). In psychotherapy, the focus is on emotional health and behavioral change. With few exceptions, such as the behavioral approach of contingency contracting (Hansen & L'Abate, 1982), most therapeutic paradigms do not utilize written agreements or documentation.

The Role of Confidentiality

Maintaining confidentiality is a critical element of both mediation and therapy. Confidentiality promotes honesty, an open exploration of the issues in question, and a greater acceptance of the interventionist.

The issue of confidentiality in mediation continues to be one of the most significant policy issues confronting the complementary dispute resolution field (Prigoff, 1988). In mediation, the confidentiality of the mediator–client relationship is legally protected in only a few states (Emery & Wyer, 1987). It has not gained the more widely accepted protection of the therapist–client or doctor–patient relationship. The ethical standards of both mediators and therapists specifically address the issue of confidentiality. (For more information on this subject, the reader is directed to the ethical standards of such organizations as the Academy of Family Mediators, the Society of Professionals in Dispute Resolution, the American Psychological Association, and the American Association for Marriage and Family Therapy.)

Since there is no uniformity in the protection of the mediator–client relationship, mediators need to be aware of any relevant rules and laws governing confidentiality in mediation. Is there information, such as knowledge of a crime or child abuse, that the mediator is legally obligated to report to the appropriate authorities?

Mediators, like therapists, have an ethical obligation to advise their clients of the limits of confidentiality and to obtain an informed consent. The mediator may be expected to make a report or recommendation to an outside agency or jurisdiction, based on information revealed in the mediation process. The record or contents of the mediation or the mediator's notes may be subject to subpoena. The court may require the mediator to give testimony regarding the dispute if the parties have not reached a resolution. In an unsuccessful mediation, the mediator may be required to conduct an investigation of the matter (Forlenza, 1988).

Until there is a consistent pattern of protection of confidentiality of mediator–client communications (Prigoff, 1988), the mediator may wish to obtain such written permission from the parties in the form of a "consent to mediate" document. This consent may also contain a statement that the parties agree not to subpoena the mediator, as well as any records or notes of the process. Saposnek (1983) offers examples of such forms used in child custody disputes.

ROLE CONFLICT AND CLIENT EXPECTATIONS

Mediators who are known primarily as mental health professionals may cause clients to have false expectations of the mediation process. This may be particularly true with highly conflicted interpersonal disputes, such as parent–child and child custody conflicts. The participants may enter the process believing they are coming for a range of therapeutic services, including family, marriage, or divorce counseling. Parties may believe or may wish to believe that they are attempting a marital reconciliation. For the clients, the distinction needs to be clearly established that mediation, though sharing common characteristics and techniques with other helping professions, is not designed to be therapy nor counseling nor any other such intervention.

ROLE STRESS

Mediation work has been acknowledged to be considerably more stressful than counseling or therapy (Gold, 1985). The mediator is constantly managing conflict. He or she attempts to contain emotions, to listen actively, to promote a rational approach, and to develop a resolution—all within a relatively brief time frame and within the constraints necessary for continued acceptance by the parties. The climate in a mediation session is typically more intense and hostile than in psychotherapy. While being rational and task focused, the mediator is in the center of the conflict, managing and at times absorbing the clients' angry and hostile feelings. This is done in order to keep the process moving. The affective component is ignored or minimized and is used primarily to advance an agreement. The mental health professional who is a mediator may find it difficult to ignore feelings without a very conscious effort. The transition from therapist to mediator requires some significant role shifts. It necessitates a major change in thinking and behavior, while still taking advantage of one's therapeutic skills. Essentially, it requires the therapist not to seek behavioral change, to resist the temptation to explore feelings, and to refrain from offering insights or interpretations (Gold, 1985).

Since the field of mediation is still in its infancy, there are fewer mediators than mental health professionals. Mediators are more likely to be isolated and to have only limited contact with other mediators (Kressel, Butler-DeFreitas, Forlenza, & Wilcox, 1989). Supervisors and peers are not as readily available for consultation in difficult cases. For these reasons, mediators may want to join the appropriate mediator organizations and to develop informal support networks. Attendance at workshops and conferences can also be helpful. Mediators may wish to work as teams or to develop a schedule of regular case conferencing with peers or consultants (Kressel et al., 1989). Many therapists who are mediators offer both services and do not wish to be limited only to mediation work (Gold, 1985).

CAUTIONS AND ETHICAL CONSIDERATIONS

Certain caveats and ethical issues should be considered in any discussion of mediation and therapy. Mediators may resolve a wide range of dispute types. These may include some very uncomplicated small-business–consumer complaints, landlord–tenant conflicts, or complex divorce mediations. Mediators are urged to recognize the limits of their expertise, training, and experience. As managers of conflicts, they promote options and alternatives, develop resolutions, improve communications, empower clients, and at times perform a host of diverse activities. Mediation is not a substitute for therapy, legal counsel, or financial advice. Mediators do not act as lawyers or financial planners or even as therapists, but do make such referrals when appropriate.

It would seem very natural for the mediator with legal or clinical background and training to be tempted to offer legal advice or therapeutic services. The therapist or attorney may easily cross the professional role boundaries. Likewise, this may occur for mediators who possess other expertise or training. However, this is not in the interest of either the client or the interventionist, and will only serve to blur the already vague and ambiguous distinctions between mediation and other interventions.

The mediator should not attempt to intervene therapeutically between two parties in a case where he or she has previously established a relationship with one of the parties. This will only tend to undermine the neutrality of the mediator. Therapists will want to avoid mediating with therapy clients. A therapist who has been a client's advocate in therapy is expected to assume the role of an impartial third person in mediation. This will probably seem to be a betrayal to the client and will destroy the client–therapist relationship.

SUMMARY

Mediation and psychotherapy have been compared and have been found to be parallel processes in several dimensions. The interventions share certain common elements, such as the need for confidentiality, but have distinctly separate goals.

Mediation resembles psychotherapy and at times may seem indistinguishable from therapy. It shares aspects with traditional psychodynamic therapies as well as with behavioral approaches. It has also been found to be similar to strategic family therapy. Techniques and strategies from these therapies can be effectively transferred to mediation.

Each of the two processes is based on an interpersonal, helping relationship. The therapeutically trained mediator will want a clear understanding of these parallel processes and their separate goals. Such an understanding is vital for effective service delivery. The parties will need to understand the process for which they are contracting. Dual relationships—that is, acting as both therapist and mediator—with clients are to be avoided.

The clinician/mediator may find mediation to be a more stressful process than therapy. The mediator is constantly dealing with conflict, anger, resentment, and hostility. Being continually in the midst of such emotions and absorbing them is taxing and stressful.

Clinically trained mediators will have to decide for themselves to what extent they are comfortable and effective utilizing their clinical skills in the mediation process. This will be influenced by their approach to psychotherapy as well as by their model of mediation. They will need to determine which clinical techniques and strategies lend themselves most productively to their style of mediation. They will find that certain common elements of the parallel processes will need to be constrained, while other elements will be expanded in their new role as mediator.

The therapist/mediator brings valuable knowledge and experience to the mediation setting. The challenge is to integrate his or her therapeutic background and skills into the mediation process without losing sight of the separate goal of mediation and without allowing mediation to become a distorted form of psychological treatment.

REFERENCES

Brown, E. M. (1988). Divorce mediation in a mental health setting. In J. Folberg & A. Milne (Eds.), *Divorce mediation: Theory and practice* (pp. 127–141). New York: Guilford.

Brown, S. M. (1985). Models of mediation. In S. C. Grebe (Ed.), *Divorce and family mediation*. Rockville, MD: Aspen.

Emery, R. E., & Wyer, M. M. (1987). Divorce mediation. *American Psychologist, 42*, 472–480.

Fisher, R., & Ury, W. (1981). *Getting to yes*. Boston: Houghton Mifflin.

Folberg, J., & Taylor, A. (1984). *Mediation: A comprehensive guide to resolving conflicts without litigation*. San Francisco: Jossey-Bass.

Forlenza, S. G. (1988). *The mental health professional as mediator*. Paper presented at the annual meeting of the Eastern Psychological Association, Buffalo, N.Y.

Gilliland, B. E., James, R. K., Roberts, G. T., & Bowman, J. (1984). *Theories and strategies in counseling and psychotherapy*. Englewood Cliffs, NJ: Prentice-Hall.

Girdner, L. (1986). Family mediation: Toward a synthesis. *Mediation Quarterly, 13*, 21–29.

Gold, L. (1985). Reflections on the transition from therapist to mediator. *Mediation Quarterly, 9*, 15–26.

Grebe, S. C. (1986). A comparison of the tasks and definitions of family mediation and those of strategic family therapy. *Mediation Quarterly, 13*, 53–59.

Haley, J. (1976). *Problem-solving therapy*. New York: Harper Torchbooks.

Hansen, J. C., & L'Abate, L. (1982). *Approaches to family therapy*. New York: Macmillan.

Haynes, J. M. (1981). *Divorce mediation: A practical guide for therapists and counselors*. New York: Springer.

Herron, W. G., & Rouslin, S. (1982). *Issues in psychotherapy*. Bowie, MD: Robert J. Brady.

Kelly, J. B. (1983). Mediation and psychotherapy: Distinguishing the differences. *Mediation Quarterly, 1,* 33–44.

Kelly, J. B., Zlatchin, C., & Shawn, J. (1985). Divorce mediation: Process, prospects and professional issues. In C. Ewing (Ed.), *Psychology, psychiatry and the law: A clinical and forensic handbook*. Sarasota, FL: Professional Resource Exchange.

Kressel, K. (1985), *The process of divorce*. New York: Basic Books.

Kressel, K., Butler-DeFreitas, F. M., Forlenza, S. G., & Wilcox, C. (1989). Research in contested custody mediations: An illustration of the case study method. *Mediation Quarterly, 24,* 55–70.

Kressel, K., Forlenza, S. G., Butler, F. M., & Wilcox, C. (1988). Interim report: Essex County Family Division custody mediation project. In *Supreme Court of New Jersey Task Force on Dispute Resolution: Research and evaluation*. Trenton, NJ: Administrative Office of the Courts.

Lam, J. A., Rifkin, J., & Townley, A. (1989). Reframing conflict: Implications for fairness in parent–adolescent mediation. *Mediation Quarterly, 7,* 15–31.

Milne, A. (1985). Mediation or therapy—Which is it? In S. C. Grebe (Ed.), *Divorce and family mediation*. Rockville, MD: Aspen.

Prigoff, M. (1988). Mediation confidentiality. Toward candor or chaos: The case of confidentiality in mediation. *Seton Hall Legislative Journal, 12,* 1–15.

Prochaska, J. O. (1984). *Systems of psychotherapy: A transtheoretical analysis* (2nd ed.). Homewood, IL: Dorsey Press.

Saposnek, D. T. (1983). *Mediating child custody disputes*. San Francisco: Jossey-Bass.

Strupp, H. (1978). Psychotherapy research and practice: An overview. In S. Garfield & A. Bergin (Eds.), *Handbook of psychotherapy and behavioral change: An empirical analysis* (2nd ed.). New York: Wiley.

Strupp, H. (1986). Psychotherapy: Research, practice and public policy (how to avoid dead ends). *American Psychologist, 41,* 120–130.

Yale, D. (1988). Metaphors in mediating. *Mediation Quarterly, 7,* 15–25.

PART IV

BEYOND NEIGHBOR
DISPUTES: EXTENSIONS
OF MEDIATION

As the field of community mediation has grown, so too has the number of problem areas to which mediation can be successfully applied. Whereas once the use of mediation may have been limited to fairly simple (although not necessarily easy-to-solve) problems, such as tenant–landlord disputes, today mediation has found a place in helping to resolve an impressive variety of complex, community-based problems. This final section is intended to illustrate the many settings in which the process of mediation has been applied, as well as to suggest areas where mediation may play an increasingly larger role in the future.

The section begins with a chapter by Elsje van Munster, who looks at the rapidly expanding area of family mediation in terms of fundamental dilemmas faced by mediators and program coordinators alike. These dilemmas include the choice between mediation and arbitration in family cases, the role of legal representation, the use of signed versus nonsigned agreements, and the decision as to when mediation may be inappropriate for a particular family case. Case studies are used to illustrate the complexity of the factors that mediators must consider in resolving these dilemmas.

Next, Michael Van Slyck and Marilyn Stern investigate the impact of a peer mediation program in an educational setting. Although the use of alternative dispute resolution techniques in schools can be traced back to the 1960s, little systematic research has been performed. The authors discuss both the short- and long-term effects of a peer mediation program on participating students, on the mediators themselves, and on the overall disciplinary climate in the school.

Victim–offender reconciliation programs (VORPs) are the subject of Stephen Woolpert's chapter on another growing area of mediation. In VORPs, a victim of a crime and the perpetrator (or offender) sit down with a mediator and work out an agreement that compensates the victim for any losses that occurred because of the crime. Equally important, the offender is

241

held personally accountable for his or her actions and is encouraged to see the crime from the viewpoint of the victim. Woolpert discusses VORPs from the perspective of the victim, the offender, and the mediator, and provides a much-needed historical context from which to understand the different types of VORPs that are currently in use.

In the next chapter, Arthur Best introduces the area of consumer mediation and describes a nationwide program initiated by General Motors (GM) and the Federal Trade Commission to handle disputes involving GM cars that contain defective components. Best points out that consumer mediation, unlike other forms, often does not involve a continuing relationship between the parties and may involve significant power inequities. He provides a critical evaluation of the GM program from the perspective of both the car company and the consumer.

Finally, Susan Carpenter gives us a sense of the broad range of problems to which mediation can be applied when she discusses attempts to resolve environmental and other types of public disputes. As Carpenter notes, public disputes, because of their complex nature and the presence of many competing interest groups, do not lend themselves to the type of standardized, formal procedure that is often associated with other types of mediation. Based on her many years of experience, she describes the difficult issues and decisions that a mediator faces when handling a public dispute.

Taken together, the chapters in this section illustrate how different types of mediation require different knowledge, training, hearing procedures, and consideration of special concerns unique to each particular type of mediation. However, all the chapters have in common the conviction that mediation can, if properly implemented, serve as a useful alternative to traditional methods of dispute resolution.

15

Dilemmas in Family Mediation: Practical Applications

ELSJE H. van MUNSTER
Center for Dispute Settlement,
Rochester, New York

The last decade has seen a considerable increase in the use of family mediation in the United States and Canada. This increase is evident in several areas: (1) a general increase in the number of referrals from a variety of sources; (2) expansion of existing programs and blossoming of associations of family mediators; and (3) an increase in both the number and size of conferences on the topic at the local, state, and national levels. Because of the increase in this extremely young field, it is essential for family mediators to examine certain dilemmas more closely. A field in which one can practice without a license must police itself and set high standards of practice and moral conduct in order to protect those who are to benefit from the process of mediation. This is not to imply that there are no standards, such as those set forth by the American Bar Association and by the Academy of Family Mediators, but to suggest that there is a need for more universally accepted standards of practice and that noncompliance with those standards should have negative consequences for the practitioner.

In general, it is fairly safe to state that mediation of family issues can be beneficial for families under certain circumstances and that under other circumstances the usefulness of family mediation is rather limited. The usefulness of this practice is evident from both empirical and anecdotal data. The latter are often more convincing, both because there are limited empirical data available as yet and because it is difficult to measure the success of a field that does not lend itself easily to scientific evaluation.

In order for family mediation to be successful, it should be used in conjunction with legal proceedings; it is not meant to be a substitute for the legal protections afforded parties. However, the legal, adversarial procedure of dealing with family disputes is often totally inadequate and can have dire financial and personal consequences for one or more members of a family. Mediation, as an alternative to the adversarial process, can provide parties with a peaceful means to resolve their disputes and can give them the power

243

to make decisions about their lives that are too often left to strangers, such as lawyers and judges. No matter how well-meaning these decision makers may be, it is unlikely that they possess adequate knowledge and information to make permanent decisions about entire families' lives.

Family mediation should be distinguished from divorce mediation, in that family mediation can include the mediation of separation or divorce as well as single issues, such as custody, visitation, maintenance (alimony), support, division of property, modification, and parent–child disputes and other intergenerational conflicts.

This chapter deals with four major dilemmas in family mediation: (1) mediation versus arbitration; (2) signed versus nonsigned agreements; (3) legal representation versus no legal representation; and (4) to mediate or not to mediate. Solving these dilemmas requires a multipronged approach and involves consideration, on a case-by-case basis, of a number of variables. Among the variables to be considered are the following: (1) who is the referral source (clients themselves, an attorney, a court, a department of social services); (2) what is the purpose of the mediation (temporary or permanent agreement, modification, resolution of a single issue or of multiple issues); and finally (3) what socioeconomic factors come into play (the parties' ability to afford legal counsel, education as it relates to a knowledge of legal rights, economic stability).

In addition to considering the variables listed above, the mediator must determine whether any court orders are in effect that limit either the power of the mediator or that of the parties to make their own agreement. Finally, the mediator must determine whether there is any abuse of the mediation process by one or more of the parties and whether there is equality of bargaining power among the parties to the mediation. Sometimes a slight inequality of bargaining power can be remedied through minor adjustments, whereas in other instances inequality may mean that the mediation has to be halted for the protection of the "less equal" party.

The case studies used in this chapter to explore and illustrate both procedural and ethical considerations indicate that the dilemmas above can be solved appropriately if all the relevant variables are taken into consideration by mediators who maintain the highest ethical standards. Despite the fact that the dilemmas and the variables are listed separately, in practice they are most often integrally related and therefore are treated in combination with each other.

It should be pointed out that all the case studies in this chapter are actual cases that have been mediated (or not mediated, as the case may be), although the names and certain identifying details have been changed to protect the parties' privacy. The cases cover individuals from the entire socioeconomic spectrum, ranging from extremely poor and/or uneducated to wealthy and/or well-educated parties. As a result of special funding, the poor were able to have access to the same mediation services as the wealthy and middle-class families.

MEDIATION VERSUS ARBITRATION

It may seem odd to discuss the issue of mediation versus arbitration as a dilemma in family mediation; however, parties frequently come to a family mediation program and request that someone else make the decisions relative to the issues in dispute. In most instances parties should be encouraged to opt for the mediation process, since arbitration will deny them the benefit of maintaining control over their own future; if the award is final and legally binding, the legal protection of individual counsel is also dispensed with.

The Johnson case was referred for arbitration, after protracted litigation, from the New York State Supreme Court. The judge ordered the parties to participate in arbitration to settle the issue of property division, which neither the parties, their attorneys, nor the court had been able to solve. Initially, the neutral third party attempted to mediate this case; however, soon it became evident that these two people would not be willing to cooperate, and the matter was arbitrated. The couple signed a submission to arbitration in accordance with the Civil Practice Law and Rules of New York State (N.Y. Civ. Prac. L. & R. 75, McKinney 1990), which meant that any award would be final and legally binding on both parties to the arbitration. Since both Mr. and Mrs. Johnson had discussed this matter with their individual counsel, there was no concern about adequate legal protection. The parties were in disagreement about almost every single item in dispute, and the personal animosity was such that mediation would have been impossible; therefore, arbitration was the appropriate method of resolving this dispute. The arbitrator rendered an award, and the long battle between the couple finally came to an end.

The facts of the Sanders case were more complicated and involved modification of previous visitation arrangements. Mr. and Mrs. Sanders also were referred from court, and the judge in this case had made it clear that he did not wish to have the matter brought before him again. The attorneys in this case even recommended that the parties arbitrate instead of mediate because they could not agree, mostly because neither party wanted to give an inch. During the time that the Mr. And Mrs. Sanders were arguing back and forth, they had totally lost track of the best interest of their children. In general, any matters involving custody or visitation should be mediated, but in this case it was possible to do "med/arb," which is a hybrid of mediation and arbitration. Basically the case was mediated, providing the parents with as much control as necessary, but the final result of the session was an arbitration award. Knowing that the "final decision" was up to the arbitrator relieved each parent of the pressure of giving in to the other spouse, and as a consequence they both were more reasonable than they had managed to be up to that point. The award was one that was beneficial to the children and provided relief for the parents and their attorneys. Follow-up inquiries have shown that the Sanders have not been back in court for any reason and that the visitation schedule has worked well for all.

The dispute over custody in the Jeffries case came to the office as a request for arbitration from the wife, who told the intake person that her husband was willing to submit to arbitration as well. The parties were asked to come in for a personal intake session to evaluate what their needs were, and it became evident almost immediately that neither parent wanted to take control. These parents had very different notions as to how children should be reared and educated. Unwilling to compromise on these issues, they would rather have an arbitrator decide that the children should live with, and be under the complete control of, one parent than take control, possibly compromise, and feel guilt. The latter was important because the mother thought she would "win" the case, but her concern was that the children would be resentful. Being able to explain to them that it was someone else who had made the decision would leave her free from that type of guilt. In this case it was necessary to explain to the parties that the matter could not be arbitrated, but that mediation would be an option for them to consider.

After Mr. and Mrs. Jeffries were confronted, both individually and together, with their fear of taking control and the fact that the reason for wanting arbitration was really an abuse of the process, they slowly came around and decided to mediate. During the mediation, the mediator was able to help the parties realize that custody did not have to be an all-or-nothing proposition. As it turned out, Mrs. Jeffries was much more concerned with the children's education and exposure to cultural activities, while Mr. Jeffries's primary concern was the children's religious upbringing. Once each parent realized that it was possible to have the one thing that was most important to him or her, both were willing to compromise on areas of secondary importance, and the children ended up with a better overall package.

The Johnson, Sanders, and Jeffries cases illustrate the dilemma of mediation versus arbitration quite well. In the Johnson case the referral came from court, and the parties had more than adequate legal representation. In addition, they were well educated and fully aware of their legal rights, and their previous interaction made it abundantly clear that mediation would not be productive. Arbitration was the appropriate method to resolve the long-standing property dispute between the Johnsons, in a manner that was final and legally binding in the courts of New York State without harming any of the parties involved. Had the Johnson case been self-referred, and had the parties lacked the benefit of legal representation, then it would have been incumbent upon the arbitrator to encourage the parties to seek legal counsel. The fact that the Johnson case involved property as opposed to custody or visitation made it less problematic to arbitrate the case.

Since the dispute between Mr. and Mrs. Sanders affected their children, it was extremely important for the parents to make as much of the decision as possible by taking control. If the couple had submitted to arbitration, instead of the "med/arb" hybrid, they might as well have left the decision to the presiding judge; they would have missed the benefit of taking an active part in the process. The mediator/arbitrator was able to bring the focus back to the best interest of the children and to show each parent that it was possible to communicate with the other parent without the use of a judge and two attorneys. Mr. and Mrs. Sanders were court-referred; they had excellent legal representation; and the bargaining power between them was quite equal. If mediation had been used solely in this case, it might have been difficult to conclude the matter, and the pattern that had developed in court might have been continued in mediation. The "med/arb" hybrid was perfect for Mr. and Mrs. Sanders because it forced them to take control and reach their own agreement, yet provided them with the finality and external security of an arbitration award.

The custody case of Mr. and Mrs. Jeffries was clearly inappropriate for arbitration, for a number of reasons. First and foremost is the fact that determining permanent custody should be a judicial matter if the parents cannot come to an agreement; it is not within the scope of an arbitrator's authority to exercise judicial powers in matters of custody. (Some readers may disagree with this statement.) Second, the couple had not consulted with counsel as frequently as they should have, and therefore might not have been fully aware of the consequences of an arbitration award in regard to their custody battle. Since there was no inequality of bargaining power between these two parents, mediation was by far the most desirable alternative and put the decision-making responsibility regarding the children back into the hands of the parents. The compromises made in mediation provided the parents with the items they needed, and the children with a much richer and more well-rounded upbringing that involved both parents rather than just one.

SIGNED VERSUS NONSIGNED AGREEMENTS

Once the mediation is concluded successfully and the issues have been resolved, there remains the dilemma of whether the parties should sign the resulting document or not. The discussion below is based on the assumption that the mediator will conclude his or her task and that the parties will have separate private counsel to complete the legal process. There are individuals who act both as mediators and as "lawyers" (or as scribes); however, the issues raised by such representation are beyond the scope of this chapter. These issues are sufficiently complicated to require detailed treatment elsewhere.

The document resulting from a successful mediation is called many different names; the Center for Dispute Settlement in Rochester, New York, prefers to refer to this document as the "preliminary plan for the resolution of issues." It is preliminary in nature because it is not final or legally binding until the parties' individual attorneys have reviewed the document and incorporated it as part of the "legal documents." Other mediators prefer the term "memorandum of understanding" or "agreement of the parties." In many instances these documents are signed by the parties even if they have not had the benefit of receiving legal counsel. The preference should be, no matter what the name, for the document *not* to be signed until the parties' attorneys have a chance to review the plan. Some mediators prefer the signing ceremony as a means of bringing closure to the mediation process. However, since the end of the mediation does not generally mean the end of the entire process (in a divorce or a separation), it seems that one can have closure without signing and then send the parties on to their attorneys to complete the dissolution. Thereby the mediator is able to provide the parties with a resolution of the issues in dispute, but also to ensure that they have the advantage of final legal protection from their individual advocates.

There are times, however, when the needs of the parties require some flexibility, and a signed document serves the purposes of the couple more fully than a nonsigned document. One example of this is the Gordon case. The Gordons came to the office because their current living situation was no longer tolerable, but they had no idea what the future would hold for them. They were unsure even as to whether a separation would eventually lead to a permanent separation or divorce, or whether perhaps they would resume a married life if the "contract" between them worked out. The Gordons were both working, were well educated, and had no children. They had each spoken with their attorneys, but wanted to take control and not to involve the attorneys any further at that particular time. The attorneys had given the Gordons the green light to go ahead and mediate their "preliminary separation," and to sign the "contract" between them without further consultation of counsel. After several mediation sessions, the Gordons' issues were resolved; the preliminary plan was written up, reviewed by the parties, and signed. All issues in anticipation of a dissolution of the marriage were resolved, and the parties had all intentions of living by this "contract" until they had clearer ideas about the future. Since there were no children involved in the Gordon case and the parties were well informed about their respective rights, the signed contract posed no threat to anyone involved in the case. Neither party sought support from the other spouse, and the bargaining power between the spouses was comfortably equal.

The Naughton case, referred by family court, consisted of a parent–child conflict that had escalated sufficiently for the family to end up in family court on several occasions and for the 16-year-old son to be subject to a "person in need of supervision" (PINS) petition. The father had given the mother an ultimatum in regard to the son: "Either he goes or I go!" The mother was unwilling to make that choice; when the judge suggested that the family try mediation, the mother was able to convince both the father and the son to give mediation a chance, since all else had failed. Initially, the mother sat on one side of the table with the son, and the father sat by himself on the opposite side. The mediator spent hours trying to bring the parties together and eventually succeeded in having them listen to one another. In fact, it was the first time that the father had actually really listened to the son, and the first time also that the son had heard what the father was feeling.

After the mediator spent some time in caucus with each of the parties, something interesting happened. The mother, upon her return to the hearing room, took a seat at the end of the table opposite the mediator and helped (consciously or unconsciously) to mediate the case. She had watched the mediator break through to these two men in a way that no one had been able to do before, and somehow she was able to use some of those same skills to help in bringing about a solution to this case. The judge who referred the case had requested that a consent agreement to be drawn up and signed by the parties. Despite the fact that the parties were not represented by counsel, it was proper to have a signed agreement in this case because the judge would still review it. As it turned out, both the family and the judge were sufficiently pleased with the final result that the consent agreement became a permanent part of the court order.

The visitation matter in the Sheffield case was also referred from family court because existing visitation arrangements were no longer adequate. There was some concern initially that the parties should not sign their agreement because they could not afford counsel, but after discussions with the family as well as the judge, it appeared that a signed agreement was more desirable in this case. The problem for the Sheffields was that both parents worked, but their hours were extremely irregular and the shifts quite complicated, making it all but impossible for them to stick to any kind of visitation schedule set up by the court. Each parent did want the children to see the other parent, but they could not manage to figure out a schedule that would work for both. The mediator literally made up a visitation schedule for every possible combination of shifts the parents might be assigned for the next 9 to 12 months. At the conclusion of the mediation sessions, the parties signed a consent agreement, and the judge incorporated the visitation schedule in the court order. Follow-up revealed that the parties were able to live comfortably with the visitation schedule. Approximately a year and a half later, the parties called the mediation center to request a modification because the father had changed jobs, and they wanted the help of the mediator to set up an equally successful schedule.

LEGAL REPRESENTATION VERSUS
NO LEGAL REPRESENTATION

Perhaps the question should not simply be *whether* the parties should be represented by counsel, but *when* it is appropriate for the parties to seek counsel. Mediation practice in regard to this dilemma is mixed. As a general rule, parties should be advised to seek their own individual counsel, preferably *prior* to the first mediation session. The benefits of early representation include the following: (1) Parties are able to participate in the mediation process with an awareness of their legal rights; (2) if an attorney objects to mediation, the parties can decide not to mediate or can switch attorneys without wasting additional time and money; and (3) if the parties have legal questions during the mediation or between sessions, they are able to consult with their own counsel as needed. There are mediators who believe that early representation is a disadvantage, because often attorneys do not like mediation, and therefore the clients may not mediate. This approach seems to be somewhat short-sighted if the parties involved in the process are supposed to receive the benefits from mediation. As long as the parties have been fully informed about the benefits of mediation as well as of early representation, the decision to mediate or not should be left up to them, unless there is a compelling reason to change that general rule.

The Marks case was self-referred, and the couple wanted to mediate a separation agreement without benefit of attorneys. At the intake session, it was explained to Mr. and Mrs. Marks that it would benefit them to consult with legal counsel prior to the mediation as well as at the conclusion of the mediation. It soon became evident that the parties were not only well educated, but also well informed about their legal rights. As professional people they each had considerable contact with their own counsel, but they refused to get counsel involved at that time. Since (1) there were no children involved in the Marks case, (2) the bargaining power was equal, and (3) their decision to proceed without counsel was informed, there was no reason to deny this couple access to the mediation process. Because of the amicable relationship between Mr. and Mrs. Marks, the issues were resolved quickly to the satisfaction of both.

A well-educated young couple by the name of Weiss came, referred by friends, to the center for mediation; they, too, decided that they did not wish to retain counsel prior to mediation. Although they liked each other, continuing disagreements about money had brought them to the conclusion that they did not wish to continue living as husband and wife. They had no children, and since both were at the beginning of their careers, they had very little money or property. The couple intended to find *one* attorney after the mediation to file the legal papers, despite the recommendation of the mediator to the contrary. The parties were told that the mediator's role is that of a neutral third party who can provide guidance to the couple, but that the mediator (or an attorney who acts as a "scribe") is not and cannot be an advocate for either party. Despite these warnings, the couple decided to proceed without counsel; the mediation took place, and the parties left with an unsigned preliminary plan in hand.

The relatively uncomplicated nature of the Marks and Weiss cases made it possible for the mediator to go ahead with the mediation after appropriate warnings had been issued to the parties relative to their retaining individual counsel. There are instances, however, when the mediator must say no when the dilemma of representation comes up, even if it means halting a mediation in progress or never starting one. The following three cases illustrate both the dilemma of representation and that of mediation versus no mediation.

TO MEDIATE OR NOT TO MEDIATE

The Cantor case was referred to mediation by another couple that had used the process successfully. The Cantors had been married for 20 years, had two children, and owned a business as well as extensive property. In view of the length of the marriage as well as the amount of property in dispute, the parties were strongly advised to consult with counsel prior to the first mediation session. Despite this advice, the Cantors came to their first session without having spoken with counsel; after being urged once again by the mediator to consider doing so, the couple showed a united front and insisted that they wanted to mediate because of the children. Several sessions took place, and the parties showed a considerable amount of cooperation on matters involving the children and certain aspects of the property division. Unfortunately, when it came to the business, the parties were suddenly in total disagreement as to what it was worth, who owned what share, and how it should be divided. A careful look at the tax returns for several years showed zero income for all the years that returns were available.

Considering the Cantors' lifestyle and the amount of property in dispute, the mediator knew that something did not add up. It was obvious that not all the cards were on the table and that both parties were fully aware of that fact. The mediator once again emphasized that full financial disclosure was not a matter of *whether* one discloses, but rather a question of *when;* in addition, it was made clear that if the parties did not disclose all assets and liabilities, the mediator would be forced to halt the mediation on ethical grounds. The wife was willing to go along with the husband on certain points if she could get a piece of real estate that was of utmost importance to her. Something seemed wrong, and the mediator proceeded to caucus with the parties separately to determine what was really going on. Mrs. Cantor knew her husband was hiding assets, but the real estate she wanted could only be had if she moved immediately on several other pieces; otherwise, the whole deal would fall through. She was willing to go along with the husband's game on the assumption that once she had what she wanted she could, in her words, "point out to the judge what was really going on and get that son of a bitch." The husband in the meantime had his own agenda, and the mediator was forced to tell the parties that under the circumstances the mediation would have to be halted.

The parties still insisted that they wanted to go ahead with the mediation. The mediator was not at liberty to discuss with either party what had been discovered in caucus with the other spouse, but made it clear that under the rules of good faith and full disclosure, the center could not and would not continue with the mediation. There was some indication that Mrs. Cantor was not merely afraid to lose out on the real estate deal, but was also concerned about her own legal liability, since she had signed all those tax returns. Both parties were given the bar association's lawyer referral number as well as a list of local attorneys. The agreements reached between the parties in regard to the children and some other matters were written up and mailed to them. Clearly, the Cantors' attempts to abuse the mediation process and the lack of legal protection for the parties made it necessary for the mediator to halt the mediation, for the good of the parties as well as for the integrity of the mediator and the mediation process.

Another case that exemplifies the to-mediate-or-not-to-mediate dilemma is the "mail-order bride" case. This couple requested mediation after being referred by the husband's attorney. The marriage had lasted approximately 10 years, and the couple had two young children. During the intake session, both parties seemed exceedingly willing to participate in the mediation process, although the husband seemed to do most of the talking. Even when questions were addressed to the wife, the husband jumped in and answered for her. When the question of legal representation came up, he answered quickly that they had sought legal counsel and were "all set" on that score. Such symptoms as these may indicate that there is inequality of bargaining power and/or some type of abuse in the relationship.

The mediator explained to the parties that occasionally it is necessary to speak with each party separately in a caucus, and the wife was asked to leave the room first. In the caucus the husband was not very helpful in shedding light on the situation, other than showing that he was extremely eager to get the process going—maybe just a little too eager. Then the husband was asked to leave and the wife returned for her caucus, which was a great deal more revealing. As it turned out, the wife spoke English quite well for a foreigner, but she lacked any knowledge of the American legal system and her rights in it. Her understanding, which came strictly from what her husband had told her, was that because she wanted the divorce she had no right to anything; she could leave, but she would have to leave with nothing other than whatever it was that he would "let" her have. When asked whether *she* had spoken with the "family attorney" who had referred them to mediation, she indicated that she had never talked with him. Since the husband handled all the money and she had been a "work-at-home" wife, she believed that she had absolutely no means or right to retain her own counsel. Although she felt ashamed to talk about it, the evidence suggested that there was some form of abuse (emotional and/or physical) going on in the relationship as well.

Not only was this a case where mediation was totally inappropriate for ethical reasons, but it was essential that the wife leave the center with sufficient information to get protection, legal and otherwise. Before she left, the wife was given the numbers of the local battered women's shelter, legal assistance and other legal aid societies, attorneys who would provide free consultations, and the bar association referral service. In addition, it was explained to "the bride" that she should not let herself be talked into going to another mediator, but should seek legal counsel immediately. It was difficult to convince her that she did have legal rights. When the intake session continued with both spouses in the room, the parties were told that the center would not commence a mediation unless both parties had retained their own counsel, and that after both had done so, the mediation could take place. The husband was furious that the center declined to mediate his case.

Many of the variables discussed earlier came into play in the "mail-order bride" case: (1) The referral source did not provide added protection; (2) the purpose of the mediation was for permanent arrangements; (3) socioeconomic factors such as inability to afford counsel and lack of knowledge about legal rights were major obstacles; and (4) there was no equality of bargaining power between the two parties. Because of the combination of all of these variables, the mediator had an affirmative duty, based on ethical considerations, not to go ahead with the mediation and to provide the "bride" with sufficient information to seek adequate protection for herself.

The third case in which the to-mediate-or-not-to-mediate dilemma came to the fore was the Miller case. Mrs. Miller heard about mediation from a friend who had been happy with the process a year and a half prior to that time. She had spoken with her husband about getting a divorce, but he refused to accept the inevitable and took no action at all. Mrs. Miller came to the Center for Dispute Settlement to obtain the necessary information, despite the fact that her husband refused to participate. It should be emphasized that an intake with both spouses simultaneously is preferred to meeting with only one spouse.

During the initial intake session, it became evident that Mrs. Miller had not consulted with an attorney, and that because of many years of abuse there was a power imbalance between the spouses. The mediator explained to Mrs. Miller that because of her circumstances, mediation might not be appropriate. Since during the two decades of marriage the husband had dominated the relationship, there was a good possibility that the same domination would take place in the mediation. Mrs. Miller had given all of those considerations a great deal of thought and had come to the conclusion that it was "necessary" for her to "do this and take charge for once" in her life. If Mr. Miller could be convinced to come to mediation, the center would consider doing the mediation, on the conditions (1) that Mrs. Miller would retain her own attorney and consult with him or her prior to the first session; and (2) that she would contact someone at a local shelter for battered women. In addition, if the power imbalance between the spouses could not be eliminated, the center reserved the right to terminate the mediation. Initially Mrs. Miller insisted that she could not afford an attorney, but the mediator was able to convince her that she could not afford *not* to see one; she then agreed to the conditions and proceeded with the onerous task of convincing her husband to participate.

It took several months before the couple came in for their first mediation session, and the husband's reluctance made it all but impossible to mediate. After two sessions, he accepted the inevitability of the separation and determined that perhaps mediation would be the lesser of two evils. In the meantime, Mrs. Miller had retained an attorney and had also spoken with one of the caseworkers at a local shelter for victims of domestic violence. Mr. Miller did attempt to dominate the mediation sessions; however, Mrs. Miller was more than able to hold her own with the help of the mediator. It appeared that as long as the third party neutral was present to intervene if necessary, Mrs. Miller felt safe and was able to assert herself in a way that she was unable to accomplish when alone with her husband. As the mediation progressed, the need for the mediator to intervene became less frequent as the power imbalance between the parties became increasingly less pronounced. Throughout the process, both parties consulted with their attorneys in accordance with the conditions set by the center. After all the issues, including custody, visitation, and financial and property division, were resolved, the preliminary plan was drafted and mailed to the attorneys.

The Miller case is an excellent example of the fact that at times flexibility on the part of mediator can be beneficial to the participants. If the center had turned away Mrs. Miller because of the abuse in this case, she would not have been able to take charge of her life. Instead, an attorney would have taken care of the case for her, as her husband had taken care of her during the marriage. It was essential for Mrs. Miller to take control and to convince herself that she could do it. At the same time, it is clear that if Mrs. Miller had not been represented by counsel, the center should not have mediated the case. The conditions set at the start of the mediation provided sufficient protection for Mrs. Miller that it was reasonable to give mediation a chance.

By the same token, the mediation should have been terminated if the power imbalance between the Millers had persisted throughout the mediation.

An interesting follow-up occurred in this case. Approximately 2 years later, the program director received a call from a person who wished to interview the director about the family mediation program. A time was arranged, and the interviewer turned out to be Mrs. Miller, who by then had changed her name. She was studying to become a social worker and was doing her honors thesis on divorce mediation. Prior to conducting her interview, Mrs. Miller spoke about her own experience of submitting to the mediation process. She felt that her participation in mediation had been the most important event in helping to turn her life around, and that without it she might still have been a "helpless victim."

It is likely that Mrs. Miller was giving too much credit to mediation and too little to her own inner strength and determination, but it does illustrate a point for those who insist that cases in which there is any type of abuse should never be mediated. The point is that each case has to be evaluated on its own merits, and that the mediator must take into consideration all of the variables discussed in this chapter. If mediation is not conducted for the benefit of the parties involved, it simply should not take place.

GENERAL QUESTIONS FOR MEDIATORS

In determining whether mediation should take place and what form it should take, certain questions must be considered by the mediator. First, will the parties benefit from the process of mediation? If the answer is no, then mediation is inappropriate, and the parties should be informed accordingly.

Second, are the parties adequately represented by their own legal counsel? If the answer is yes, in most instances the mediation should go forward if the parties so desire. If, however, the answer is no, the mediator must advise the parties to seek counsel at the earliest possible time. As some of the case studies above indicate, mediation can take place under certain circumstances even if the parties are not represented, as long as adequate warnings have been provided and there are no ethical impediments that render the process inappropriate.

Third, is there equality of bargaining power? Once it is established that there is no equality, it becomes essential to determine whether the inequality is sufficient to decide against mediation, or whether a balance can be achieved with some intervention. Again, this dilemma must be resolved by examining all of the variables and the abilities of the parties, as well as the intervention skills of the mediator. In these types of cases, the mediator walks a fine line between acting as a neutral third party and intervening to provide the necessary power balance.

Fourth, although related to equality of bargaining power, is the question of abuse. In many cases where abuse is a part of the relationship between the parties, it is often inappropriate to mediate because the abuse itself has created a power imbalance that cannot be overcome during the mediation process. However, even these cases must be evaluated individually to determine their appropriateness for mediation, as long as it is clear that any doubt is to be resolved by a decision not to mediate.

Fifth, is there attempted abuse of the mediation process itself by one or more of the parties? If there is, the mediator must be willing to terminate the mediation if the party or parties persist in these attempts.

Sixth, can a mediator handle a particular case? Is the mediator sufficiently skilled to help the parties resolve their issues? It is essential to know one's limitations as a mediator and to accept or decline cases accordingly.

Finally, in answering these questions and in conducting mediations, is the mediator able to maintain the highest ethical standards? A mediator must always act in accordance with the best interest of the parties who wish to participate in the mediation process. The beginning family mediator may find it helpful to consult Coogler (1978), Haynes (1981), Marlow and Sauber (1990), Wallerstein and Kelly (1980), and Folberg and Milne (1988) prior to answering this question and the others posed here.

Appropriate resolution, after careful deliberation, of all of the dilemmas faced by practicing mediators will eventually help mediators win the respect and recognition they deserve. As a result, mediation of family disputes will gain greater acceptance as a viable alternative to the adversarial process.

REFERENCES

Coogler, O. J. (1978). *Structured mediation in divorce settlements: A handbook for marital mediators*. Lexington, MA: Lexington Books.

Folberg, J., & Milne, A. (Eds.). (1988). *Divorce mediation*. New York: Guilford Press.

Haynes, J. (1981). *Divorce mediations: A practical guide for therapists and counselors*. New York: Springer.

Marlow, L., & Sauber, S. R. (1990). *The handbook of divorce mediation*. New York: Plenum Press.

N.Y. Civ. Prac. L. & R. 75 (McKinney 1990).

Wallerstein, J., & Kelly, J. (1980). *Surviving the breakup: How children and parents cope with divorce*. New York: Basic Books.

16

Conflict Resolution in Educational Settings: Assessing the Impact of Peer Mediation Programs

MICHAEL VAN SLYCK
Research Institute for Dispute Resolution, Buffalo

MARILYN STERN
State University of New York at Albany

The application of conflict resolution principles and techniques to educational settings consists of two primary forms, which are distinct but related. On the one hand are efforts concerned with curriculum development and implementation. This application ranges from full-scale semester-long curricula to more time-limited workshops, seminars, and presentations. The objective of this application is to teach students about nonadversarial conflict management and dispute resolution techniques, such as negotiation, mediation, and problem solving (e.g., Einstein, 1985; Loescher, 1983). The other major area of application consists of the implementation of actual dispute resolution programs as an alternative mechanism to standard disciplinary methods for resolving student conflicts. Most often these are peer mediation programs, in which students are trained in conflict resolution techniques to mediate disputes between other students.

In general, these applications have been undertaken separately. Most often, conflict resolution curricula and workshops are implemented without the development of actual conflict resolution programs. These efforts in curriculum implementation are usually limited to practice exercises such as role plays and workbook assignments. Similarly, conflict resolution programs are often implemented without the context of a comprehensive curriculum. A principal area of overlap is that conflict resolution programs necessarily include training components (e.g., workshops) that provide basic instruction in the concepts and skills of dispute resolution. These efforts, both curriculum development and program implementation, are currently being conducted at all levels of education—primary, secondary, and higher education.

The principal but not exclusive focus of the application of conflict resolution to educational settings is on the student (Lam, 1989). The goal of curriculum implementation is generally conceptualized as global and long-term in nature. The aim is to educate the student in conflict management concepts that can be applied to most aspects of the student's life, both in the present and in the future (e.g., Arnett, 1980). The implementation of actual dispute resolution programs includes this element, but has a more pragmatic, short-term goal of teaching specific techniques that can be actively used to resolve disputes between other students in a formal school-based setting.

A primary focus on the student can be contrasted with two other manifestations of the application of conflict resolution to educational settings. One involves the training of teachers in conflict management techniques to serve as mediators between students in conflict (Dana & John, 1986). The other approach focuses on the mediation of disputes between teachers and students (Kriedler, 1984). To date, only limited activity has been reported concerning these applications. An additional manifestation of the use of conflict resolution in educational settings that differs sharply from those delineated above can be noted: Specifically, alternative dispute resolution techniques are being used increasingly on a national level for resolving conflicts between parents and schools over such issues as the placement of children in regard to special education needs (Singer & Nace, 1985). The most recent count indicates that 28 states are currently using a program involving mediation services for resolving special education disputes (Achenbach, 1987).

The focus of this chapter is on peer mediation programs, in which students at the primary and secondary levels are trained to mediate disputes between other students. This focus has been chosen because this application constitutes the greatest area of activity and the one in which major portion of research has been conducted on conflict resolution in educational settings. Virtually no research has been conducted on programs in which the teacher is the mediator or in which teacher–student disputes are the focus. In addition, only limited research has evaluated the impact of curriculum implementation (Edleson, 1981; Kalmakoff & Shaw, 1987). Some research has examined other applications, such as the development of dispute resolution programs in higher education (Miller & Ledbetter, 1987) and special education mediation programs (Singer & Nace, 1985). However, these can be seen as distinct from primary and secondary peer mediation programs and more on a par with standard adult dispute resolution programs, in which the disputes are between adults and are mediated by adults.

Finally, an additional reason can be suggested for our focus on peer mediation at the primary and secondary levels. It can be argued that this application of conflict resolution to educational settings has the greatest potential for impact and therefore raises the most interesting and important questions. The nature of the impact of peer mediation, and issues associated with it, are delineated in the balance of this chapter.

HISTORICAL BACKGROUND

The application of conflict resolution to educational settings has a number of historical roots. Initial activity in this general area began in the middle to late 1960s, stemming from two distinct orientations. One orientation is what is generally referred to as the "peace and justice movement," which takes a broad view of conflict and is concerned with such issues as global peace and community violence (Davis, 1986). Another early orientation emerged from the field of academic educational psychology as the concept of cooperative learning in the classroom (Deutsch, 1974; Johnson & Johnson, 1983). This orientation suggests that cooperative experiences will promote higher academic and social achievement. These two orientations are still evident, with their impact predominantly in the area of curriculum development and implementation.

The growth of what is generally referred to as the "community dispute resolution movement," which began in the 1970s and burgeoned in the 1980s, resulted in a focus on the development and implementation of actual dispute resolution programs in schools (Davis, 1986). This more recent trend in the use of conflict resolution in educational settings came together in a more organized fashion in the mid-1980s—first in the form of a special conference of educators interested in this field, and subsequently in the form of the National Association for Mediation in Education, which serves as the major resource center, clearinghouse, and focal point for activity in this area (Davis, 1986). No precise statement of the number of schools that have developed peer mediation programs can be made. However, based on a general reading of the literature, it can be estimated that as many as several hundred such programs are currently operating across the country. Similar programs have also been developed on an international basis, primarily in English-speaking countries (e.g., Canada, Australia, New Zealand, England).

Two of the earliest peer mediation programs were developed in San Francisco and New York City (Davis, 1986). The San Francisco Community Boards program is community-based, is not generally involved with the criminal justice system, and focuses on issues of community development. The Community Boards School Initiatives Program, begun in 1982, has developed training and program models for elementary schools ("Conflict Managers") and secondary schools, and more recently has developed a full curriculum. In contrast, the SMART program in New York City operates under the auspices of a dispute resolution program that has a strong link to the criminal justice system. The auspices of these agencies are reflected in their orientation to the development of their programs. The Community Boards program can be characterized as a consultation model in which program staff members provide training for and assistance in implementing individual schools' programs, but generally do not engage in administration. In contrast, the SMART program institutionalizes and runs the programs in each school, monitoring their impact on such factors as suspension rates.

Other programs across the country embrace one or the other of these models, or vary on a continuum between them in terms of their independence from outside auspices; some programs change their orientation over time. One example comes from the school that served as the site for the principal research reported in this chapter. In this case, the peer mediation program was originated and implemented by a community dispute resolution program funded in large part by the New York State court system. Initially, cases processed at the school were counted as part of the statewide caseload. Subsequently, the school has largely withdrawn from this relationship and continues the program independently.

GOALS AND OBJECTIVES OF
PEER MEDIATION PROGRAMS

An examination of the goals and objectives of peer mediation programs is best undertaken in the broader context of community dispute resolution, from which it has emerged. It has been suggested (McGillis, 1986) that the community dispute resolution movement has to a large extent failed to achieve many of its initial goals, such as reducing court caseloads and backlogs, and delivering speedier and more cost-effective justice. However, it has been argued (McGillis, 1986) that these initial goals and objectives may well have been inappropriate expectations and thus unattainable. In line with this, it has been suggested (Roehl & Cook, 1985) that the community dispute resolution movement has been successful in achieving a number of its goals and objectives, when allowances are made for initial overenthusiastic and perhaps unwarranted expectations.

This context provides a basis for the examination of the goals and objectives that have been articulated for peer mediation programs—both reasonable and unreasonable. Clearly, the goals articulated for a program will influence the focus of any research conducted to examine its impact. To the extent that goals are broadly defined, and cannot be easily translated into observable and measurable events, they are less subject to meaningful scrutiny. In contrast, when goals are articulated in terms of observable and measurable events, research can be designed to produce evidence to determine the nature and quality of the impact of a program. A delineation and understanding of the goals, objectives, and expectations of peer mediation programs is therefore a necessary prerequisite for an analysis of research that attempts to elucidate and evaluate the impact of these programs.

The two historical roots of the application of conflict resolution in schools noted earlier can be differentiated by their respective emphasis on long-term, global goals versus short-term, pragmatic goals. From the "peace and justice" perspective, it is argued that it is the responsibility of schools to model the skills and techniques of peaceful and nonadversarial conflict resolution (Davis, 1986) and to involve children in peacekeeping alternatives before they become violent members of society. Indeed, it has been suggested that the learning of conflict resolution skills should become the "fourth R" (Davis, 1986). Thus, this orientation focuses chiefly on general issues of conflict in society, and its goal can be characterized as long-term and global in nature. This perspective suggests that exposure to conflict resolution principles will produce empowered citizens and therefore a more harmonious world. In contrast, the cooperative learning orientation places a primary emphasis on the short-term, pragmatic impact of conflict resolution activities. Its specific focus is on the potential benefits for education, with a goal of promoting academic and social achievement (Johnson & Johnson, 1983).

The community dispute resolution movement has brought with it goals that are in line with each of the categories outlined here—that is, short-term and pragmatic as well as long-term and global. Examples of long-term goals include having students learn citizenship and develop critical thinking skills (Davis & Porter, 1985). Examples of short-term goals include helping students to take more responsibility for discipline and to improve communication (Davis & Porter, 1985); teaching negotiation skills to resolve conflicts (De Cecco & Schaeffer, 1978); and producing positive and safe school discipline climates, thereby promoting school effectiveness (Purkey & Smith, 1982).

Clearly, these goals, objectives, and expectations vary from rather broad and abstract "hopes" for general but profound impact to more narrowly defined goals with more specific outcomes. The former, often value-laden, global, and long-term in nature, are therefore not easily amenable to quantitative measurement and validation. The latter are more pragmatic in nature, seek immediate impact, and are therefore more amenable to quantitative measurement and validation.

This analysis of the goals and objectives of the application of conflict resolution in schools can be related to the discussion of the goals and objectives of the broader community dispute resolution movement offered earlier. To the extent that the purpose of conflict resolution in the schools is based on such goals as promoting world peace and reducing community violence, it may be a long time, if ever, before evidence can be generated to assess success. Such an approach is analogous to what we have described earlier as the overly enthusiastic and therefore inappropriate initial goals of the community dispute resolution movement. To the extent that the goals and objectives embraced by advocates of conflict resolution in the schools are narrowly defined and pragmatic in nature, there will be a greater likelihood of developing a sound data base concerning the impact of such programs. Such a data base is necessary both to further our understanding of peer mediation and to generate the support and funding for further research and program development.

INITIAL RESEARCH ON PEER MEDIATION

To date, only limited research has been conducted that examines the nature or scope of the impact of school mediation programs (Lam, 1989). The first empirical study reported on a school-based peer mediation program was one we conducted with a colleague (Stern, Van Slyck, & Valvo, 1986). This study is reviewed in detail in this section. The purpose of this research was to establish an empirical basis upon which to make judgments concerning the impact of the program. Three areas of potential impact were selected for examination. These were the impact on "school discipline climate," defined as the perceptions of students and faculty concerning such issues as discipline and violence in the school setting, as well as the actual number of disciplinary problems and violent incidents; the effect on student peer mediators, including aspects of self-image; and the effect on student disputants, including the number and nature of disciplinary problems experienced subsequent to participation in a mediation. These areas were selected as the most likely indicators of a short-term, measurable impact of the program.

The program studied was implemented in a middle school (sixth through eighth grades) in New York State. The school is in one of the "target" areas in the state for a special education curriculum. It is thus made up of a disproportionate number of students enrolled in a compensatory remedial program. The majority of the students in the study had minority backgrounds and were from low-income families, and nearly one-half were welfare recipients. Adolescents (average age = 13.1 years) were trained as peer mediators in a 3-week program. These sessions were conducted by a professional trainer and focused on the acquisition of basic mediation skills. The participants trained as peer mediators were chosen by the administration so that they would represent a cross-section of the school population. Approximately one-half of the peer mediators scored below grade level on standardized tests of basic skills. Over one-third were enrolled in the compensatory remedial program at the time of the training. At the other end of the continuum, over one-third of the peer mediators were involved in the school council and were viewed as positive role models with leadership potential. In contrast, some of the peer mediators were considered negative role models by the administration.

The study employed a pre- and postintervention measurement design. To examine the overall impact of the mediation program on the school discipline climate, a questionnaire was distributed to all students and faculty prior to the start of the mediation program and at the end of the school year. This questionnaire was abstracted from the Discipline Context Inventory (Wayson, 1982). It was designed to assess attitudes concerning, and approaches to, such issues as conflict, discipline, and citizenship as they related to the quality of school life. In addition, a survey seeking general reactions to the program was administered to faculty members at the end of the school year.

To examine the impact of the program on students selected to be peer mediators, a battery of questionnaires was administered prior to training and at the end of the school year. This assessment battery included two of the self-image scales (Morals and Vocational–Education) from the standardized Offer Self-Image Questionnaire (OSIQ; Offer, Ostrov, & Howard, 1977). This instrument is a multidimensional measure of self-image, with higher scores indicating positive adjustment. Three subscales (Denial, Self-Blame, and Active Mastery/Problem-Solving) derived from the widely used Ways of Coping Scale (Folkman & Lazarus, 1985) were also employed. This instrument assesses preferred coping strategies used in dealing with a particular conflict or stressor. In addition, a questionnaire focusing on aspects of mediation training, leadership, and perception of self in relation to peers and family was completed by the participants. Finally, to evaluate the effectiveness of the program on disputants, their ratings of satisfaction with the mediation process, their compliance with the agreement, and subsequent disciplinary problems were assessed.

The results from the school discipline climate questionnaire for peer mediators showed a significant increase in positive attitudes several items. The peer mediators reported an increase in students' on being able to take responsibility in the school and being able to express their problems. In addition, the results for the faculty also showed positive increases in ratings on a number of the more pertinent questions relating to school discipline. Specifically, ratings of students' participation in solving school problems, feelings of school involvement, responsibility for enforcing rules, and perceptions of school discipline as good, as well as of staff–student ability to discuss problems, showed positive increases. In addition, the majority of respondents to the faculty evaluations reported a perception that conflict had decreased in the school. However, the results of the school discipline climate questionnaire for the student body did not show the predicted increases from first to second administration in students' perceptions of their involvement in school discipline matters.

The potentially most interesting results concerned the impact on peer mediators' self-image. The average OSIQ pretest standard scores on the Morals subscale for the trained mediators indicated a lack of any significant disruption for both males and females, with the scores falling almost exactly

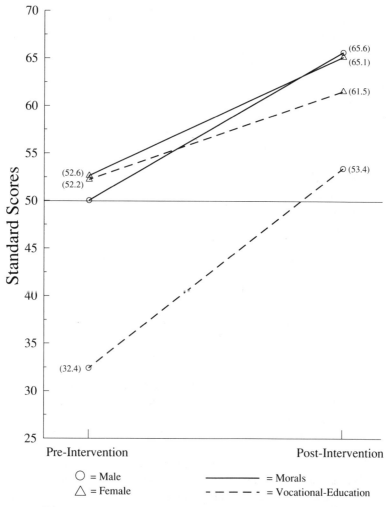

FIGURE 16.1.   Offer Self-Image Questionnaire (OSIQ) mean profile: Morals and Vocational–Education subscales. From *Enhancing Adolescents' Self-Image: Implications of a Peer Mediation Program* by M. Stern, M. Van Slyck, and S. Valvo, 1986, August, paper presented at the meeting of the American Psychological Association, Washington, DC.

at the standardized normed mean (see Figure 16.1; mean/average = 50). The average posttest standard scores were significantly higher for both males and females (representing an increase of 1.5 standard deviations) from prior to mediation training to the end of the school year. (The standards deviation is a measure of variation used to express how far any given score is from the average of a set of scores.) This substantial gain in scores indicated that the peer mediators developed a greater sense of "duty, responsibility, and concern for others" over the course of the mediation program (see Figure 16.1).

The average OSIQ standard score for females on the Vocational–Education subscale was within the standardized normed range (i.e., the average score). However, males exhibited a significantly poorer self-image than females (scoring nearly 2 standard deviations below the standardized mean). As Figure 16.1 indicates, the increase in scores for males was greatest. OSIQ scores for males increased from a significantly low self-image score to a score slightly above the standardized norm mean (a positive increase of over 2 standard deviations). Females also increased from an average self-image score on this dimension to a significantly above-average score (see Figure 16.1). This substantial gain in scores indicated that the peer mediators developed a greater sense of the personal importance of vocational and educational attainment over the course of the mediation program.

The preintervention profile for the peer mediators showed a somewhat greater reported preference for the use of denial and self-blame styles of coping, rather than active mastery, in dealing with their conflicts. These preferred styles are emotionally based and have been found to be associated with poorer functioning (Zevon, Tebbi, & Stern, 1987). It was hypothesized that training in and experience with mediation would enhance the development of the active mastery/problem-solving coping style. However, no change in coping style preference (e.g., higher scores on the Active Mastery/Problem-Solving subscale) was found from pre- to postintervention administration of the scales. It is not clear from this finding whether mediation does not have an impact on coping style preference or whether this particular measure is not sensitive to potential changes in this area.

In response to questions concerning their experiences in the program, peer mediators reported that they were more eager and more enthusiastic about becoming peer mediators at postintervention than at preintervention administration of the questionnaire. Interestingly, males were much less eager and enthusiastic about becoming mediators than females at the beginning of the program, but were somewhat more eager and enthusiastic than females by the end of the school year. A significant increase also was found in the peer mediators' perceptions of the importance of being a good leader from prior to the start of the program to the end of the school year. Finally, the peer mediators reported that they felt their talent for mediation increased from prior to the start of the program to the end of the school year.

A total of 81 cases were mediated by student mediators. Nearly one-half of the cases brought to mediation were characterized as involving rumors of a "he said she said" quality. The other half of the cases involved harassment or an actual physical fight. Of the disputants involved in the program, 75% reported that they would have had a fight if they had not been referred to mediation. Year-end school-wide data on reported fights also were examined. The data showed a decrease (16.7%) in the number of reported fighting incidents from the year prior to the implementation of the mediation program.

The results from this study suggest that the peer mediation program had an impact on all three areas examined. The positive increase in teacher ratings of student attitudes about school discipline, and the positive increase in peer mediators' perceptions on this same dimension, suggest a generally positive impact on school discipline climate, but one perhaps limited to those most actively involved in or aware of the peer mediation program. However, the subjective reports of fewer conflict incidents by faculty, the indication by disputants that a fight would have occurred in 75% of the cases referred to mediation, and the decrease reported in actual physical fights from the year before all suggest a broader impact on school discipline climate, as well as providing some support for the contention that the peer mediation program reduced violence. Possibly the most exciting aspect of the results are those concerning student mediators' self-image. The dramatic positive increases in self-image in the areas of social morality and vocational–educational attitudes suggest that the most important impact of peer mediator programs may be on those students who function in the capacity of peer mediators.

In conclusion, the results of this research effort indicate that the implementation of a peer mediation program had a positive impact on aspects of overall school discipline climate, reduced the level of violent disciplinary problems, and had potentially important beneficial effects on those students who participated as peer mediators. However, the methodological shortcomings of the research project clearly limit the certainty of any causal inferences that can be drawn. The full range of methodological problems found in peer mediation research is delineated in the next section. The major limitation of the study reported here was its failure to use a comparison or control group. The logistical constraints of the particular research setting prevented this possibility.

In this study, the failure to establish and use comparison control groups limits the validity of the results. Thus, any changes found over time may perhaps be attributed to other factors, such as what is referred to as the "Hawthorne effect" (i.e., a positive change in performance due to simple attention) or, in the case of adolescents, maturation. One effort used to counter this loss of methodological rigor was the use of standardized instruments to assess the impact of the program on peer mediators. The use of standarized measures allowed for comparison between the current adolescents' scores and those of a normed group of adolescents. This approach provides support for an attribution of a positive impact to the program. Finally, we should note that this was not a long-term study, although it was longitudinal in nature. Further data collection for a period of 1 or more additional years would have been necessary to investigate possible long-term effects, such as the enhancement of academic performance.

ASSESSING THE EVIDENCE ON PEER MEDIATION

With the growth of the number of peer mediation programs in the last 5 years, there has been a concomitant increase in efforts to describe them and to evaluate their impact. These efforts are limited in both quantity and quality, and virtually none has been published. Lam (1989) has reviewed and synthesized the results of the 14 extant efforts that have examined the impact of peer mediation (including the study reported in full above). These efforts vary both in the purpose of, and in the expertise brought to the study of, peer mediation programs (Lam, 1989). In fact, few of these qualify as acceptable research projects, with most best characterized as limited evaluation efforts. Overall, this body of research is devoid of a theoretical orientation and of methodological rigor.

The key issue in assessing the impact of peer mediation is the quality of the evidence concerning this impact. A lack of methodological rigor has a negative impact on the quality of evidence generated by research. A number of important methodological shortcomings in dispute resolution research have been noted (Kressel, Pruitt, & Associates, 1989). All of these are found in the research on peer mediation reviewed by Lam (1989). These include the lack of appropriate control groups (i.e., no comparison of students who are trained as peer mediators with those who are not trained); the failure to control for pretreatment differences (i.e., failure to ensure that the two groups of students compared are equivalent on important variables); the ignoring of possible placebo effects (i.e., failure to examine the impact of simply receiving attention); the failure to use standardized, reliable, and valid quantitative instruments (i.e., those measures with established norms that yield consistent results and measure what they intend to); and over-reliance on unvalidated, qualitative data (i.e., open-ended impressions of the program's impact). An additional problem is the consistency with which potential areas of impact are defined and examined. As Lam (1989) notes, few studies assessing the impact of peer mediation programs have examined the same variables. Even when the same impact is examined, it is often defined and operationalized in different ways. These methodological shortcomings limit the validity and generalizability of findings on peer mediation and its impact.

However, an examination of Lam's (1989) review and synthesis indicates that the results of these various research efforts are generally consistent with those of the initial study on peer mediation reported here (Stern et al., 1986) as well as with those of one another. This consistency lends credibility to the findings. In general, there is evidence that peer mediation programs have a positive impact on peer mediators, school discipline climate, and the amount of violence. There have been no findings of any school-wide positive impact on general attitudes toward school, and, with one exception (the New York City SMART program), no evidence for a decrease in the actual number of suspensions and detentions has been found.

Clearly, the broadest and most consistent findings on the impact of peer mediation programs are those concerning the peer mediators. Of these, the most important would seem to be the enhancement of aspects of self-image or self-esteem. This finding is supported by reasonably reliable, quantitative data from two studies and qualitative data from an additional four studies. Other areas of impact on the peer mediators that have been found with some consistency include positive effects on their general attitude toward conflict, their knowledge concerning and/or development of problem-solving skills, their perceptions of school discipline climate, their general attitude toward school, and their leadership experience (Lam, 1989). Support for one or more of this group of indicators is found in all but two studies. This evidence consists of both quantitative and qualitative data.

The other area of impact of peer mediation programs that has demonstrated some consistency is on what is referred to as "school discipline climate." Some limited and mostly qualitative data indicate an impact on school discipline climate, in that students and teachers report a generally better atmosphere in the school concerning these issues. These subjective reports are bolstered by indications of lessened actual violence. The evidence for the level and the extent of actual violence in the school consists of objective behavioral data (i.e., number of recorded violent incidents), as well as subjective reports by teachers of lessened violence and reports by students that a number of fights were prevented by the availability of mediation services.

These results indicate that the major impact of peer mediation programs is on the students who are selected, are trained, and go through the experience of being peer mediators. There is little evidence indicating a broader impact on general attitudes and skills of those students not going through this "core" experience. Even where an attitudinal effect is reported for the general student body (e.g., school discipline climate), it is strongest for the peer mediators. The recorded and reported reductions in the amount of violence are not supported (with the one exception noted above) by recorded decreases in actual detentions, suspensions, or expulsions. Concomitantly, to the limited extent that it has been examined, no positive impact has been reported in the area of delinquency prevention. Finally, virtually no evidence indicates a positive impact on academic performance for peer mediators, student disputants, or the general student body.

Yet another area of impact that has been examined by peer mediation program research is the actual resolution of student disputes. The majority of the studies reviewed by Lam (1989) examined this issue. The results are consistent with those reported in the broader community dispute resolution literature (Kressel et al., 1989) in finding a generally high rate of successful resolution. As Lam (1989) notes, however, this component has received little specific attention and seems to have been relegated to an ancillary issue in this area.

In conclusion, the results of the research on peer mediation conducted to date suggest two major points. On the one hand, the overwhelming majority of these research efforts did not employ acceptable methodological rigor. Specifically, the general failure to employ comparison groups, either within or across schools, makes the validity of any of the findings questionable. The use of nonstandardized measures and a reliance on unvalidated qualitative data also detract from credibility. On the other hand, there is a general consistency in the results of the research. The findings cluster in two areas, indicating a specific positive impact on peer mediators and a more general positive impact on school discipline climate and levels of violence. This consistency adds to the credibility of the findings.

Future research should replicate and extend the initial studies of peer mediation, using more rigorous methodology. The design of future research should address the methodological problems noted here through the implementation of a longitudinal, multidimensional, randomized controlled study. The principal areas examined in research to date—the effect on peer mediators, and the impact on school discipline climate and levels of violence—produced the strongest findings in our initial research (reported in the preceding section) and the strongest results in all subsequent research. Thus, they should constitute the primary areas of investigation in future research. In addition, potential areas of impact that have received only limited scrutiny should be more fully investigated. These include the short-term impact on the number of actual disciplinary actions and possible long-term effects on academic achievement and delinquency prevention.

DEVELOPING A THEORETICAL CONTEXT FOR PEER MEDIATION

As emphasized in the preceding section, methodological rigor is needed to produce a creditable data base for assessing the impact of peer mediation programs. However, the lack of methodological rigor is not the only problem with peer mediation research. An additional lack of a theoretical orientation limits the validity of these findings. The development of a theoretical orientation, as well as implementation of methodological rigor, is necessary both to advance our fundamental understanding of mediation and to foster programming efforts.

The majority of activity in, and most of the research on, peer mediation takes place with adolescents. This fact suggests the source of a potential theoretical framework—adolescent development. A principal issue in adolescent development is the resolution of what is referred to in the literature as the "independence–dependence" conflict (Erikson, 1968). Adequate resolution of this important developmental task is deemed necessary to the formation of the healthy adult personality. Successful resolution is fostered by an environment that allows for—indeed, encourages—the acquisition and development of adaptive, active, problem-solving-oriented coping skills (Stern & Zevon, 1990; Zevon et al., 1987). In turn, the development of more adaptive styles of coping both enhances and fosters the development of positive self-esteem.

A principal goal of the dispute resolution movement in general, and of mediation specifically, is the empowerment of the individual to address and resolve conflict without recourse to or dependence on authoritarian conflict resolution mechanisms. This orientation is manifested through mediation, which encourages individuals to take responsibility for resolving their conflicts by embracing a problem-solving approach. Thus, the prevailing orientation of dispute resolution, as well as its specific approach through mediation, is congruent with the necessary conditions for optimal resolution of the independence–dependence developmental task of adolescence.

This analysis suggests a theoretical explanation for the findings concerning the positive impact of peer mediation programs on peer mediators. Specifically, the development of the problem-solving skills associated with peer mediation is linked theoretically to research findings indicating that an enhancement of self-esteem results from the acquisition of such skills. This theoretical explanation also suggests why a more consistently positive impact is found for peer mediators and not for other students. It suggests that the actual acquisition and practice of skills, not mere exposure to concepts, are necessary for such an impact. The explanatory power of this theoretical framework for the findings on the impact of peer mediation can be useful for the generation of hypotheses to be tested in future research.

This theoretical analysis may be particularly relevant for students from "at-risk" populations. As noted, the population of student mediators examined in the initial study, in which the strongest impact on self-image was found, had an overrepresentation of disadvantaged, minority-group youths (Stern et al., 1986). This type of population constitutes the samples examined in over one-half of the research efforts conducted to date (Lam, 1989). Adolescents from disadvantaged backgrounds have been found to be at greater risk for problems in successfully resolving the independence–dependence task. To the extent that independence is achieved, it is often done by embracing negative models, which can result in greater use of drugs (Stern, Northman, & Van Slyck, 1984), higher dropout rates, and earlier sexual activity and unwanted pregnancies (Stern & Alvarez, 1987). Thus, peer mediation programs may have their greatest potential for impact on these populations as a method of primary prevention.

CONCLUSIONS AND IMPLICATIONS

The last decade has seen an increasing interest in and use of peer mediation programs. Numerous goals for and benefits of these programs have been articulated, but only a limited number have been documented or supported by creditable research (Lam, 1989). In this chapter, we have reviewed the development of peer mediation programs and the various goals advanced and claims made for them. In this regard, we have suggested that these goals for peer mediation can be divided into two categories—those that can be characterized as long-term and global (e.g., producing better citizens and a more harmonious world), and those which can be characterized as more short-term and pragmatic in nature (e.g., producing more engaged students and a more positive school discipline climate). We have suggested that the latter will be more easily observable and measurable than the former in any research that attempts to examine the impact of peer mediation.

In this context, we have reviewed the extant research on peer mediation, both our own and that of others. This limited body of research is circumscribed by distinct methodological flaws, which hamper inference and generalization. We have indicated the necessary steps to ensure methodological rigor in future research on peer mediation. However, the findings that have emerged to date are fairly consistent and suggest a real and positive impact of peer mediation programs on what can be regarded as short-term and pragmatic factors (e.g., enhancing the self-esteem of peer mediators, reducing the amount of physical violence, and promoting a more positive school environment).

We also have offered a theoretical framework that is consistent with the research findings and suggests an explanation for the impact found for peer mediation to date. Taken together, the theoretical framework offered, the methodological approaches suggested, and the areas of consistency in the research results provide the basis for the future direction of the study of peer mediation. Future research should further investigate the short-term effects that have been demonstrated by previous research, as well as the possibility of long-term effects in such areas as academic performance and delinquency prevention. The information generated from such research will provide a basis for determining the validity of the claims made for peer mediation.

Throughout this chapter, we have emphasized the necessity of establishing clear-cut, observable, and measurable goals as a basis for implementing and evaluating peer mediation programs. Only through such an approach can creditable information be generated to provide an understanding of the impact of peer mediation as a basis for making policy decisions concerning its use, implementation, and funding. Adherence to amorphous, global, and long-term goals is not likely to produce such evidence and may hamper the growth of this field. Specifically, we suggest here that an emphasis on this orientation may well produce some of the same negative experiences currently being manifested in the general dispute resolution field, in which the failure to meet initial overly enthusiastic goals has often resulted in a loss of credibility.

The contention that dispute resolution per se should become the "fourth R" in schools (Davis, 1986) may be unwarranted. Not surprisingly, the research findings that have emerged as creditable to date support the claims for short-term, pragmatic impact, with little evidence for long-term and global effects. Indeed, the results suggest that the simple exposure to dispute resolution concepts (i.e., "the fourth R" approach) may have little or no measurable or meaningful impact on students. In contrast, the evidence suggests that the acquisition and use of dispute resolution concepts and skills are the necessary components of achieving an impact.

Specifically, the peer mediators, and not student disputants or the general student body, are the ones who seem to benefit most from a peer mediation program. This is consistent with the assertion by Merry and Rocheleau (1985) that in the long term, the greatest positive impact of the dispute resolution movement will be on those individuals trained as mediators. This suggests that curriculum development and peer mediation program implementation should be fully integrated in such a way that all students are given the opportunity to practice their skills on a regular basis. The evidence suggests that only through this approach can peer mediation programs have the positive impact claimed for it by its proponents.

Acknowledgments

We take this opportunity to thank several people who were instrumental in conducting the research for the principal study reported in this chapter. Terry Funk-Antman, executive director of the Community Dispute Resolution Center of Dutchess County, New York, provided the impetus for this research. We were assisted greatly by Darshano Alba, former school project director; Chuck Kortz, former assistant principal; and Marva Clark, current assistant principal, all of the Poughkeepsie Middle School, Poughkeepsie, New York. Special thanks go to Nellie Mann, director of the School Mediation Project, who was instrumental in the collection of the data. We also would like to thank the National Association of Mediation in Education and Julie Lam for providing us with some of the resource information on the current status of mediation in educational settings presented in this chapter.

REFERENCES

Achenbach, G. (1987, Winter). Pennsylvania's special education mediation services, *N.A.M.E. News, 9*, pp. 3–4.

Arnett, R. (1980). *Dwell in peace: Applying nonviolence to everyday relationships.* Elgin, IL: Brethren Press.

Dana, D., & John, C. (1986). *Teacher mediation: Skills for settling conflicts between students.* Bloomfield, CT: Mediation Training Institute.

Davis, A. (1986). Dispute resolution at an early age. *Negotiation Journal, 2,* 287–297.

Davis, A., & Porter, K. (1985). Dispute resolution: The fourth 'R.' *Missouri Journal of Dispute Resolution, 1,* 121–139.

De Cecco, J., & Schaeffer, J. (1978). Using negotiation to resolve teacher–student conflicts. *Journal of Research and Development in Education, 2,* 64–77.

Deutsch, M. (1974). The social psychological study of conflict: Rejoinder to a critique. *European Journal of Social Psychology, 4,* 441–456.

Edleson, J. (1981). Teaching children to resolve conflict: A group approach. *Social Work, 26,* 488–493.

Einstein, V. (1985). *Conflict resolution.* St. Paul, MN: West.

Erikson, E. (1968). *Identity, youth, and crisis.* New York: Norton.

Folkman, S., & Lazarus, R. (1985). If it changes it must be a process: A study of emotion and coping during three stages of a college examination. *Journal of Personality and Social Psychology, 48,* 150–170.

Johnson, D., & Johnson, R. (1983). The socialization and achievement crisis: Are cooperative learning experiences the solution? In L. Bickman (Ed.), *Applied social psychology annual.* Beverly Hills, CA: Sage.

Kalmakoff, S., & Shaw, J. (1987). *Final report of the school peacemakers education project.* Burnaby, British Columbia.

Kressel, K., Pruitt, D. G., & Associates. (Eds.). (1989). *Mediation research: Studies in the process and effectiveness of mediation.* San Francisco: Jossey-Bass.

Kriedler, W. (1984). How well do you resolve conflict? *Instructor, 93,* 30–33.

Lam, J. (1989). *The impact of conflict resolution programs on schools: A review and synthesis of the evidence.* Amherst, MA: National Association for Mediation in Education.

Loescher, E. (1983). *Conflict management: A curriculum for peace K–12.* Denver, CO: Cornerstone: A Center for Justice and Peace.

McGillis, D. (1986). *Community dispute resolution programs and public policy: Issues and practices.* Washington, DC: National Institute of Justice.

Merry, S., & Rocheleau, A. (1985). *Mediation in families: A study of the children's hearing project.* Cambridge, MA: Cambridge Family and Children's Services.

Miller, J., & Ledbetter, C. (1987). Liberal arts faculty as mediators: The Pulaski County program. *Arkansas Political Science Journal, 7,* 1–7.

Offer, D., Ostrov, E., & Howard, D. (1977). *A manual for the Offer Self-Image Questionnaire for adolescents and parents.* Chicago: Michael Reese Hospital and Medical Center.

Purkey, S., & Smith, M. (1982). Too soon to cheer? Synthesis of research on effective schools. *Educational Leadership, 40,* 64–69.

Roehl, J., & Cook, R. (1985). Issues in mediation: Rhetoric and reality revisited. *Journal of Social Issues, 41,* 161–178.

Singer, L., & Nace, E. (1985). Mediation in special education: Two states' experience. *Ohio State Journal on Dispute Resolution, 1,* 55–98.

Stern, M., & Alvarez, A. (1987, April). *Adolescent mothers: Relationship between coping, self-image, and family environment.* Paper presented at the biennial meeting of the Society for Research in Child Development, Baltimore.

Stern, M., Northman, J., & Van Slyck, M. (1984). Father absence and adolescent "problem behaviors": Alcohol consumption, drug use, and sexual activity. *Adolescence, 19,* 301–312.

Stern, M., Van Slyck, M., & Valvo, S. (1986, August). *Enhancing adolescents' self-image: Implications of a peer mediation program.* Paper presented at the annual meeting of the American Psychological Association, Washington, D.C.

Stern, M., & Zevon, M. (1990). Stress, coping, and family environment: The adolescent's response to naturally occurring stressors. *Journal of Adolescent Research, 5,* 290–305.

Wayson, W. (1982). A stimulus for positive faculty action: The Discipline Context Inventory. In W. Wayson, G. S. De Voss, S. C. Kaser, T. Lasley, & G. S. Pinnell (Ed.), *Handbook for developing schools with good discipline.* Bloomington, IN: Phi Delta Kappa.

Zevon, M., Tebbi, C., & Stern, M. (1987). Psychological and familial factors in adolescent oncology. In C. Tebbi (Ed.), *Major topics in adolescent oncology* (pp. 325–349). Mount Kisco, NY: Futura.

17

Victim–Offender Reconciliation Programs

STEPHEN WOOLPERT
St. Mary's College

HISTORICAL BACKGROUND

Underlying the current growth of interest in victim–offender reconciliation programs (VORPs) is the confluence of two justice reform movements: one seeking greater concern for the plight of crime victims, and the other seeking alternative dispute resolution through "informal" or "neighborhood" justice. The idea of victim–offender reconciliation, however, originated in an impromptu experiment undertaken without a defined set of objectives. The "Elmira case," generally regarded as the progenitor of VORPs, began in 1974 as a routine case of teenage vandalism in the town of Elmira, Ontario. When the case reached provincial court in nearby Kitchener, Mark Yantzi, the probation officer assigned to the case, suggested an unusual idea to the presiding judge: "[T]here could be some therapeutic value in these two young men having to personally face up to the victims of their numerous offences" (quoted in Peachy, 1989, p. 15). To everyone's surprise, Judge Gordon McConnell acceded to his request. The probation officer proceeded to escort the two boys to 21 sites where they had caused damage; at each location the boys identified themselves as the culprits and explained that they had come to determine the costs of their misdeeds. They were subsequently fined $200 and placed on probation for 18 months, on the condition that they make restitution to the victims for their uninsured losses, which amounted to nearly $1,100. Within 3 months, the youths had personally delivered the money to each victim.

Mark Yantzi's interest in experimenting with alternatives to the formal criminal justice process stemmed from his earlier work with the Mennonite Central Committee (MCC). The Mennonites' long-standing interest in noncoercive conflict resolution made victim–offender mediation an attractive idea. The following year, Yantzi and his MCC colleagues formalized the Kitchener experiment into a program proposal called the Victim/Offender Reconciliation Project. In 1978, the Mennonite Church and the Prisoner and

Community Together (PACT) organization in Elkhart County, Indiana, established the first VORP in the United States. By 1986, 46 other programs had been created. The most recent inventory (Gehm & Fagan, 1989) identified 67 programs in operation in the United States, 35 in Canada, 18 in West Germany, and 12 in the United Kingdom. The National VORP Resource Center, created by PACT, serves as a nationwide clearinghouse for information, training, and technical assistance.

As Christie (1977, p. 1) points out, criminal conflicts "have been taken away from the parties directly involved and thereby have either disappeared or become other people's property." Offenders and especially victims are almost completely peripheral to the criminal justice process; attorneys, probation officers, and judges assume responsibility for processing the case. In the VORP process, by contrast, the parties meet voluntarily in a neutral setting away from the agencies of the government, in the presence of a lay member of their community, in order to deal informally with the entire range of issues involved—psychological, economic, and legal. VORPs seek outcomes that are individualized to meet the unique circumstances of each case. The primary objectives are reconciliation and restoration rather than deterrence and retribution.

The typical VORP is operated by a nonprofit (often church-based) organization rather than by a criminal justice agency. Community volunteers play a central role in most VORPs: receiving referrals from the criminal justice system, making the initial contacts with victims and offenders, scheduling and serving as neutral mediators at the face-to-face meetings, drawing up written statements of the nature of restitution agreed to, and monitoring subsequent progress toward completion of the agreements. The Dallas, Texas, Mediation and Restitution Program is the largest, with an annual caseload of 700. The more recently established VORPs have smaller caseloads (usually 20 to 40 per year); the average program caseload is 109. In 1989, VORPs in this country handled 4,692 cases, typically operating with one or two paid staff members and budgets of about $31,000 (Gehm & Fagan, 1989).

RATIONALE

Although the practice of reconciling criminal conflicts through personally arranged and performed restitution was originally developed by the MCC for reasons related to the historical pacifism of the Mennonite Church, each of the following nonsectarian justifications has been offered in support of the VORP concept. Some of these point to the superiority of VORPs over the *process* of adjudication, whereas others assert that it produces *outcomes* preferable to the conventional court-imposed sanctions of probation, fines, and incarceration. Some goals are common to all mediation programs; others are unique to the criminal justice context.

1. VORPs improve the conflict-resolving capacity of those involved. Mediation empowers people to participate in solving their own problems, rather than depending on the coercive power of the state's judicial and administrative apparatus to impose sanctions. The use of volunteer mediators promotes social integration and self-reliance by encouraging the use of cooperative problem-solving techniques.

2. The venting of feelings, the exchange of viewpoints, and the making of amends all help bring closure to the criminal event. Mediation is collaborative, not adversarial. By personalizing the conflict resolution process, VORPs attempt to alter the stereotypical notions that victims and offenders who are strangers often hold about each other. In cases where the crime is the consequence of an underlying conflict between the parties, mediation strives to get to the root of such problems by permitting the parties themselves to identify the issues involved. Each party comes to have a better understanding of the significance of the crime for the other party, why it occurred, and its impact.

3. Victims receive material compensation for their losses. But unlike state-supported victim compensation programs, mediated restitution allows the parties themselves to determine appropriate and often creative methods by which the offender can personally contribute to the victim's well-being, generally through direct service or earned money.

4. Restitution has a reformative effect on criminals. In addition to the educational benefits of hearing the victim's experience of the event, VORPs provide offenders with a chance to take responsibility for the consequences of their actions and to make amends, thereby assuaging guilt and enhancing feelings of self-worth. Voluntary mediation also lessens the labeling and alienating effects of traditional punishments.

5. By achieving reconciliation rather than mere punishment, VORPs prevent further trouble. Insofar as crime represents a breach in the bonds that hold the community together, mediated restitution serves as a social healing process. Hence, the level of fear and tension in the community at large is reduced to a degree not attainable through the operation of the formal criminal justice system.

6. VORPs divert cases away from the court system. By relieving overburdened criminal justice personnel of a portion of their caseload, they free scarce resources for other disputes.

7. The VORP procedure is speedier and less costly than the more formal and cumbersome adjudication process.

8. The outcomes of mediated restitution are fairer than those of the formal criminal justice system. The goal of restorative justice is attained to

the extent that offenders are held accountable for the damage done to their victims, victims are able to attain closure regarding the crime, and community ties are strengthened.

The multiplicity of goals has proven to be both a help and a hindrance in the spread of VORPs. On the one hand, different constituencies may be attracted to the program for different reasons, creating a broad potential base of support. Unfortunately, it is not possible to optimize all of these goals simultaneously; each program makes tradeoffs, pursuing some subset of goals to the neglect of others, or seeking a compromise that partially fulfills many objectives but achieves none satisfactorily. Lack of agreement about a VORP's precise aims also confounds attempts at evaluation, since its success can only be measured against a predetermined set of purposes.

In reviewing the principal theoretical and practical issues concerning the operation of VORPs, I begin by considering each of the major participants in the process: the victim, the offender, and the mediator. I then consider the relationship between VORPs and the social context in which they operate—that is, the criminal justice system and the community at large.

PARTICIPANTS IN THE PROCESS

The Victim

One of the most striking features of the VORP model is the active role that the victim plays in determining the disposition of the case. Several obstacles have traditionally prevented victims from participating in the criminal justice process. First, our system of jurisprudence regards crimes as offenses against the public order, and so it is the state, not the victim, that levies charges and imposes sanctions. Second, as criminal cases proceed through the stages of adjudication, the actors in the system have progressively less information about the harm inflicted on the victim. Third, case outcomes are influenced more by the evidence, the offender's prior record, and the values of criminal justice officials than by the crime's impact on the victim (Hernon & Forst, 1984).

It is no longer accurate to say, however, that victims are ignored by criminal justice officials. The President's Task Force on Victims of Crime (1982) made numerous recommendations for improved treatment of victims. The Victim and Witness Protection Act became law. A special Office for Victims of Crime was created within the Justice Department's Office of Justice Assistance, Research and Statistics. Changes in state and local practices have also occurred, spurred by such groups as the National Organization for Victim Assistance, the Victims Assistance Legal Organization, and the Victim's Committee of the American Bar Association.

Despite these developments, however, there remain two common objections to the idea of including victims in the criminal justice decision-making process (Galaway, 1985): (1) Victims do not want to participate, and (2) victims will be vindictive toward offenders. The available evidence, although incomplete, casts doubt on each of these assertions.

The most important issue, both theoretically and administratively, is the question of whether victims are willing to engage in the process of mediation. On the one hand, participation offers both psychological and economic benefits: the chance to discover the criminals' identity and motivation, the opportunity to receive an apology and to experience ownership of the conflict, the opportunity to tell their story and possibly prevent further crimes by helping offenders appreciate the harm they have caused, and the recovery of monetary losses. On the other hand, meeting an offender may evoke painful memories and arouse feelings of fear or anger that a victim would prefer to avoid. Since many offenders are unable to make more than modest restitution and are given time to pay, victims may be justifiably skeptical about the prospects of receiving comprehensive compensation. Others may be insulted by the idea that they can ever be "made whole" by the offenders. Even though many victims want to be better informed about the progress of their cases, they may not wish to share the responsibility of deciding what should happen to the offenders.

Several studies of VORPs have shown that a majority of victims contacted are willing to engage in face-to-face meetings with their offenders (Galaway, 1985; Reeves, 1989). The VORP in Elkhart County, Indiana, for example, reported that from 1978 to 1982 between 60% and 70% of victims contacted took part in mediation. In Umbreit's (1986) study of burglary victims referred to the VORP in Hennepin County, Minnesota, 62% of those interviewed elected to meet with their offenders. Far less information is available on the types of victims who are most likely to participate. The victims in Coates and Gehm's (1989) sample were fairly diverse in terms of age and education. Launay and Murray (1989) indicate that elderly women are more likely to have difficulty confronting burglars than are other burglary victims, and O'Brien (1987) reports that victims of more serious offenses and victims who know the offenders well are less interested than others are in mediation.

Evidence on the reasons for victims' participation or nonparticipation is also scanty, but Reeves (1989) reports that the desire to know more about offenders and their motives was the paramount reason for participating, followed by the desire to let offenders learn the consequences of their actions and the desire to ventilate feelings. Coates and Gehm (1989), by contrast, found that victim's primary goals were recovering their losses, helping the offenders, and participating meaningfully in the criminal justice process. Umbreit (1989a) reports that the victims in his study were more interested in fairness than in retribution. The components of fairness mentioned most frequently were meeting the offenders' need for rehabilitation and holding the offenders accountable for the consequences of their conduct. Despite isolated instances of victims' attempting to victimize their offenders (McKnight, 1981), for the large majority of victims the importance of financial restitution appears to be based on their desire for restorative justice rather than private gain. This runs counter to the expectation of those who fear that victims would be vindictive.

Clearly, much remains to be learned about the attitudinal and circumstantial correlates of victim participation. The amount of time elapsed between the crime and the invitation to meet the offender is likely to be influential, particularly in more traumatic cases. Program characteristics may also be important (e.g., whether the meeting occurs before or after adjudication, the conduct of the mediator, etc.).

As important as obtaining such information, however, is ensuring that the information is available for use by those who refer cases to VORPs. In most cases, eligibility criteria are based on characteristics of the offender and/or the offense, in part because victim data are not available to prosecutors, judges, and probation officers. Since the program is intended to meet some of the victim's needs, it is appropriate to take victim data into account when referring cases for mediation.

Ensuring the voluntariness of victims' participation is another potentially difficult issue. Usually an offender's willingness to meet a victim is ascertained first, to avoid the risk of disappointing a willing victim whose offender refuses to seek reconciliation. When the initial contact with the victim takes place, therefore, the victim usually is told that the offender has already agreed to meet. This, coupled with the VORP staff member's temptation to encourage participation by "selling" the benefits of mediation, may put undue pressure on an unwilling victim. Those who choose not to participate may feel guilty or angry at such pressure. Particular attention needs to be given to the design and evaluation of the initial VORP contact with the victim, to assure that participation is genuine and to minimize the psychological costs of refusal to participate.

For certain classes of victims it may be desirable to modify the structure of the program. Both the Oklahoma Department of Corrections and the Genesee County Sheriff's Department in Batavia, New York, for example, have extended the VORP model from nonviolent property offenses to crimes of violence, such as robbery, assault, rape, and manslaughter (Umbreit, 1986, 1989b). Victims in such cases require a longer period of time between the offense and the initial VORP contact, more extensive pre- and post-mediation contacts, and the provision of additional victim services.

Another variation has been developed in England. Group sessions are arranged between victims of unsolved burglaries and youths convicted of burglary (Launay & Murray, 1989). Such meetings, called Victims and Offenders in Conciliation, are held at the detention center where the offenders are serving their sentences. They are not aimed at producing restitution agreements, but at positive attitude change and better understanding on both sides. The Minnesota Restitution Center also works with prisoners, providing a halfway house for parolees to live in while they make reparations to their victims (McGillis, 1986).

The final issue regarding victims in the VORP process is that of the benefits they actually receive from participating. Victims should be able to claim all relevant losses associated with the crime (repair and replacement of property, medical expenses, lost work time, etc.). However, even though 90% of property crimes involve losses of less than $250, it is unrealistic for victims to expect that full restitution by offenders is guaranteed.

According to the *Victim–Offender Reconciliation and Mediation Program Directory* (Gehm & Umbreit, 1986), over 90% of victim–offender meetings result in a mutually acceptable restitution agreement. Studies of the amount of restitution actually paid by offenders do not generally distinguish between VORPs and other restitution programs. For example, the National Juvenile Restitution Initiative conducted by the U.S. Department of Justice (Schneider, Schneider, Griffith, & Wilson, 1982) observed some 10,000 delinquent youths from various restitution programs in 85 communities over a 2-year period. Of these youths, 88% successfully completed restitution to their victims and/or communities. In all, over $1.5 million and over 200,000 hours of unpaid work were received. The average victim received about $180. McGillis's (1986) survey of 27 adult restitution programs, including eight VORPs, also found that in a substantial majority of cases full restitution was made, with payments generally ranging from $200 to $250. In the absence of more accurate and complete data, it is difficult to determine the success of VORPs in making victims whole in economic terms. In many cases even partial payment may be worthwhile in defraying the costs of crime, whereas payments in others may be marginal and insufficient.

Victims' attitudes toward the fairness of restitutionary punishments are generally favorable (Hudson & Galaway, 1980). Umbreit (1989a) reports that victims who took part in mediation were twice as likely to have experienced fairness as those who declined to participate. Hughes and Schneider (1989) sampled representatives of 79 VORPs for juvenile offenders. Their respondents strongly agreed that the outcomes were both satisfactory and fair to victims, but the basis for such evaluations is not clear.

Victims' satisfaction with the VORP process is not solely a function of the financial compensation received. Even a sincere apology can have a therapeutic effect. The *Guide to Juvenile Restitution* (Schneider, 1985) states:

> It is very important to highlight the fact that the focus of the VORP process is reconciling the conflict between the victim and offender. The actual restitution agreement that is worked out by both is a tangible byproduct of the reconciliation. (p. 53)

There is, in fact, evidence that the psychological benefits are viewed by victims as more important than restitutionary payments. Coates and Gehm (1989) report that 83% of the 37 victims interviewed were satisfied with the VORP process. The personal meeting with the offender was seen as the most satisfying aspect of the experience. Similar results have been obtained by Ruddick (1989), Launay and Murray (1989), and Marshall and Merry (1988). Reasons for victims' dissatisfaction include the length of time between the offense and the meeting, and the failure of some offenders to provide restitution as promised.

The best study to date of the broader psychological effects of mediated restitution on victims is that by Davis, Tichane, and Grayson (1980) of a Brooklyn, New York program dealing with felonies among acquaintances. In a random assignment experiment, some cases were assigned to mediation and others to routine court procedure. Among the major findings were the following:

1. Sixty-two percent of mediation case victims felt that the behavior of the defendants had improved after the session, compared with 40% of court case victims.
2. Forty-eight percent of court case victims remained angry at their victims following the conclusion of their cases, compared with 23% of mediation case victims.
3. Confusion regarding the offenders' motives was expressed by 50% of court case victims, but only 38% of mediation case victims.

Finally, Zehr (1985) reports an evaluation of five VORPs in Indiana and Ohio, in which improved attitudes toward the criminal justice system were indicated by nearly half the victims.

The Offender

VORPs are designed not only to empower and repay victims, but also to hold criminals personally accountable for the damage their crimes cause. Unlike conventional sanctions, in which criminals' only responsibility is to submit obediently to state control, mediated restitution presupposes an obligation on criminals' part to make at least symbolic amends to their victims; reconciliation can occur only if the offenders agree to accept that obligation. As with other restitutionary sentencing programs, the underlying goal is neither retribution nor prevention of future crimes (though these may also result), but restorative justice (Abel & Marsh, 1984; Barnett, 1977; Schafer, 1970).

In principle, the VORP model is applicable to a wide variety of offenders. In practice, few programs accept every case referred to them; most have selection criteria that target particular offender subgroups. Of the 67 programs listed in the latest VORP directory (Gehm & Fagan, 1989), 29 accept only juveniles, whereas 14 are exclusively for adults. In a 1983 survey by Coates and Gehm (1989), 73% of participating offenders were under age 18. Hughes and Schneider (1989) report that violent offenders are most often excluded from juvenile VORPs, but sex offenders, child abusers, substance abusers, and the mentally retarded or disturbed are also ineligible in some jurisdictions. The most common offenses accepted for mediation are nonviolent property crimes (e.g., burglary, theft, and vandalism), although, as mentioned above, violent offenders have been targeted in Oklahoma and upstate New York. Eight of the programs listed in the latest VORP directory (Gehm & Fagan, 1989) take only misdemeanor cases, and five take only felonies.

Hardened criminals, those who deny their guilt, and those who show no remorse are unlikely to be predisposed to seek reconciliation with victims; consequently, they are often considered inappropriate for VORPs. In addition, since the face-to-face meeting requires at least some communication skills, those who have difficulty expressing themselves may be hampered in their efforts to achieve reconciliation, even with the help of a skilled mediator. Offenders deemed most likely to benefit include naive or first-time offenders and offenders whose ongoing relationship with their victims is such that future offenses may occur if the air is not cleared between them. Coates and Gehm (1989) found that only 20% of victims in their survey had prior convictions and that only 17% had previously been sentenced to jail or prison. Empirical data on the relative willingness of various offender subgroups to meet their victims and make restitution are needed.

Despite the hope of proponents that VORPs may serve as an alternative to incarceration, most cases referred to such programs involve offenders who would otherwise have received probation (McGillis, 1986). There is some evidence, however, that VORP participation may reduce the courts' reliance on confinement as a sanction. Coates and Gehm (1989) compared matched groups of VORP participants and nonparticipants in terms of postconviction incarceration. About equal numbers were incarcerated from each group, but the VORP group served shorter sentences and were more likely to be sentenced to jail rather than state prison.

However, for those offenders who would otherwise have been placed on probation with no restitutionary obligation, taking part in the VORP process represents a greater intrusion of the justice system into their lives. This underscores the need for close scrutiny of selection criteria. As with so many innovative justice reforms, there is a danger of "creaming"—that is, selecting cases with the most favorable prognosis, thereby widening and strengthening the net of social control (Dittenhoffer & Erikson, 1983).

Participation by offenders in the reconciliation process is never compulsory. Those who deny their guilt, of course, retain the right to seek acquittal or dismissal of charges in court. But even when guilt is not an issue, some elect not to participate. Umbreit (1986) states that 21% of the juveniles referred to the Minneapolis VORP declined to take part; about half of the youths randomly assigned to the Washington, D.C. program chose probation instead (Schneider, 1986).

Why do offenders agree to engage in the reconciliation process? Unlike victims, offenders often face more than just subtle psychological pressure to participate. Most referrals come from criminal justice authorities who are in a position to bring coercive pressure to bear on offenders. Some see a VORP as merely the lesser of two evils. McKnight (1981) and Ruddick (1989) discuss instances in which offenders agreed to mediation in order to avoid prosecution or harsher sanctions. Offenders in the Coates and Gehm (1989) evaluation believed they had little choice but to take part. Although some do agree to take part out of a sincere desire to reconcile the dispute, or at least to mitigate their sense of guilt by offering an explanation, not enough is known about offenders' reasons for entering the mediation process, nor about the relationship between initial motivation and the probability of a successful outcome.

The conciliatory manner in which VORPs handle disputes is seen by some as their primary virtue. Nonetheless, it is important to examine the consequences they produce. A critical factor influencing the outcomes of victim–offender mediation is criminals' earning capacity. A significant number of offenders are unemployed or earn too little to make meaningful financial restitution. Many VORPs respond to this problem by helping indigent offenders find work. This can be accomplished in several ways. A few programs arrange for jobs with employers from the private sector. The leading example of this strategy is the Earn-It program in Quincy, Massachusetts, which works with the local Chamber of Commerce to provide employment opportunities for juveniles who are making restitution (Klein & Kramer, 1981). Some employers with high turnovers come to rely on referrals from the justice system; others participate out of a civic-minded commitment to aid victims and offenders in their community.

Other VORPs arrange for jobs in public or nonprofit agencies or on work crews supervised by program staff. In some cases, third-party funding, grants, or corporate contributions are used to subsidize such employment. A third strategy is to provide training programs in job search and employment skills. Employers often prefer to hire offenders who apply on their own after completing job training, rather than court-referred applicants (Schneider, 1985).

Each of these strategies is the cause of some concern. In areas where unemployment is high, objections may be raised when convicted criminals receive help that is not available to law-abiding job seekers. Conversely, there is the risk of offenders' being exploited as a source of cheap labor. Finally, offenders in custody are not helped by any of these approaches, so that only those deemed not to be a threat to public safety are in a position to make financial restitution. Some authors (Abel & Marsh, 1984; Cannon,

1982; Hickey & Scharf, 1980; Smith, 1963) have argued that incarcerated criminals (excluding the mentally and physically incompetent) should be given the opportunity to repay their victims while in confinement by performing meaningful work at prevailing wages. Their release would be contingent upon completion of the restitution agreement. However, the cost of incarceration is already so high that there is little political support for increasing the wages paid to prisoners. Organized labor also opposes the idea of providing work for prisoners that could otherwise be done by union workers.

On the other hand, it should not be assumed that financial reparation is required for reconciliation to occur. Personal service to the victim, an agreement to change certain behaviors, or even a formal apology may be satisfactory. Given the evidence cited above that victims place greater value on the psychological than on the monetary benefits of meeting their offenders, symbolic restitution is by no means a secondary goal of mediation.

The effect of mediated restitution on offenders' attitudes and subsequent behavior has not yet received the careful attention it deserves. Tittle (1978) has speculated that restitution agreements may motivate offenders to commit further crimes in order to repay their original victims, but there is no empirical evidence to support this concern. Like victims, offenders generally express the belief that mutually agreed-upon restitution is fair (Hudson & Galaway, 1980). Those who work in VORPs tend to share that belief and to view their programs as having a rehabilitative effect on offenders (Hughes & Schneider, 1989). Offenders in Coates and Gehm's (1989) evaluation reported satisfaction with discovering that their victims were willing to meet them and with the opportunity to "make things right." About half reported a change in their attitudes about crime, particularly increasing awareness of its lasting impact on victims. Eighty percent agreed that justice had been served in their cases.

Most of the evidence regarding the favorable behavioral impact of VORPs on offenders is impressionistic and anecdotal (Umbreit, 1989b; McKnight, 1981; Schneider, 1985; Zehr & Umbreit, 1982). However, one quantitative study of the relationship between reconciliation and recidivism (Schneider, 1986) in the Washington, D.C. VORP shows promising results. Serious juvenile offenders (i.e., offenders with at least one felony conviction) who were randomly assigned to victim–offender mediation had a significantly lower recidivism rate than comparable offenders receiving straight probation. However, youths who were selected for restitution but who refused to participate also had lower recidivism rates than those assigned to probation. The authors speculate that all those selected for restitution were given an opportunity to participate in determining their disposition, whether they agreed to mediation or not, and that this allowed them to choose the option best suited to their motives and circumstances.

But positive findings are not universal. A Vera Institute of Justice study of criminal disputes between acquaintances (Davis et al., 1980), also using random case assignments, found no significant differences between mediation and adjudication in reducing subsequent hostilities. A similar conclusion was reached by Felstiner and Williams (1979–1980) in their follow-up investigation of the community mediation program in Dorchester, Massachusetts.

The methodological difficulties associated with recidivism research, coupled with the paucity of relevant data that most VORPs collect about offenders, had hindered assessment of their effectiveness in this area. One should not expect exposure to a VORP by itself to have a major impact on offenders, whose lives are typically beset by countless personal problems and repeated instances of failure and antisocial behavior. For some, participating in a VORP may be the first socially approved act they have successfully performed. Any program that shows evidence of even slight improvement in the outlook and conduct of offenders, however, is welcome. There are good theoretical reasons to investigate the extent of VORPs' success in this regard. It is particularly important to determine which program models are most effective with which types of offenders—a question about which little is currently known.

The Mediator

Despite the concerns of some criminal justice professionals regarding the use of volunteers in VORPs, many programs rely on trained community laypersons to facilitate the face-to-face meetings between offenders and victims. Two-thirds of the sessions reviewed by Coates and Gehm (1989) were conducted by volunteer mediators. However, Hughes and Schneider (1989) found that only 45% of the programs in their survey used volunteers at all, and only 8% relied exclusively on volunteer mediators. Programs that deal primarily with violent crimes rely on professional mediators, because the effects on the victims tend to be far more traumatic (Umbreit, 1989b).

In programs that do not use volunteers, staff members from the nonprofit organization or local probation department operating the program serve as mediators. However, even these may use volunteers to help with fund raising, publicity, clerical work, transportation, or locating jobs and community service placements for offenders (Schneider, 1985). There are several benefits to using nonprofessional mediators. It prevents the parties from deferring to a paid expert in the negotiating process. It underscores the neutrality of the process by excluding the presence of those responsible for supervising offenders. And it gives an active role in the management of conflicts to members of the community, who are more likely than justice system professionals to share the same values and outlook as the disputants.

The training of mediators generally requires between 16 and 32 hours in the classroom, followed by apprenticeship to an experienced mediator for two or three cases. The median training time in programs reviewed by Hughes and Schneider (1989) was 20 hours, plus 9 hours of in-service work. Such training ordinarily includes information about the nature and purpose of victim–offender mediation; the operation of the criminal justice system; the experience of victims and offenders in the justice system; and mediation principles, procedures, and techniques. Presentations of videotapes and role plays are typically included. A few programs, however, reported no formal mediator training at all.

Some programs also help the trainees understand their own motives for becoming mediators (Felsteiner & Williams, 1982). Grønfers (1989) identifies three general types of motivations: Some trainees are critical of the criminal justice system and seek alternatives to it; some support the system and want to help it operate better; and some wish to make a personal contribution to their community, without considering broader issues of principle or organization. The mediators studied by Coates and Gehm (1989) mentioned humanizing the system, increasing offenders' accountability, and providing a larger role for victims as their main goals.

Mediators are trained to be nonjudgmental, objective, active listeners who gain the trust of both sides. They are also urged to emphasize the difference between mediation and adjudication by not interrupting or interrogating the disputants. Instead, they learn to elicit information through reflective and nonverbal prompts. Patience, flexibility, quick absorption of information, and assertiveness skills are useful traits.

The first task that a mediator faces after a case has been referred to and accepted by the program is to contact the offender and victim separately, in order to introduce them to the VORP concept and determine their willingness to meet the other party. At this time each party is encouraged to tell his or her story, not only to provide the mediator with information about the crime but also to establish rapport with the mediator and to lower the emotional level at the subsequent mediation session. The role of the mediator and of each participant in the face-to-face meeting is explained, and the potential benefits are outlined. It is advisable to conduct the initial meeting with the offender first in order to determine possibilities for restitution. This information can then be conveyed to the victim to prevent unrealistic expectations from developing. Finally, the mediator seeks an agreement from the victim to meet the offender at a specific time and place; many victims prefer a neutral setting such as the VORP office, whereas others want the meeting to be held in their homes. Some encouragement on the part of the mediator is considered permissible, but overselling the program is dangerous, and the parties' freedom to decline must be respected. The consent of the parents of juvenile offenders and victims may also be necessary.

Reconciliation is possible even in the absence of a face-to-face meeting. Harding (1989) and Ruddick (1989) describe programs in which mediators engage in "shuttle diplomacy," serving as intermediaries for parties who do not wish to engage in direct negotiations. This approach retains some of the benefits of personal confrontation (e.g., exchanging information and feelings, working out mutually acceptable reparations contracts) with less emotional strain. However, given the evidence cited above that many participants consider the face-to-face meeting to be the most satisfying part of the reconciliation process, mediators should serve as go-betweens only if no other form of negotiations is acceptable to the parties.

Mediation is often most effective if it occurs as soon as possible after the offense, when memories are freshest (Veevers, 1989). If mediation takes place after a case has been adjudicated, the adversarial process may polarize the conflict and inhibit reconciliation (Shaw, 1989). Delays may also frustrate victims, further complicating the mediation process. Victims of violent crimes, however, often need a considerable period of time and several advance meetings with the mediator before they are psychologically ready to face their offenders (Umbreit, 1989b).

Ideally, the mediator opens the meeting by introducing everyone and explaining the ground rules of the process. The victim and offender then discuss facts and feelings concerning the crime, followed by negotiations about possible restitution. If agreement is reached, both parties sign a written statement of the terms. In cases where juveniles are involved, their parents also sign the agreement. A follow-up meeting is then scheduled to review progress toward completing the agreement.

In practice, a number of difficulties may arise. Both the victim and the offender are likely to walk into the mediation session with some apprehension, despite the reassurances they have received ahead of time. Communication may be slow and awkward. In "status offense" cases involving adolescents who have run away from home or are beyond parental control, the "victim" is the parent or guardian, who also has legal authority over the offender. The task of the mediator is more complicated in such disputes.

If there is a disparity in status or power between the two, such as in crimes by indigent criminals against wealthy individuals or corporations, the weaker party is apt to be at a disadvantage. An objectively fair settlement in these cases may reinforce an offender's belief that the powerful get what they want while the weak suffer what they must. The danger of this is especially great if such cases dominate the program's caseload; for example, a study of the Columbus, Ohio, Night Prosecutor Program found that 61% of the cases involved business complaints against customers for bad checks (McGillis & Mullen, 1977). Moreover, defendants may feel obligated to acquiesce to their victims' demands in order to avoid a harsher sentence in court. Alternatively, a persuasive offender may talk a nervous victim into accepting an unfair settlement. An offender may also conclude from the victim's acceptance of an apology that the crime was not blameworthy.

In such situations, the mediator must walk a fine line between regulating the interaction in order to maximize the benefits for both parties and maintaining neutrality regarding the reasonableness of a victim's request for restitution. A superficial agreement that only buries underlying conflicts may be worse than none at all. The mediator is expected to aid the communication process, focus the discussion on areas where interests converge, and ensure that both parties genuinely "own" the agreement.

The mediator is also responsible for monitoring the offender's compliance with the terms of the agreement and submitting a final report. In approximately 20–25% of cases, the offender fails to complete the terms of the restitution agreement. This may necessitate additional victim–offender meetings. If possible, the same mediator is present at each session. In some cases, noncompliance results from a restitution agreement that is beyond the offender's ability to pay or that is perceived by the offender as excessive— both of which indicate that the mediator failed to guide the initial negotiations satisfactorily. In other cases, however, the offender may simply have become unemployed or suffered personal misfortune.

The follow-up meeting addresses these issues and searches for realistic, mutually acceptable modifications to the agreement. Compliance rates are higher in programs that monitor offender performance closely and in which courts have tools for enforcing compliance, such as liens; garnishments; and revocation of probation, parole, or suspended sentences (McGillis, 1986). However, reliance on coercive sanctions runs counter to the goal of voluntariness, which is argued to be an integral part of genuine reconciliation (Tomasic & Feeley, 1982).

Considerable research is needed on the relationship among mediator characteristics, mediation styles, and VORP outcomes. Is reconciliation more likely to result if mediators share some of the same social background characteristics as the parties? Do volunteers actually share the same values as victims and offenders? Do justice system professionals and volunteers achieve similar results as mediators? In what kinds of cases, if any, is active intervention by the mediator preferable to passive facilitation? Such information is needed to improve our understanding of the dynamics of mediated restitution.

THE CONTEXT OF VICTIM–OFFENDER MEDIATION

Relation to the Justice System

Face-to-face mediation and making amends to attain reconciliation are essential components of all VORPs. Implementation of these generic characteristics, however, takes place in a variety of ways. Underlying these differences in program design are divergent philosophies about the role that victim–offender reconciliation should play in the social system. The first question that needs to be answered before a new program is begun is whether it is intended to be an alternative to the criminal justice system or a part of it. The former position emphasizes its noncoercive, informal, deprofessionalized qualities, whereas the latter stresses its potential for improving the system's flexibility, responsiveness, and efficiency.

Closely related to this issue is the determination of the program's primary objectives. Those who view VORPs as alternatives to the system see improved understanding and reconciliation between offenders and victims as the major goals. Those who view VORPs as part of the system give greater weight to victim restitution and reform of the offenders. Several organizational issues are affected by these divergent orientations. Should the program be operated by a private nonprofit agency using trained volunteers, or by the probation department using paid staff? Is the mediated agreement that is reached by a victim and an offender independent of legal sanctions, or should it be aimed at influencing the sentencing of the offender and therefore enforced by the court? Will the program accept disputes directly from the public or only from the justice system? Should the outcomes be determined by the parties' subjective perception of fairness or by objective criteria (i.e., the actual harm suffered by the victim)?

Coates and Gehm (1989) distinguish four idealized VORP models:

1. *The normalized community conflict resolution model*. Local residents voluntarily bring their disputes, both criminal and noncriminal, to a reconciliation program funded and operated independently of the criminal justice system. Improvement in interpersonal relations is the primary goal.

2. *The diversion model*. Working closely with criminal justice officials, the program targets predelinquents or minor offenders prior to their trials, striving to steer them away from criminal careers.

3. *The alternative-to-incarceration model*. Convicted offenders who are likely to receive jail or prison sentences are referred to the program prior to sentencing. A successful mediation agreement is intended to reduce reliance on incarceration by providing the court with an intermediate criminal sanction between probation and confinement.

4. *The justice model*. Working within the formal justice system but with an emphasis on restorative justice, this program emphasizes victim restitution as the appropriate sanction for virtually all criminal conduct. This model seeks to incorporate the goal of personal accountability to victims into the entire range of sanctions, from probation to imprisonment.

Most programs combine elements from two or more of these types. Every program, however, needs a clear statement of its scope and guiding philosophy. Where multiple objectives are sought, priorities must be established. Otherwise, the allocation of resources within the program and its relationship with the justice system will surely suffer.

Administrative arrangements also depend upon the program's mission concept. VORPs that operate through nonprofit agencies outside the justice system (as most do) may have difficulty developing large caseloads without strong support from criminal justice practitioners. Independence from the system, in other words, probably reduces the scope and impact of the program, since frequent voluntary referrals from the public are unlikely. In practice, probation officers and courts are the most frequent sources of referrals, although cases do come from the police, victim assistance agencies, and schools as well (Hughes & Schneider, 1989). These referral sources may not share the same concept of the VORP's purpose and may have different agendas from the VORP staff. Probation officers, for example, may see VORP as part of a larger program of offender rehabilitation, whereas victim assistance agencies may be more interested in securing financial restitution.

Programs that view mediated restitution as a means of diverting offenders from extensive exposure to the criminal justice system operate in a pretrial setting. Those that seek to expand the sentencing options of judges function best when cases are received after conviction but before imposition of punishment. A report of a successful reconciliation meeting may lead to a reduced sentence for the offender, in addition to providing the judge with more detailed information about the victim's losses. If, on the other hand, the central goals are voluntary reconciliation and improved interpersonal understanding, it is best for mediation to occur when the outcome can have no effect on the behavior of criminal justice professionals (i.e., either before a dispute enters the system at all, or after sentencing). Postsentencing victim–offender meetings take place a considerable time after the criminal incident, which may be desirable for traumatic crimes but less therapeutic in other cases.

Pretrial and presentencing programs are likely to have an above-average percentage of offenders who are willing to participate, in the hopes of earning leniency from the court. Pretrial programs have the additional feature of dealing with cases before the adversarial process has polarized the parties and fixed blame. This is particularly attractive in cases where each party bears some responsibility for the occurrence of the crime.

Starting up any new program produces short-term costs; savings appear in the longer term, if at all. Identifying and securing a stable funding base are chronic problems facing all innovative programs. VORPs receive their financial support from various sources: government funding, religious organizations, businesses, civic organizations, and foundations (Hughes & Schneider, 1989). Their cost-effectiveness is related to several program design features. Savings are most likely to accrue to the criminal justice system if the program serves as a true alternative to incarceration; case-handling costs for VORPs are far below those for confinement. Whether a program actually succeeds in reducing prison and jail sentences depends on several factors, including case selection criteria, the willingness of parties to participate, the percentage of successful mediations, and the attitudes of sentencing magistrates toward mediated restitution as a sanction.

Reconciliation programs may also reduce the number of cases entering the justice system, either by lowering recidivism or by providing an alternative forum for the resolution of conflicts. For example, a report on the Cleveland Prosecutor's Mediation Program (Cincinnati Institute of Justice, 1984) documented a significant drop in the number of citizen-filed misdemeanor cases during its first full year of operation, easing the workloads of police, prosecutors, and courts. Disposition of cases took place within 15 days of the complaint, compared with the court average of 105 days.

However, merely diverting offenders who admit their guilt from probation or suspended sentences to VORPs is unlikely to be faster or less expensive, although the use of volunteers rather than probation officers helps lower per-case costs. Considerable time and planning are often needed to coordinate the needs of victims, offenders, and the justice system professionals involved in cases. Monitoring compliance with restitution agreements and conducting follow-up meetings also add to program costs.

Some VORPs may, in fact, actually *increase* the overall expenses of the justice system by widening the net of social control, especially if failure to complete the restitution agreement results in revocation of probation, contempt of court, or execution of a suspended sentence (McGillis, 1986). Moreover, victims who receive restitution from their offenders may in the future be more likely to report crimes and to testify in court, adding to the system's caseload. In return, however, VORPs often provide advantages in terms of victim compensation, community service work, and therapeutic benefits that traditional dispositions do not offer.

Most programs have rather limited data-collecting procedures (e.g., case intake, progress, and closure forms). In view of the difficulty of measuring the net impact of VORPs on justice system costs and the intangible quality of many of the benefits, it is unlikely that such programs can produce evaluations that will justify themselves in cost–benefit terms alone. Hughes and Schneider (1989) found that only 41% of the VORPs they surveyed had conducted an evaluation during the 5 years prior to their study (many, however, had not been in operation long enough for an assessment to be warranted).

Relation to the Community

The communities in which VORPs operate are as diverse as the organizational arrangements by which they are implemented. Counties ranging in population from 3,000 to over 2 million currently have VORPs (Hughes & Schneider, 1989). The degree of community involvement in a program's operation varies considerably. In part this reflects differences in program design, and in part differences in the nature of each community. Indeed, some programs operate in geographic areas that could scarcely be called "communities" in the sense the Mennonites understood the term when they envisioned reconciliation as a way to restore the bonds of shared existence.

Merry (1982) makes an important distinction between the social context of contemporary America and the situations in which mediation has historically served as a primary method of conflict resolution (i.e., primitive, small-scale societies; socialist people's courts; and commercial and labor arbitration). American residential areas are characterized by a high degree of mobility, openness, and heterogeneity. Norms and values are pluralistic and therefore do not provide a uniform set of shared understandings about what constitutes customary and deviant behavior. Litigiousness and the deeply held belief in individual legal rights encourages "win–lose" rather than "win–win" thinking, which in turn discourages reliance on conciliation as a method of resolving disputes. It is therefore often unwise to equate modern social systems with traditional, cohesive communities. Merry (1982) observes:

> The extent and condition of ongoing relationships, the role of consensus and shared values, the need to settle, and the availability of avoidance and court as culturally acceptable and socially possible alternative solutions to conflict all seriously influence the way mediation functions. (p. 177)

Furthermore, it is not always meaningful to apply the notion of "mending the community fabric" to the anomic environment of modern urban and suburban life, because it implies a return to a state of affairs that may never have existed in the first place. Finally, the underlying assumption of VORPs that conflict per se is a disturbance of the social order, and that the reaching of agreement by the disputants is therefore a return to normality, may be naive (Felstiner & Williams, 1982).

VORPs that are fully integrated into the criminal justice system, relying on professional staff and using mediation to expand the flexibility and efficiency of formal mechanisms of control, need not be highly dependent on community involvement and support for their success. The support of justice professionals is more critical in such instances. But those programs that emphasize voluntariness, empowerment of the community at large, and reintegration of offenders into society need broad support from the lay population as well as from justice professionals. The use of trained volunteer mediators is one of the principal methods of ensuring active community participation and support. Another is the recruitment of community members to serve on the advisory board that oversees the program. Maintaining a high profile through public relations activities is also needed to ensure sufficient interest among local residents.

Because many VORPs are small and innovative, with precarious funding arrangements, their existence may not be well known in the community. The difficulty of documenting their cost-effectiveness further hinders their efforts to gain public support. However, most victims and offenders who participate express a willingness to engage in mediation in the future (Coates & Gehm, 1989). VORP personnel also report satisfaction with the operation of their programs (Hughes & Schneider, 1989). Public opinion research shows that the idea of restorative justice is generally viewed as an appropriate goal for the justice system (Hudson & Galaway, 1980). If reconciliation continues to build a positive reputation among those involved, increased community support appears likely, particularly in light of the widespread dissatisfaction with the inadequacies and expense of conventional criminal justice practices (Woolpert, 1988).

CONCLUSION

The principles of restorative justice and offender accountability on which VORPs rest represent a significant departure from the retributive and deterrent philosophies of punishment that have traditionally guided our criminal sanctions. Rather than relying on universal and eternal standards of right and wrong, restorative justice is closer to the relational, contextual concept of justice that Gilligan (1982) describes as integral to feminine thought. Her research on women and morality reveals a propensity for women to connect justice to ideas of responsibility and care in sustaining relationships, while men think of justice more in terms of autonomy and individual rights. Similarly, VORPs represent a movement away from categorical and uniform rules of fairness toward a notion of fairness that is framed in the context of a personal dialogue between victim and offender.

Movements for criminal justice reform in this country have a long history (Walker, 1980). Like the Mennonites of today, the Quakers of the 18th century sought to make their society's response to crime more humane. They conceived the penitentiary in hopes of reforming rather than brutalizing the criminal. The subsequent history of that innovation is eloquent testimony to the way in which noble ideas become distorted in practice.

Consequently, despite the major differences between VORPs and conventional criminal justice processes, their net impact is likely to be modest. Most crimes will still go unsolved. The poor offender and the poor victim will continue to be at a serious disadvantage in relation to the well-to-do. Abuse of the reconciliation process is always a possibility. Our knowledge of VORPs' dynamics is still meager. At worst, VORPs may be a passing fad, utilizing poorly trained volunteers, widening the net of social control, manipulating parties into "quick-fix" agreements that mask underlying problems, and adding to the costs of the justice system. The current alternatives, however, are increasingly hard to justify in terms of cost-effectiveness, public safety, fairness, or humane treatment. The preliminary evidence of

VORPs utility provides sufficient grounds to justify further expansion and evaluation of this approach.

REFERENCES

Abel, C., & Marsh, F. (1984). *Punishment and restitution*. New York: Greenwood Press.

Barnett, R. (1977). Restitution: A new paradigm of criminal justice. *Ethics, 87*(4), 279–301.

Cannon, M. (1982). Correcting our corrections system: Alternative sentencing and prison industry programs. *Vital Speeches of the Day, 48*(24), 758–762.

Christie, N. (1977). Conflict as property. *British Journal of Criminology, 17*(4), 1–15.

Cincinnati Institute of Justice (1984). *Report on the Cleveland Prosecutor's Mediation Program*. Cincinnati, OH: Author.

Coates, R., & Gehm, J. (1989). An empirical assessment. In M. Wright & B. Galaway (Eds.), *Mediation and criminal justice* (pp. 251–263). London: Sage.

Davis, R., Tichane, M., & Grayson, D. (1980). *Mediation and arbitration as alternatives to criminal prosecution in felony arrest cases: An evaluation of the Brooklyn Dispute Resolution Center (first year)*. New York: Vera Institute of Justice.

Dittenhoffer, T., & Erikson, R. (1983). The victim offender reconciliation program: A message to correctional reformers. *University of Toronto Law Journal, 33*(3), 315–347.

Felstiner, W. F., & Williams, L. (1979–1980). *Community mediation in Dorchester, Massachusetts*. Washington, DC: U.S. Government Printing Office.

Felstiner, W. F., & Williams, L. (1982). Community mediation in Dorchester, Massachusetts. In R. Tomasic & M. Feeley (Eds.), *Neighborhood justice: Assessment of an emerging idea* (pp. 111–153). New York: Longman.

Galaway, B. (1985). Victim participation in the penal–corrective process. *Victimology, 10*(1–4), 617–630.

Gehm, J., & Fagan, H. (1989). *Victim–offenders reconciliation and mediation program directory*. Valparaiso, IN: Prisoner and Community Together Institute of Justice.

Gehm, J., & Umbreit, M. (1986). *Victim–offender reconciliation and mediation program directory*. Valparaiso, IN: Prisoner and Community Together Institute of Justice.

Gilligan, C. (1982). *In a different voice: Psychological theory and women's development*. Cambridge, MA: Harvard University Press.

Grønfers, M. (1989). Ideals and reality in community mediation. In M. Wright & B. Galaway (Eds.), *Mediation and criminal justice* (pp. 140–151). London: Sage.

Harding, J. (1989). Reconciling mediation with criminal justice. In M. Wright & B. Galaway (Eds.), *Mediation and criminal justice* (pp. 27–43). London: Sage.

Hernon, J., & Forst, B. (1984). *The criminal justice response to victim harm*. Washington, DC: National Institute of Justice.

Hickey, J., & Scharf, P. (1980). *Toward a just correctional system: Experiments in implementing democracy in prison*. San Francisco: Jossey-Bass.

Hudson, J., & Galaway, B. (1980). A review of the restitution and community service sanctioning research. In J. Hudson & B. Galaway (Eds.), *Victims, offenders and alternative sanctions* (pp. 173–194). Lexington, MA: Lexington Books.

Hughes, S., & Schneider, A. (1989). Victim–offender mediation: A survey of program characteristics and perceptions of fairness. *Crime and Delinquency, 35*(2), 217–233.

Klein, A. R., & Kramer, A. L. (1981). *Earn it: The story so far*. Washington, DC: U.S. Department of Justice, Office of Juvenile Justice and Delinquency Prevention.

Launay, G., & Murray, P. (1989). Victim/offender groups. In M. Wright & B. Galaway (Eds.), *Mediation and criminal justice* (pp. 113–131). London: Sage.

McGillis, D. (1986). *Crime victim restitution: An analysis of approaches*. Washington, DC: National Institute of Justice.

McGillis, D., & Mullen, J. (1977). *Neighborhood justice centers: An analysis of potential models*. Washington, DC: U.S. Department of Justice.

McKnight, D. (1981). The victim–offender reconciliation project. In B. Galaway & J. Hudson (Eds.), *Perspectives on crime victims* (pp. 292–298). St. Louis: C.V. Mosby.

Marshall, T. F., & Merry, S. (1988). *Crime and accountability: Home Office research study*. London: Her Majesty's Stationery Office.

Merry, S. E. (1982). Defining "success in the neighborhood justice movement. In R. Tomasic & M. Feeley (Eds.), *Neighborhood justice: Assessment of an emerging idea* (pp. 172–192). New York: Longman.

O'Brien, E. (1987). *"Asking the victim": A study of the attitudes of some victims of crime to reparation and the criminal justice system*. Gloucester, England: Gloucester Probation Service.

Peachy, D. (1989). The Kitchener experiment. In M. Wright & B. Galaway (Eds.), *Mediation and criminal justice* (pp. 3–17). London: Sage.

President's Task Force on Victims of Crime. (1982). *Final report*. Washington, DC: U.S. Government Printing Office.

Reeves, H. (1989). The victim support perspective. In M. Wright & B. Galaway (Eds.), *Mediation and criminal justice* (pp. 44–55). London: Sage.

Ruddick, R. (1989). A court-referred scheme. In M. Wright & B. Galaway (Eds.), *Mediation and criminal justice* (pp. 82–98). London: Sage.

Schafer, S. (1970). *Compensation and restitution to the victims of crime*. Montclair, NJ: Patterson Smith.

Schneider, A. L. (Ed.). (1985). *Guide to juvenile restitution*. Washington, DC: U.S. Department of Justice, Office of Juvenile Justice and Delinquency Prevention.

Schneider, A. L. (1986). Restitution and recidivism rates of juvenile offenders: Results from four experimental studies. *Criminology, 24*(3), 533–552.

Schneider, P. R., Schneider, A. L., Griffith, W., & Wilson, M. (1982). *Two-year report on the national evaluation of the juvenile restitution initiative: An overview of program performance*. Eugene, OR: Institute of Policy Analysis.

Shaw, M. (1989). Mediating adolescent/parent conflicts. In M. Wright & B. Galaway (Eds.), *Mediation and criminal justice* (pp. 132–139). London: Sage.

Smith, K. (1963). *A cure for crime: The case for the self-determining prison sentence*. London: Routledge & Kegan Paul.

Tittle, C. (1978). Restitution and deterrence: An evaluation of compatibility. In B. Galaway & J. Hudson (Eds.), *Offender restitution in theory and action* (pp. 223–248). Lexington, MA: Lexington Books.

Tomasic, R., & Feeley, M. (Eds.). (1982). *Neighborhood justice: Assessment of an emerging idea*. New York: Longman.

Umbreit, M. (1986). Victim/offender mediation: A national survey. *Federal Probation, 50*(4), 53–56.

Umbreit, M. (1989a). Victims seeking fairness, not revenge: Toward restorative justice. *Federal Probation, 53*(3), 52–57.

Umbreit, M. (1989b). Violent offenders and their victims. In M. Wright & B. Galaway (Eds.), *Mediation and criminal justice* (pp. 99–112). London: Sage.

Veevers, J. (1989). Pre-court diversion for juvenile offenders. In M. Wright & B. Galaway (Eds.), *Mediation and criminal justice* (pp. 69–81). London: Sage.

Walker, S. (1980). *Popular justice*. New York: Oxford University Press.

Woolpert, S. (1988). Applying humanistic psychology to politics: The case for criminal restitution. *Journal of Humanistic Psychology, 28*(4), 45–62.

Zehr, H. (1985, September). VORP evaluated. *Center for Community Justice Newsletter*, pp. 2–4.

Zehr, H., & Umbreit, M. (1982). Victim–offender reconciliation: An incarceration substitute? *Federal Probation, 46*(4), 63–68.

18

Mediating Consumer Complaints

ARTHUR BEST
University of Denver College of Law

Making mediation available and enabling it to operate successfully for the resolution of buyer–seller disputes would serve a number of important goals. It would make marketing more efficient, since unresolved consumer problems undermine the discipline of honest competition, which the free enterprise system uses to stimulate producers and sellers to make well-designed products available at prices that reflect their worth. It would help individual buyers get their money's worth in transactions that are important to them, either because large amounts of money are involved or because the subject matter of the transaction has special significance. And it would make a small step in the direction of replacing brute strength with justice, since consumer disputes often do not get resolved at all (Best, 1981) because of the power inequities present in the typical buyer–seller relationship. Experience with mediation's potential to replace force with fairness could well influence the lives of participants in particular buyer–seller disputes beyond the scope of specific issues concerning shortcomings in products or services.

This chapter describes some of the typical attributes of consumer problems that affect their suitability for treatment through mediation. It also identifies potential strengths and weakness of buyer–seller mediation, in the context of a brief case study of a large-scale consumer mediation program currently operated by General Motors. At present, mediation of consumer problems ordinarily takes place at state and local law enforcement agencies (such as the offices of state attorneys-general or local consumer affairs departments); at Better Business Bureaus (private business-sponsored local trade organizations); in single-industry complaint resolution programs; and—infrequently—at general-purpose community mediation programs (McGillis, 1987). The General Motors program is administered at Better Business Bureau offices, under the terms of a consent settlement with the Federal Trade Commission.

EVALUATING THE SUITABILITY OF BUYER–SELLER DISPUTES FOR MEDIATION

Consumer problems may be more difficult to bring to mediation than some other types of disputes, because the parties may have no perceived interest in maintaining a continuing relationship. Also, they may know each other only in the context of their buyer–seller relationship; they may have drastically unequal power; and they almost certainly do not share a tradition that recognizes a role for mediation in the resolution of consumer disputes. When a consumer problem does become the subject of mediation despite these impediments, additional obstacles may appear. Buyers may have difficulty defining their goals, since consumer problems typically become more and more complex over time, and grievances about prior failed attempts at handling the complaint may be added to grievances about the underlying failure of a product or service. Facts are sometimes difficult to identify, either because (as in billing disputes) they are highly complicated, or because a good deal of time has passed since the events in controversy, or because the buyer had no way of knowing the names of people with whom he or she dealt in initial efforts to resolve the problem. Finally, both buyers and sellers may be ignorant of societal or legal standards that relate to their dispute. In the absence of some degree of certainty about external norms, the buyer and seller will need to rely on their own (probably disparate) views of fairness in the marketing context.

Scholars have suggested that alternative dispute resolution (ADR) will ameliorate the problem of overloaded court dockets (Edwards, 1986; Lieberman & Henry, 1986); that avoiding the delays of the judicial system will save money for disputants and the government (Feinberg, 1989; Sander, 1984); and that the results it produces will be better than those achieved in other ways, since procedural issues are not likely to be determinative (Nyhart & Dauer, 1986). However, a risk in applying mediation techniques to consumer problems is that expediency may supplant justice as the fundamental goal (Alschuler, 1986; Subrin & Dykstra, 1974). Disputants may derive benefits from participating in standard litigation that cannot be equaled in alternative systems. Also, important society-wide benefits of traditional litigation may be lost when disputes are treated in alternative processes (Fiss, 1984). Substituting mediation for standard litigation, for example, may deprive disputants of important aspects of fairness and justice, and concentrating on measures such as speed of resolution of numbers of cases resolved may distract attention from this fundamental shortcoming. If mediation becomes more prevalent in the consumer context, as it is likely to do, observers need to identify ways to measure its accomplishments. Criteria may include participant satisfaction, the furthering of social justice, empowerment of the parties, facilitation of the parties' abilities to acknowledge each other's perspectives and common humanity, individual autonomy, social control, social justice, and social solidarity (Bush, 1989; Luban, 1989).

For *all* conceptions of the role that ADR may play in promoting or delivering just orderings of societal relationships, an important set of questions involves identifying the disputants who enter the processes and the types of disputes for which they consider them appropriate. For consumer disputes, analysis should begin with identifying flaws that buyers perceive in purchases (Best, 1981). Research has shown strikingly little use of third parties by people involved in consumer disputes (Ladinsky & Susmilch, 1983). Some have sought to explain this avoidance by examining how much knowledge potential complainants have about techniques of complaining, or by pointing to the costs involved in making complaints (Felstiner, 1974; Nader, 1980). In some settings, antipathy toward disputing can itself be a central attribute of people's notions of how to conduct themselves in society (Greenhouse, 1986).

GOVERNMENT-ORDERED MEDIATION AND ARBITRATION BY GENERAL MOTORS

The GM program, available to owners of particular GM cars, was begun in 1984 under the terms of an FTC consent order settling charges that GM had deceptively failed to inform buyers that particular models of cars contained components with unusually low durability (FTC, 1983). GM offers owners of vehicles with the specified components the opportunity to participate in a combined mediation and one-way-binding arbitration program, operated by a BBB in each of a large number of cities. The program has two parts. The owner of a car within its coverage who presents his or her problem to a participating BBB is asked to quantify the redress he or she wants. GM then has the opportunity to offer a settlement payment. GM, the FTC, and the BBBs characterize this process as "mediation." For a consumer who rejects the mediation offer, the program provides arbitration that will be binding on GM but not on the consumer. The FTC could have litigated its case and sought to impose a requirement that GM make uniform payments to the owners of the affected cars. Its decision to rely on a mediation/arbitration program raises the issue of how the results of buyers' use of that program measure up to the results that might have been achieved in traditional litigation.

The homogeneity of the consumer problems involved in the case is relevant to evaluating the success of the mediation program. The allegedly low-durability components were used over many years in different models of vehicles. Thus, poor performance could have had different consequences for various owners of the vehicles in which they were installed. On the other hand, the instances of possible consumer abuse in this case must have much

less variation than would have been found if the universe of purchases had
been *all cars*, and the flaws had been in *any features* of the cars. The
components covered by the settlement are, in fact, three narrowly defined
automobile parts that can fail in ways that are less numerous than potential
failures of all automobile parts. In the FTC-GM settlement, the definition of
"specified components" highlights its narrowness. The specified components
are as follows: "THM 200 automatic transmissions"; "camshafts or lifters in
305 or 350 cubic-inch displacement (CID) gasoline engines" produced in
Chevrolet plants; and "fuel injection pumps or fuel injectors in 350 CID
diesel engines" produced in Oldsmobile plants (FTC, 1983, p. 1742). This is
obviously a small proportion of the parts and systems that are contained in a
typical car.

The FTC has released data (FTC, 1988a) showing that in 144 cities from
October 1985 through July 1987, 81,480 consumers participated in the
program, and GM made payments totaling approximately $22 million. (A
context for the $22 million figure is GM's estimated sales volume of $126,932
million for a recent 12-month period; "The Forbes Sales 500," 1990). Of the
cases presented, 70,340 were resolved in mediation. Mediation required a
consumer to prepare a claim and present it in person or by mail to a BBB
office, and required GM employees to analyze the case and present an offer
to the consumer through the medium of a BBB employee. Of the cases that
went to mediation, 11,140 were pursued beyond the mediation stage to
arbitration. Arbitration required in-person appearances by the consumer
and a GM representative, and also required the work of a volunteer arbitrator to conduct the hearing and write an opinion. A number of consumers
(23,707 individuals) requested redress but did not accept a mediation offer or
choose to participate in arbitration.

In material released along with the statistical information, the FTC's
chairman has described the program as an "overwhelming success" that
"shows government, private industry, consumer groups, and individual
consumers working together for the common good" (FTC, 1988b, p. 1). The
staff report noted a wide range in individual settlements, and stated that
"[s]ince each case is a unique set of circumstances and is decided on an
individual basis, this variation of payments was foreseen. Consumers seek a
wide range of payments and receive a wide range of compensation" (FTC,
1988a). The FTC's position, however, ignores a fundamental issue that
should have been suggested by a straightforward examination of the data:
Large unexplained differences have appeared among the participating cities.
Although varied *individual* results in different *cases* would be expected,
varied *average* results in different *cities* are surprising, unless there are large
differences in the types of cars or types of car owners from city to city. For
example, a comparison can be made between two cities with similar caseloads: Houston, which processed 1,016 cases from October 1985 through
July 1987, and Akron, which processed 1,026 cases. The mean mediation

settlement in Houston was $352.39, compared with a mean in Akron of $240.56. The mean arbitration award in Houston was $223.26, whereas the mean in Akron was $113.08. Mediation represented 68.0% of the caseload in Houston, and 90.0% of the caseload in Akron.

If the program has treated cases equitably, individual *cities* in which it operates should have roughly similar records in terms of all the important measures of their operation. In particular, cities with relatively high case-loads should produce results similar to those of cities with relatively low caseloads. Proportions of cases resolved in mediation (and therefore pro-portions of cases resolved in the postmediation phase of arbitration) should be similar among the program's cities. Variations from city to city (with statistical significance) among the means for various measures of the pro-gram's work would suggest that there have been systematic failures to provide resolutions tailored to the unique circumstances of particular cases. Because types of consumers and types of vehicle deficiencies can be assumed, on average, to be similar from place to place, data showing that consumers have received more money in some cities than in others could indicate that mediation has overpaid some consumers and underpaid some others.

The published data cover a number of aspects of the program for each city in which GM makes the program available, such as the mean amount requested by the consumer, mean settlement amount, mean settlement as a percentage of mean request, the total number of cases, and the overall consumer recovery in both mediation and arbitration as a percentage of the total amounts requested. The FTC has reported means, summary per-centages, and total numbers of cases, but no individual case data, for each city. This precludes a typical statistical significance analysis, such as one that would consider whether individual cities had significantly different charac-teristics, because only means or totals for the values in each city (and not the standard deviations) have been released. An analysis can, however, group the cities according to certain attributes, calculate the means of each group's means for various program attributes, and then explore the statistical signifi-cance of variations among those means of "means" (or the averages of those reported "average" values). The mean, then, for any city is a characteristic of that city with respect to a specific attribute. For example, a typical hypoth-esis in this study is that cities where dispute settlement is dominated by mediation (and arbitration is therefore infrequent) have different characteris-tics from cities where mediation is less prevalent. Grouping cities by high and low mediation ratios allows us to determine the significance of differ-ences between the mean mediation ratios of the two groups of cities.

Table 18.1 illustrates statistically significant differences between groups of cities for every important variable associated with this program. When the cities are ranked according to the mean mediation amounts requested in each city, the mean mediation request in the 36 cities in the highest quartile

TABLE 18.1.   Mean Values of Selected Program Attributes among Each Attribute's
Top- and Bottom-Quartile Cities

Attribute	Bottom quartile ($n = 36$)	Top quartile ($n = 36$)
Mean mediation request ($)	460.80	666.90
Mean mediation settlement ($)	236.90	377.70
Mean mediation settlement as percentage of mean request (%)	47.1	61.3
Mean mediation offer refused by arbitrating claimant ($)	17.80	107.70
Mean arbitration request ($)	407.80	871.02
Mean arbitration award ($)	70.82	342.23
Percentage of caseload resolved in mediation (%)	70.4	94.1
Mean arbitration award as percentage of mean request (%)	11.5	57.4
Percentage of cases with repairs obtained by owner	0.7	2.6

Note. Means of means in cities in top and bottom quartiles for each attribute. Differences in each row are statistically significant at the .05 level, according to a t test (two-tailed) with 70 degrees of freedom.

is $666.90. The mean mediation amount request in the 37 cities in the lowest quartile is $460.80. Of greater importance than amounts requested, however, are amounts actually received. The mean for cities in the highest quartile with respect to that variable is $377.70. The mean of the means for cities in the lowest quartile is $236.90. The difference of about $140 is huge, in the context of a $236–$377 range. It represents about 60% of the $236 figure for the lowest-quartile cities.

An initial hypothesis to explain these variations may be that programs with high caseloads develop patterns different from those in programs with low caseloads because intake personnel become familiar with the results in past cases and may communicate encouragement or discouragement to claimants. In the GM program, mediation does not require an in-person appearance by a GM representative, since GM makes its offer in writing or by telephone to a BBB employee. Arbitration, however, requires attendance at a hearing by the claimant and by a GM employee. It is possible that a high volume of cases may lead the GM personnel to make more generous initial offers than they would otherwise make, whereas low overall case volume may decrease the risk that frequent appearances at arbitrations will be required. Another consequence of high caseload may be that the representatives of GM become conditioned to participation in the program and thus more willing to approve payments that may seem unusual to less habituated representatives.

When cities are grouped into the bottom and top quartiles with respect to total caseloads, there are statistically significant differences between each quartile's values for the following: amount received in mediated settlements, the percentage of claimants' requests obtained in mediated settlements, the percentage of all claimants' requests obtained through both mediation and arbitration, and the proportion that mediation represents of the cities' total caseloads. As an example, the mean of the mean mediation settlement amounts received by consumers in the cities in the lowest quartile of caseload size was $289.38. The corresponding amount for cities in the highest quartile of caseload size was $327.45. This suggests that many cases processed in the system may have been subject to variation in the range of ±10%, merely as a result of their having been presented at a low- or a high-volume location. Table 18.2 shows the values for the means of the variables for which there are statistically significant variations between cities in the high- and low-caseload-volume quartiles.

The significance of a program's total caseload is also shown when the programs are grouped according to the mean settlements in mediation. Cities in the highest quartile on that measure had mean mediation settlements much higher than the mean mediation settlements in cities in the lowest quartile. Although there is no reason why cities that process many cases should handle cases deserving higher payments than the cases in cities that process relatively fewer cases, the mean total number of mediated cases in the cities with low settlement payments was 327.6, compared with 687.9 for the same measure in cities with high settlement payments.

Another attribute in which there is statistically significant variation among cities is the percentage of caseloads resolved in mediation, which ranged from a low of 14.3% to a high of 100%. Cities in the lowest quartile on

TABLE 18.2.   Variables with Statistically Significant Variation, According to Cities' Total Caseloads

Variable	Bottom-quartile cities (137 or fewer cases; $n = 36$)	Top-quartile cities (715 or more cases; $n = 36$)
Mediation settlement accepted ($)	289.38	327.45
Mediation settlements as percentage of request	51.7	56.7
Total awards as percentage of total requests	46.6	53.0
Mediated cases as percentage of total cases	78.1	86.0

Note. The differences are all statistically significant at the .05 level, according to a *t* test (two-tailed) with 70 degrees of freedom.

this measure resolved 78.1% of their cases in mediation, whereas cities in the highest quartile resolved 91.1% of cases that way. The cities where mediation more strongly dominated the dispute resolution program reported values that show statistically significant differences from the corresponding values for cities where mediation was less prevalent. The differences show that those cities granted consumers an overall higher percentage of their requests than consumers received in the cities where mediation was less dominant. The comparable percentages are 46.5% and 51.5%, representing a typical difference of about 5%. That percentage is important, given that consumers in the program from 1985 to 1987 typically requested at least $500. There is also a large difference in the mean caseloads, with mediation dominant in cities where caseloads were, on average, about twice as large as the caseloads in cities where mediation was somewhat less dominant. These data are shown in Table 18.3.

Two other groupings of cities are defined here, to permit further exploration of any other statistically significant differences between the results for various program attributes among different cities. Each of these groups of cities processed, in total, about one-quarter of the whole program's caseload. One group consists of the cities with the lowest individual caseloads, which processed, as a group, about one-quarter of the program's total caseload. The other consists of the cities with the highest individual caseloads, which processed, as a group, about one-quarter of the total program caseload. As is shown in Table 18.4, the two groups have statistically different mean values for total awards as a percentage of total requests, for mediation awards as a percentage of total mediation requests, and for the ratio of mediation cases to total cases processed. These results further support the likelihood that aspects of the operation of the program in high-volume locations favored consumers, or, correspondingly, that it hurt consumers to have their cases treated at the lower-volume locations.

The pattern of operation at the various program locations suggests that

TABLE 18.3.   Variables with Statistically Significant Variation, According to Cities' Percentages of Caseloads Resolved in Mediation

Variable	Bottom-quartile cities (78.1% of cases resolved in mediation; $n = 36$)	Top-quartile cities (91.1% of cases resolved in mediation; $n = 36$)
Total awards as percentage of total requests	46.5	51.5
Total caseload	295.7	629.3

Note. These differences are statistically significant at the .05 level, according to a t test (two tailed) with 70 degrees of freedom.

TABLE 18.4.   Variables with Statistically Significant Variation between the Low-Volume City Group and the High-Volume City Group

Variable	Lowest-volume cities processing approximately 25% of program caseload ($n = 94$)	Highest-volume cities processing approximately 25% of program caseload ($n = 7$)
Mediation awards as percentage of mediation requests	53.2	58.7
Total awards as percentage of total requests	48.8	55.7
Percentage of caseload resolved in mediation	82.9	87.3

Note. These differences are statistically significant at the .05 level, according to a *t* test (two-tailed) with 99 degrees of freedom.

although a lot of money has been distributed, there is considerable reason to question the fairness of its allocation. Variations between groups of cities *cannot reasonably be attributed to variations in the cars or car owners found in them.* Only a few types of components have been involved in all of the 81,480 cases analyzed. Vehicle age, vehicle initial cost, individual styles of driving, and individual style of response to consumer problems could be expected to be distributed randomly among participating cities. Finally, if variation in results could be explained by variation in the condition of the cars that were the subjects of the cases, there would be no link between a city's total caseload and the results achieved in the city, in terms of mean mediation settlement or other factors. Yet total caseload and percentage of caseload treated through mediation seem to have had a positive influence on the absolute amounts of recoveries consumers received and on the relationship of those amounts to the claims consumers presented. These relationships suggest that factors in the programs, rather than in the problems presented to the programs, have caused disparate treatment of similar cases. Mediation, which can produce results well tailored to the desires of particular disputants, has apparently been influenced by factors beyond the control or knowledge or the consumers who have used the GM program.

MEDIATION'S STRENGTHS AND WEAKNESSES, ILLUSTRATED IN THE GENERAL MOTORS EXPERIENCE

An advantage often ascribed to mediation is economy. For the FTC-GM settlement, however, a full accounting of all expenditures suggests that cost savings have not been accomplished. It cannot be known what the total expense of formal litigation of an FTC action seeking uniform redress would have been. However, the costs expended in the GM program under the settlement can be described. Each mediated case required a personal visit or detailed correspondence and telephone communications by the aggrieved vehicle owner, as well as analysis by GM personnel. A BBB employee communicated the GM decision to the car owner. Records were kept of these procedural stages. Since roughly 194,000 cases were involved in mediation from January 1984 through July 1987, if all this effort cost $10 a case, $1.94 million was expended. If a fair estimate would be $20 a case, then the total cost was nearly $4 million. Traditional litigation would have required FTC staff work for several years, defense costs for GM for several years, and costs of administering the agency trial process and possible judicial review of the agency's action. Huge costs might have been required for the traditional process, but it is clear that bit by bit and case by case, ADR has been extremely costly itself.

The quantitative data provided by the FTC provide very little evidence about how well users of the program liked it. Some people who made an inquiry and then did not pursue a case to mediation or arbitration were probably dissatisfied with some aspects of the program, such as the amount of effort required to obtain redress, or the amount of redress they may have anticipated would be produced for that effort. Others left the program because their complaints were suitable for treatment in a separate GM-BBB process. More than 20% of participants failed to complete the program in the period ending July 1987 (FTC, 1988a). Everyone who went past the mediation phase to arbitration was clearly dissatisfied with the mediation results. As Table 18.1 shows, the percentage of caseload resolved in mediation varied widely from city to city. For cities in the lowest quartile on that measure, the average percentage of caseload resolved in mediation was 70.4%. This suggests that, in at least some cities, a major component of the program failed to satisfy a large number of participants. The fact that some other cities were able to resolve almost all of their complaints in mediation suggests that in the cities with low mediation percentages, something was flawed in the mediation procedures. Suspecting that the process was flawed is reasonable, unless the customers and GM representatives in some cities were very different in their demands and incentives from those in other cities.

In considering user satisfaction, a vital issue is determined by the definition of "user." In one sense, this ADR process was (and is) intended to serve all victims of the alleged abuse—all purchasers of cars with the "specified components." If about 20 million vehicles were affected, the volume of participation in the program indicates that about 1 out of 100 potential victims sought redress. Serving such a small set of victims falls far short of satisfying the legitimate compensation needs of the overall group.

Delivery of redress to only a small percentage of those eligible for it is particularly unjust in the circumstance of an innovative third-party system, since it is likely that those who participated in it were disproportionately drawn from the better-educated and better-informed owners among all the owners of affected cars. Under the settlement, special notification of the ADR process was to be made to individuals who had already complained to law enforcement officials or to the FTC, and notification of the program was also required to be given to consumers who "identify a specified component" (FTC, 1983, p. 1763). These notification provisions would have favored articulate and rights-conscious customers.

CURRENT CONSUMER DISPUTE ISSUES FOR MEDIATION PRACTITIONERS AND RESEARCHERS

Expectations typically expressed for mediation seem not to have been fulfilled by the GM program during the period under study. This reflects some unique aspects of its organization, and may illustrate typical difficulties in applying mediation to consumer problems. The GM program's mediation component did not involve face-to-face discussions between car owners and GM representatives, and apparently consisted only of the communication of owners' requests and GM's settlement offers through the medium of a passive BBB employee. This prevented the parties from having the benefit of hearing each other's presentations of their points of view on past occurrences and proper future actions in response to those past events. It also prevented the parties from developing collaborative relationships in which they might have developed innovative resolutions.

Certain social factors that may facilitate successful mediation were not present in the GM disputes, and are likely to be absent in general in the buyer–seller context. For example, buyers and a car company do not have a shared perception that their relationship must continue after their dispute ends. In buyer–seller disputes between a large national seller and a local buyer, there is likely not to be any background of previous successful interactions to provide a common base for developing a solution to the present problem. The third parties involved in the GM program were either noninteractive BBB employees who conveyed information between the buyers and GM without elaboration during the mediation phase, or nonexpert volunteer arbitrators. Although these third parties were assuredly neutral, they did not bring expertise in mediation or expertise in car problems to bear on the cases in which they were involved. Where mediation is offered by community service groups or as an adjunct to consumer protection agencies or courts, its quality may similarly be influenced by the skill of the mediators. Where they are volunteers, they may share the apparent passivity of the mediators in the GM program.

The possible failure of the GM program to reach large numbers of affected consumers could have been predicted, since recourse to third parties is a highly unusual response to buyer–seller problems. Particularly where the subject matter of a dispute involves issues of judgment or difficult proof, consumers may be reluctant to invest the time and psychological resources required to participate in a mediation program, because predictable rewards for that effort are not present. These factors are generalizable to all of consumer problems, and represent a significant obstacle that any consumer mediation program must overcome. Although such benefits of ADR as individual satisfaction and self-transformation may have been realized by some of the GM program's participants, those social gains must be balanced against the failure of the system to demonstrate that it provided equal treatment to equivalent cases, and that it delivered redress to a significant portion of those eligible for it.

Participants in consumer mediation programs must be alert to the possibility that resolving cases may not be the same as providing fair and just results. The FTC's possibly overly enthusiastic descriptions of the GM program's success indicate another potential difficulty in the administration of consumer mediation: Those who have a stake in the success of the program may be inclined to overstate its effectiveness, and to ignore questions about the program's reach and the equity of the program's individual case dispositions.

The GM program affected the car owners who participated in it, but, unlike traditional litigation and regulatory processes, it could not produce authoritative decisions capable of creating broad social consequences. The GM program's operations influenced each dispute's actual participants, but cannot be characterized as having affected people who were not parties to the particular disputes it processed. It cannot be known whether the burdens GM has borne as a result of the FTC settlement have influenced GM and other car manufacturers to avoid the types of marketing practices that allegedly violated the FTC Act. However, the settlement provided no guide for future actions by GM and other sellers with regard to what disclosures should be made when marketing vehicles with components of less than typical durability. And as a deterrent to conduct that might in the future overstep the as-yet-undrawn line of legality on this topic, the settlement cannot be seen as a strong force. Handling the disputes that were presented to the program may have cost GM less than it would have spent on them had they been treated in standard corporate channels. Compared to the cost of litigation, the program probably was a bargain for the company (Widdows, 1987), and thus could not provide an incentive for changing future conduct.

If consumers' alternative to the establishment of the GM program was to obtain no recovery, the program has been a success. Mediation for the general range of consumer disputes must also be considered in the context of the alternatives available to buyers with grievances. If in the absence of the GM program, consumers might have received court-ordered payments of redress (after lengthy FTC litigation), then the program's desirability is less clear. Long-delayed uniform payments to car owners are less beneficial to them than prompt payments. Balanced against that fact, however, are two aspects of the ongoing program. First, it is not free to participants, in the sense that it requires significant expenditures of time, effort, and emotional involvement. It also has been costly to GM. Second, its lack of uniform payments may not indicate the virtue of precisely tailored responses to individual cases, but may relate more closely to other factors, such as the volume of caseload at a particular program location. Although uniformity of payment might be considered an undesirable attribute of a redress mode that seeks judicial determination of a standard reimbursement, if the varied payments produced through mediation and arbitration are themselves not closely related to the specifics of particular cases, then their variety is irrelevant to the goal of fair compensation and cannot support a preference for the case-by-case method of dispute resolution. If results in general-subject consumer mediation programs are no better, for example, than results consumers might obtain in small-claims court, then it might be unwise to devote resources to those programs.

For a mediation/arbitration program to be accepted by a government agency as an adequate means of providing a correction for past misconduct, there should be confidence that the mechanism will work fairly. Experience with the FTC-GM settlement would not justify that confidence. Where consumer mediation is part of a governmental entity's ongoing functions, or is provided by a community-based organization, its availability will be free from the risk that it is replacing a possibly more efficient group treatment of a class of problems. In those instances, its development deserves encouragement in the expectation that increased availability of avenues of redress for consumer injuries will benefit individual buyers and sellers, as well as society as a whole.

Acknowledgments

This chapter is based partly on a paper presented at the 1989 annual meeting of the Law and Society Association. Thanks are gratefully given to Professor David A. Barnes, who helped generously with (but is not responsible for) the statistical analysis. The case study described in this chapter is given fuller treatment in a forthcoming article in the *Missouri Journal of Dispute Resolution* (Best, 1990).

REFERENCES

Alschuler, A. W. (1986). Mediation with a mugger: The shortage of adjudicative service and the need for a two-tier trial system in civil cases. *Harvard Law Review, 99*(8), 1808–1859.

Best, A. (1990). Consumer problems and ADR: An analysis of the Federal Trade Commission-Ordered General Motor Mediation and Arbitration Program. *Missouri Journal of Dispute Resolution, 2*.

Best, A. (1981). *When consumers complain*. New York: Columbia University Press.

Bush, R. A. B. (1989). Defining quality in dispute resolution: Taxonomies and anti-taxonomies of quality arguments. *University of Denver Law Review, 66*(3), 335–380.

Edwards, H. T. (1986). Alternative dispute resolution: Panacea or anathema? *Harvard Law Review, 99*(3), 668–684.

Federal Trade Commission (FTC). (1983). In the matter of General Motors Corp. *Federal Trade Commission Reports, 102*, 1741–1803.

Federal Trade Commission (FTC). (1988a). *Analysis of data on results of General Motors' third party arbitration program for the period October 1985 through July 1987*. Washington, DC: Author.

Federal Trade Commission (FTC). (1988b, September 22). *Press release*. Washington, DC: Author.

Feinberg, K. R. (1989). Mediation: A preferred method of dispute resolution. *Pepperdine Law Review, 16*(S5), S5–S42.

Felstiner, W. L. F. (1974). Influences of social organization on dispute processing. *Law and Society Review, 9*(1), 63–94.

Fiss, O. (1984). Against settlement. *Yale Law Journal, 93*(6), 1073–1090.

The Forbes sales 500. (1990, April 30). *Forbes Magazine*, p. 230.

Greenhouse, L. (1986). *Praying for justice: Faith, order and community in an American town*. Ithaca, NY: Cornell University Press.

Ladinsky, J., & Susmilch, C. (1983). *Community factors in the brokerage of consumer product and service problems* (University of Wisconsin Disputes Processing Research Program Working Papers, 1983, No. 14). Madison: University of Wisconsin Disputes Processing Research Program.

Lieberman, J., & Henry, J. (1986). Lessons from the alternative dispute resolution movement. *University of Chicago Law Review, 53*(2), 424–439.

Luban, D. (1989). The quality of justice. *University of Denver Law Review, 66*(3), 381–417.

McGillis, D. (1987). *Consumer dispute resolution: A survey of programs*. Washington, DC: National Institute for Dispute Resolution.

Nader, L. (Ed.). (1980). *No access to justice*. New York: Academic Press.

Nyhart, J. D., & Dauer, E. A. (1986). A preliminary analysis of the uses of scientific models in dispute prevention, management and resolution. *Missouri Journal of Dispute Resolution, 1986*, 29–53.

Sander, F. (1984). Rhetoric and reality in the dispute resolution movement. *Missouri Journal of Dispute Resolution, 1984*, 5–8.

Subrin, S. N., & Dykstra, A. R. (1974). Notice and the right to be heard: The significance of old friends. *Harvard Civil Rights and Civil Liberties Law Review, 9*(3), 449–480.

Widdows, R. (1987). Consumer arbitration as a dispute resolution mechanism in customer–seller disputes over automobile purchases. *Arbitration Journal, 42*, 17–23.

19

Dealing with Environmental and Other Complex Public Disputes

SUSAN CARPENTER
Consultant, Riverside, California

Communities are changing the way they are conducting business. A decade ago, a handful of citizens could tackle a problem, determine a solution, and proceed to sell it to the public. Sometimes the solution was opposed, but usually it got implemented. Today diverse interests expect and demand involvement in decisions that affect their lives. Fewer deals are cut in back rooms; those deals that are risk vigorous opposition from citizens who have not been included in the process. As the number and diversity of citizens involved in decision making increases, reaching agreements becomes more difficult, and with that the appeal of using an impartial third party becomes more attractive.

The insertion of an impartial third party into a local environmental or other complex public dispute is a relatively new application for mediation skills (see Carpenter & Kennedy, 1988; Susskind & Cruikshank, 1987; Gray, 1989). As mediators from the fields of labor management and interpersonal conflict begin to work on public disputes, they find themselves confronted with a number of professional issues. This chapter explores issues raised when mediation is applied to environmental or other complex community disputes.

CHARACTERISTICS OF COMPLEX PUBLIC DISPUTES

Mediators who choose to work in the public arena must begin with an understanding of the nature of these controversies and must be prepared to respond to their special characteristics. Public disputes are messy, dynamic situations that bring together diverse interests in an intricate web of relationships; a complex set of technical information and emotions; and a context of imposing (and sometimes conflicting) local, state, and federal regulations.

Public disputes involve complex interrelated issues. Substantive issues can be highly technical, and they can represent fundamental differences in values. For example, a conflict over the siting of a new public-assisted housing project will involve technical issues of zoning, design, scale, real estate values, property rights, location, and management. The knowledge of architecture, economics, planning, and law will be required to address key issues.

Technical issues are often mixed with strong personal and community values. The same conflict over a public-assisted housing project also brings out strong statements of values from the public. The concerns for social justice that support the need for more housing are juxtaposed with the rights of individual property owners to protect their investments and maintain their current quality of life. Easy answers do not exist.

The structure of interest groups involved in a conflict vary from loose coalitions of ad hoc or membership organizations to highly structured corporate or government bureaucracies. Interest groups also use different methods for making decisions. Some groups rely exclusively on a consensus procedure; others vote and have clearly defined hierarchical lines of decision making. Legally incorporated groups with boards of directors are subject to greater accountability than are interest groups that have formed for the sole purpose of fighting a proposed project and have no intention to continue as a group beyond the immediate battle.

Interest groups also vary in their familiarity with the technical issues of a controversy and in their skills in working with one another. Groups bring different types of power to the table. Some parties represent political power; others can mobilize large groups of people to respond; others have financial resources, valuable knowledge, or useful skills.

Unlike labor management negotiations, public disputes have no formal mechanisms for convening parties and conducting negotiations. The initiative for bringing in a mediator usually comes from one or more of the parties or other concerned groups in a community. The mediator works with the parties to determine whether negotiations are appropriate, and then to identify who should participate and what form the negotiation process should take.

Public controversies are conducted in the context of government rules and regulations. Required public hearings, exparte rules preventing discussions between parties and regulators, and mandatory decision-making time frames influence how and when a negotiation process is structured. Knowledge of federal, state, and local rules is critical, with the added understanding that their interpretation may vary from administration to administration. Conflict in regulations do exist between different agencies at the same level of government and among different levels of government.

The challenge of resolving public disputes lies in the mediator's ability to structure and conduct a process that respects the diversity among parties, embraces the complexity of the issues, and understands the political context in which discussion will occur.

TYPES OF PROBLEMS

Public disputes arise over policy decisions, programs, and projects that affect a community. The topics of controversies are as varied as the people who live in communities. Efforts to revise a community's master plan, to establish a drug-abuse program, to site high-density townhouses near an affluent neighborhood, or to construct a new solid waste facility quickly draw attention and then public responses from diverse interest groups.

Conflict can focus on *whether* to proceed with a proposal, as well as *how* to proceed. Frequently these questions get blurred together. A controversial proposal to build a new freeway often has one set of interest groups debating the most appropriate route for the road and the exact location of interchanges, while other groups adamantly argue that the proposed freeway is unnecessary and marshal resources to oppose its construction under any circumstances. Mediators must work with the interest groups to establish a common definition of a problem before proceeding to develop a process or convene parties.

THE ROLE OF THE PUBLIC DISPUTE MEDIATOR

Public dispute mediators offer a range of useful third-party services. Parties involved in public disputes are less likely to be familiar and skillful with the tools of negotiations than parties who regularly participate in institutionalized negotiation procedures. They require more assistance from a mediator to structure and maintain a productive process.

A mediator may be invited to conduct an assessment of a dispute. By interviewing parties, the mediator helps a community sort out critical issues, identify stakeholders, and gain a sense of whether it would be appropriate to bring parties together—and what such a process might involve.

A community may also ask a mediator to help it design and set up a process for productive discussions. A mediator works with the parties to define the problem in a way that all parties can accept, establishes goals for the process, determines necessary roles and who should fill them, suggests a process model and specific activities within that model, determines a realistic time frame, and helps parties secure resources necessary to conduct the discussions.

Public dispute mediators are frequently asked to intervene in conflicts when other methods of reaching agreements have failed. A mediator is more likely to initiate a new negotiation than to continue with one in progress. This requires that a mediator first conduct an assessment and, on the basis of this acquired information, initiate a new negotiation that may include additional parties and expand or reframe issues to be discussed. A mediator may spend weeks assessing how to structure a process before convening any of the parties. Because efforts to resolve public disputes through the use of negotiation follow no standard convention that all parties understand and accept, the process itself may contribute to the failure of parties to reach agreements.

A public dispute mediator may also be asked to bring parties together and to conduct a productive negotiation early when an issue is first identified, before parties have staked out intractable positions. The mediator will work with the parties to assess the issue, design a process, convene representatives, and conduct the negotiations.

In addition, a mediator may be asked to design and run a difficult phase of a negotiation and sometimes a particularly tough meeting. The mediator may also be invited to conduct sessions with a concerned public in conjunction with a negotiation. Negotiators recognize that certain phases of their discussion will be more difficult than others; initial discussions of parties' issues and interests can result in an escalating series of accusations if these discussions are not carefully structured and monitored. Reaching agreement on controversial data is yet another area where the services of a mediator may be employed.

The public dispute mediator is often asked to continue to work with the parties after they have reached agreements, in order to help them sort out tasks, refine their plans, and evaluate the success of their efforts. The mediator may reconvene parties to work out a particularly sticky issue or serve on an as-needed basis to the group.

It is up to the parties to determine what role they want the mediator to play. A request for advice early in a controversy often leads to an assessment of the issues, the design of a process, and, in turn, an invitation to a mediator to conduct the negotiations.

CASE EXAMPLES

The following two cases illustrate the use of third-party assistance in two community disputes (see Ashton, 1988, 1989, for additional information regarding these cases). The first controversy involved a clash between economic development and historic preservation interests in Atlanta, Georgia. In the second conflict, the community of Fort Worth, Texas, was embattled in issues over the design of a new highway.

Atlanta Historic Preservation Program

Atlanta was struggling to preserve its historical properties and resources, and at the same time was committed to promoting economic development. Public opposition to the demolition of three apartment buildings proposed for historic designation prompted the City Council to consider several legislative initiatives, while the city's Urban Design Commission proceeded to propose the addition of 85 buildings and 16 districts to the city's inventory of designated historic structures. Seeing the potential conflicts ahead, representatives from city government, downtown business interests, and preservation advocates formed the Historic Preservation Task Force to consider acceptable options. The task force decided to engage in negotiation with the assistance of a mediator. A mediation team composed of members from two university-based mediation centers was brought in to design and conduct the process.

The mediators interviewed more than 40 community leaders to clarify the sources of conflict, the issues involved, and the parties' thoughts about possible solutions. The mediators worked with the task force to design a program and select 16 members for the Policy Steering Committee, which represented all major interests in the debate. At the same time, a resource group of professionals with expertise in the legal, programmatic, and economic aspects of historic preservation and community development was created.

Initial negotiation sessions dealt with major issues raised during the interviews and with process objectives. A national expert agreed upon by the participants led discussions and wrote a paper addressing issues raised by the participants. Additional technical information was provided by other experts during the process.

After the first four sessions, a statement of the goals and general outline of a historic preservation program emerged. The details of the program were committed to a single text. For the next 4 months, negotiations involved six plenary sessions, several caucus meetings, and eight work group sessions. Caucuses allowed the representatives of single-interest groups to discuss issues and possible revisions to the text alone with a mediator. On the basis of caucus discussions, the single text was modified.

A work group, consisting of 10 members of the Policy Steering Committee and the resource group, was created to facilitate more direct negotiations among the three interest groups. The work group debated, explored solutions, and crafted compromises. The negotiated text reflected problem solving and compromise; it included an implementation strategy with assigned responsibilities, and a timetable for translating the programmatic and planning elements of the agreement into legislation necessary to implement the program. An advisory group of the Policy Steering Committee, assisted by mediators on an as-needed basis, was selected to oversee the city staff's implementation of the program.

Fort Worth I-30 Working Group

The state of Texas proposed to extend an already existing overhead highway from four lanes to eight in Fort Worth. A community group composed of business and citizen interests objected to the proposal on the basis of its unattractive design and its proximity to a park and two historic buildings.

One group opposed the expanded overhead highway and proposed a depressed highway; another group, less concerned about design, urged a rapid completion of the project. The community polarized over solutions to the problem and proceeded into litigation.

An outside mediator was invited to help the community seek a solution to the problem. The first 4 months were spent conducting 30 interviews to gather information about the nature of the conflict, to determine the stakeholders, to educate parties about negotiations, to establish credibility for intervenors, and to encourage the parties to participate in a meeting regarding the conflict. People interviewed included city and state officials and civic leaders who represented different points of view.

A representative group of 14 people was convened in an attempt to find a solution. Their first discussions were confidential in order to begin building trust. The local press cooperated. The first meeting was spent agreeing on ground rules for the process. The group acknowledged that its efforts would be complementary with state and federal regulatory practices. Meetings took place approximately once a month for a year; consensus was used to make decisions. By the fifth meeting, the I-30 Working Group, as it had become known, opened its process to the public. The public and press were invited as observers, and the public could ask questions during breaks and after meetings.

In parallel with the I-30 Working Group, the state hired engineering consultants to develop and examine alternatives, and offered to have the consultants meet with the group for input. The group developed a document listing criteria for the new highway, as well as possible alternatives. Fifteen options replaced the original two. Design engineers studied these recommendations and came back with four alternatives within the range of acceptability. The state held three public meetings to share information and elicit comments. The consensus solutions generated by the I-30 Working Group offered alternatives to the options of an expanded overhead highway or a depressed highway, and received immediate and broad community support. An environmental impact study was conducted to consider the implications of the new design.

Although the Texas State Highway Commission had the authority to make the final decision, the decision was based on the maximum input and understanding from all concerned parties. The I-30 Working Group continued to meet on an as-needed basis.

ISSUES IN PUBLIC DISPUTE MEDIATION

Complex community disputes present the mediator with challenges and responsibilities. The remainder of this chapter examines these. The responsibilities and the issues they raise are divided into three sections:

the prenegotiation stage, the negotiations themselves, and implementation of agreements.

The Prenegotiation Stage

Mediators of complex community disputes play an active role in prenegotiation discussions. A mediator conducts an assessment of a conflict, works with the parties to design a process, and then helps the parties convene the discussions. The mediator can spend several weeks to several months with the parties preparing for a negotiations. More attention paid at this first stage of the process leads to a better negotiation and more satisfying results.

Conducting an Assessment

A mediator will find it valuable to conduct an assessment of a conflict before deciding whether to intervene and what process format to use. Such an assessment will provide information about what the history of the controversy has been, who the major actors are, who has an interest, what solutions have been proposed, and how open parties are to working together to reach agreements.

A few issues that are important to keep in mind when planning an assessment are the questions of who should conduct the interviews, who should be interviewed, and what should be the sequence of interviews. Interviews provide an opportunity to gather information about a conflict and to develop creditibility for the mediator and the process of mediation. The decision as to who should conduct interviews can affect this creditibility; for example, sending a young and inexperienced mediator to interview the president of the largest bank in town or the mayor can be viewed as an insult.

By the same token, who gets interviewed will be watched carefully. Parties will ask mediators whom else they plan to interview. They will be curious as to whether the mediator is getting the full range of views, and will be highly critical if the mediator does not appear to be doing so. Simple matters such as scheduling the interviews can also take on significance if the mediator concentrates on one group first and then proceeds to interview individuals from another interest group later. Mediators must be careful to mix the order of their visits, to be open with people about who is being interviewed, and to enlist the help of parties about who else should be contacted.

Reaching a Common Definition of the Problem

In complex community disputes, parties can have widely differing views of how the conflict should be described. Negotiating a common definition with the parties is an important prenegotiation task. If the issue has already polarized the community, definitions of the problem will look more like solutions. One side will describe the conflict as "How can development be stopped along the waterfront?"; another side will express the issue as "How can development be expedited along the waterfront?" Here the mediator may be able to reframe the issue as "What should be the future of the waterfront?" This definition will allow parties to discuss and integrate their respective interests in regard to development, the timing of change, the character of the community, features that citizens would like to see preserved, and other options to the proposed development.

In a community conflict over the siting of a new solid waste facility, some parties may view the problem as a management issue. They may argue: "If the city's office of solid waste were given more money for professional staff, the city would be able to take care of the problem." Other interests will describe the conflict as an issue of where to site the proposed facility, and still other groups may state the problem as the community's lack of interest in exploring other options to the siting of a new facility. Here a mediator might suggest framing the issue as "What is the best way for the community to handle its solid waste?"

Reaching an agreement about the definition of the conflict is necessary before determining what type of process to use and who should be at the table.

Identifying the Stakeholders and Participants

In most other arenas where mediation is applied, the parties are clearly defined. In complex public disputes, the mediator must work with interest groups to identify who should be represented and in what capacity. During prenegotiation interviews, the mediator asks each person to identify other parties. This includes both those who will be affected by the outcome of a negotiation and those who have the power and desire to influence the implementation. The mediator looks for categories of interests, such as large-scale developers, small-scale developers, historic preservationists, city officials, downtown business owners, and downtown residents. Within each of those categories, the mediator tries to identify who can represent a particular category best. Sometimes a mediator will recommend individuals on the basis of discussions with parties; in other cases, the mediator will ask an interest group to select its own representative. A list of negotiators is developed and checked with groups to ensure that all interests are represented and that each individual is knowledgeable and able to work with the other parties.

Within an organization, the question is often raised whether a senior decision maker with less detailed knowledge of the issues should participate or whether a staff member more technically competent should be the representative. It is best to decide what level is most appropriate and ask each interest group to select someone from that level. If policy-level representatives are selected, the technical experts can then be assigned to sub-groups to research issues and assess options.

Even with careful planning and checking, parties may decide after they have begun their negotiations that new people need to be added, either to fill in a missing interest or to balance other strong interests. Parties will negotiate these additions with the assistance of the mediator.

Designing the Negotiation Process

Most communities have no formal convening system and no standard format for handling complex community conflicts. In such cases, mediators may be asked to design a productive process. A mediator works with the parties to determine what format for discussion lends itself to the problem. The mediator proposes a general format, such as a roundtable discussion with a representative of each major interest at the table, or a negotiation among teams of interests (such as government, business, and citizens). Along with a format, the mediator suggests a sequence of steps that will be modified as a negotiation unfolds. The mediator also considers how to handle technical information, how to involve members of constituency groups and the public, and what a realistic time frame might be.

Educating the Parties about Negotiations

A mediator must also spend time talking with parties about the process of negotiations. Many individuals have no direct experience with the process and may have erroneous impressions of how it works and what it can accomplish. Often parties fear that they will lose power or that they will be overwhelmed by the other interest groups. Consensus decision making raises questions. People may express concerns about the value of working with individuals who have been opposing them in public, and may worry that their group lacks either the financial resources or the access to technical experts that will enable it to participate on an equal basis with other groups. An important function of a mediator is to educate parties about the process of negotiations—how negotiation works, what it can accomplish, and what it cannot.

Who Pays?

A final issue for public dispute mediation is who pays for the time and expenses. Public dispute mediation takes time. Ideally a mediator is in-volved with all three phases of negotiation, beginning with the prenegotia-tion activities, such as interviewing parties and designing and setting up a process. The second phase, the negotiation itself, covers the establishment of ground rules, the identification of issues and interests, the gathering of data, the development of options, and the preparation of agreements. The third phase is the implementation of the agreements, which includes such activities as monitoring the progress of implementation and refining points in the agreement through additional negotiations. Some public disputes can be resolved after a few months of discussions; complex situations can take a year or more. Complex disputes frequently use a team of mediators, along with additional facilitators, technical resource people, and logistical support staff.

Mediators spend most of their time in a negotiation working behind the scenes. After a difficult negotiation session, a mediator often contacts several of the parties to listen to what each individual thought happened at the previous meeting and to solicit suggestions or test ideas about how to proceed. Smaller working groups are often established by negotiators to divide tasks into manageable portions. The responsibilities for coordinating the logistics and content of negotiation sessions and task group meetings, as well as for directing the work of resource people, generally fall on the mediator.

Few mediators can afford to commit the amount of time required to handle a case without compensation, and few community disputes can be negotiated without some financial resources to cover logistics and resource needs. An important issue is that of who pays for the mediator and other expenses associated with the process. Mediators try to give a realistic estimate of what a process will cost, and work with the parties to determine where those funds can be secured. In some communities, parties have been able to get local foundations to support a mediation; in other cases, each party has been asked to contribute according to each one's ability to pay. Sometimes a government agency will offer assistance. Important guidelines in funding are that all parties must understand what resources are required and must agree that the source of the funding is fair.

The Negotiations

During the phase of actual negotiations, the mediator is engaged with the familiar tasks of helping the parties at the table reach agreements about process, identify issues and interests, gather information related to the problem, create options, and reach agreements on substance. In addition, the public dispute mediator spends as much (if not more) time working behind the scenes with individual representatives, with technical consultants, and with task groups, while also coordinating the planning for the next negotiation session.

Dealing with Technical Information

Environmental and other public disputes generally address issues that require knowledge of technical matters. Some parties may have professional training in a technical area, while others have only superficial exposure to it. A mediator works with the parties to determine what information is necessary for all parties to understand an issue, generate options, and reach agreements.

Knowledgeable parties can come to the table with serious disagreements over specific technical information, or they may polarize over the interpretation of new information. The mediator must be prepared to handle these technical disagreements, along with other matters of substance. The mediator generally consults with the parties and then gets the group members to determine whether they want to bring in outside technical support (and, if so, who would be acceptable to all parties), or whether a few people who represent different interests want to work in a smaller task group to clarify their differences and work toward agreements on technical matters.

Working with Different Skill Levels in Negotiating

The mediator must also pay attention to the different levels of skills and styles of negotiation. Often parties who have had extensive negotiation experience are brought together with representatives who have had none. Experienced parties expect certain behaviors and make assumptions about the way other groups respond, which may not be accurate. The mediator can publicly check out assumptions by asking, "When you say that you will leave the negotiation if the other side does not accept your figures, are you prepared to do so and accept the fact that it may not be possible to bring parties together again?" Inexperienced parties may not understand the significance of issuing a threat. Mediators sometimes talk with the parties between sessions about their concerns for the process. Sometimes individuals feel the discussions are moving too slowly, and sometimes they become nervous when they move too quickly. Mediators can explain why discussions are progressing the way they are, in order to avoid any dramatic or damaging moves by one party. Parties can do significant harm to their own cause by not understanding the consequences of their actions. Some mediators have found it useful to offer a training session for all negotiators prior to convening the parties.

Working with Constituents and Keeping Them Informed

If constituents are not kept informed as discussions progress, agreements risk being rejected by unsympathetic constituents. Some participants in a public dispute negotiation understand this point well; for those less familiar with negotiation procedures, it will not be obvious.

Another issue is what role the mediator should have in working with constituents and in keeping them informed. The mediator will need to make explicit the expectation that each representative is responsible for keeping his or her constituents informed throughout the talks. Many interest groups institute regular caucus meetings between negotiation sessions to convey information and to gather opinions from the group. These sessions are critical for the success of the talks. In these caucus sessions, candid discussions occur; new ideas are tried out and disagreements worked out.

Parties may request that a mediator attend a caucus session to help explain the status of the negotiations or to assist the group members in reaching agreements among themselves. Disagreements within a constituency group can be more bitter and intensely waged than those fought across the table with representatives from other interest groups. The mediator must make it clear to all parties that he or she is available to work with any constituency group that requests assistance, and must make explicit what the boundaries of assistance are. Constituency groups will ask for advice on strategy, such as whether they should threaten to leave the table. Rather than provide a direct answer, a mediator can talk about the implications of making such a decision.

Dealing with the Public

A mediator also works with the parties to determine when and how to keep the public informed about the progress of the discussions. Keeping only the parties' constituents informed is not enough to ensure that an agreement will be supported when the time comes for its implementation. If a government decision-making body is involved in a negotiation, a mediator can work closely with the agency to coordinate the timing of appropriate public meetings. If government agencies are not involved, but public support is important, the mediator working with the parties may initiate public meetings to identify general concerns about a controversy and to seek suggestions for ways to resolve the controversy. The mediator may also organize briefings for officials, in which negotiators report on the progress of their discussion and seek guidance from the officials. In some negotiations, community mediators have been responsible for drafting press releases after each session, subject to the approval of the negotiators; in some cases involving lengthy negotiations, they have been requested to send periodic mailings to update interested members of the public.

Working with the News Media

Environmental and other complex community disputes frequently attract media attention. The news media can contribute to the resolution of a conflict through careful, accurate reporting of background information and current discussions, or can be another element that generates yet more confusion and misunderstanding among the parties and the public.

A public dispute mediator must consider how to deal with the media. If an issue has attracted the local press, a mediator may brief the editors and appropriate reporters orally or in writing, about the process and about background information regarding the issue, using language that all parties find acceptable. Not all reporters will choose to use the information, but it is one way a mediator can reduce inaccurate coverage.

The mediator also works with the parties to establish ground rules for dealing with the press. Parties must decide whether they want their sessions to be open or closed to the public and press. Open sessions may be required if elected or appointed officials participate at the table in discussion of public policy. However, discussions in open sessions are generally less candid and less productive than those in closed sessions. If the sessions are to be closed, parties can adopt a ground rule that all parties are free to talk with the press, but each person can only represent himself or herself. Questions regarding another person's opinion must be referred to the source of the comment.

Implementation of Agreements

Mediators are often asked to remain involved through the implementation of agreements. Agreements are complex. They may cut across jurisdictional boundaries and require additional negotiations. Agreements also frequently include different levels of specificity, which continue to be refined by all parties or a select group of them. Mediators can help interest groups continue to work productively.

Determining whether to retain a mediator during the implementation of agreements is a decision that must be made by the parties. Agencies may be willing to take responsibility for tasks, but if they are not careful, their actions can quickly slide into politically motivated decisions rather than the decisions made in the spirit of the agreement. Nothing is more frustrating for negotiators of public disputes than investing their precious time in a negotiation, feeling the satisfaction of reaching an agreement, and then watching their hard-earned efforts evaporate in a few bureacratic decisions. At a minimum, mediators need to help the negotiators structure a process for monitoring the implementation of agreements, and to help them devise a system for making adjustments when necessary.

SUMMARY

Applying the tools of mediation to complex community disputes requires not only a knowledge of mediation, but a familiarity with the technical issues, the political context, and procedures for working with large and small groups. As communities continue to explore the use of mediation as an alternative to protracted public controversies, more lessons will be learned, and the body of knowledge regarding public dispute mediation will become more standardized.

As parties acquire more knowledge and experience with public dispute negotiation, they will gain a greater understanding of the mediator's role and will request mediation services more often. Today's ad hoc efforts to deal productively with differences in a community will evolve into different forms of institutionalized assistance.

REFERENCES

Ashton, C. (1988). *Community problem solving case summaries* (Vol. 1). Washington, DC: Program for Community Problem Solving/ICMA.

Ashton, C. (1989). *Community problem solving case summaries* (Vol. 2). Washington, DC: Program for Community Problem Solving/ICMA.

Carpenter, S. (1989). *Solving problems by consensus*. Washington, DC: Program for Community Problem Solving/ICMA.

Carpenter, S., & Kennedy, W. J. D. (1988). *Managing public disputes: A practical guide to handling conflict and reaching agreements*. San Francisco: Jossey-Bass.

Gray, B. (1989). *Collaborating: Finding common ground for multiparty problems*. San Francisco: Jossey-Bass.

Susskind, L., & Cruikshank, J. (1987). *Breaking the impasse: Consensual approaches to resolving public disputes*. New York: Basic Books.

PART V

OVERVIEW

20

Toward a Synthesis:
The Art with the Science
of Community Mediation

PAUL V. OLCZAK
State University of New York at Geneseo
Family Court Psychiatric Clinic, Buffalo, New York

JAMES W. GROSCH
Colgate University

KAREN GROVER DUFFY
State University of New York at Geneseo

> Researchers think they know how things work, but they don't;
> practitioners don't know how things work, but they do.
>   —Anonymous

Here we are, at the end of the book but not at the end of the story, so to speak. Practitioners and researchers alike have contributed chapters on a wide variety of mediation topics. In this concluding chapter we would like to review briefly the main parts of the book, discuss issues for both sets of readers to consider further, and suggest where we in the field might collectively venture next.

Our intent throughout this book has been to foster a dialogue between two sets of individuals—scientists and practitioners interested in the future of alternative dispute resolution (ADR) techniques, particularly mediation. In Part I, readers have been introduced to general background information on conflict, mediation, applied research, needs assessment, and program promotion. In Part II, the art and the science of the process of mediation have been introduced, with separate chapters on the stages of mediation, the parties, the mediators, and so on.

In Part III, both practitioners and researchers (as in the previous units) have examined issues relevant to both interest groups. Issues raised include resistance to and acceptance of mediation, perceptions of the legal profession, credentialing, and the use of mental health professionals in mediation settings. Finally, Part IV has described possible extensions of ADR techniques to family, school, consumer, victim–offender, and complex political disputes.

Throughout this volume, we hope it has become evident that the means to better service and practice is science, and that the means to more useful science is listening to the needs and concerns of practitioners. But where do we go from here? Let us look first at a few more issues in which both groups in our audience, practitioners and researchers, may be interested. We discuss the practitioner matters first.

PRACTITIONER ISSUES

As several contributors have noted, issues surrounding the practice of mediation have become increasingly complex as the field has become more widely accepted as a legitimate method of dispute resolution. Whereas once a mediator might have been content simply to find disputants willing to participate in a mediation hearing, today both mediators and program coordinators are faced with a wide spectrum of issues that are not always amenable to simple solutions. In this section, we explore further some practitioner issues that have been overlooked or underdeveloped elsewhere in this book.

Inside the Process

Intake

Let us look first at some issues related to intake, the process that generally occurs before mediation commences. At a regional conference, one of us encountered a mediator from the Southwest who was adamant that mediators should be told *nothing* about a case by the intake worker or individual who screens the case before a hearing. He felt that the mediator's neutrality could be violated by any predisclosed information. On the other hand, we know there exist practitioners who feel that any and all available information, including tidbits from the intake interview, enables them to mediate the case better and more expeditiously. Furthermore, there are some programs where at intake, when both parties are present, the intake worker actually conducts a partial mediation via the use of neutrality, turn taking, reality testing, and so on. The parties, then, having been preexposed to the process, do not come into the formal hearing naive or neutral about the process.

Practices related to procedures *before* the hearing vary from center to center, therefore, with little current knowledge as to which practice is best. The only workable solution to selecting the most valuable procedures is to conduct research and let the research guide the practice. Then and only then can practices from center to center be established and perhaps standardized in an intelligent fashion.

Another issue related to intake of cases is the screening of cases for compatibility with mediation. Elsje van Munster, in her chapter on family mediation (Chapter 15), mentions this issue in her section on whether to mediate or not. A closely related concern is whether mediation programs are obligated to attempt mediation with everyone who is referred by another agency or who is self-referred. It occurs to us that some individuals may be in need of a conflict resolution service but may not benefit from mediation, thereby wasting the dollars and time of the mediation service, the taxpayers, and themselves. Such individuals include the alcoholic, the mentally ill, and others who are impaired for one reason or another and simply cannot negotiate in their own best interests. Although some mediation centers have screening policies to prohibit such individuals from "suffering" through the mediation process, other centers do not. Again, it is our feeling that research and sharing of intelligent policies could go a long way toward providing service to those individuals who can most benefit from mediation. The "multi-door" approach mentioned in several of our chapters is another idea that provides the possibility of offering a variety of appropriate but alternative services to individuals whose current situations prevent them from being likely candidates for mediation.

The Choice of a Mediator

Another issue that is internal to mediation, and that concerns program directors, mediators, and even the parties themselves, is the question of who the mediator will be. We have discussed credentialing and mediator effectiveness elsewhere in this volume, but what merits more discussion at this point is the assignment of mediators to cases. Two issues come readily to mind: One is the motivation of mediators; the other is the match between the mediator and the parties.

There exists little research on what specifically motivates mediators. We do know that some mediators are volunteers and that some are paid. There also exist policies about volunteer versus paid mediators, but these policies vary from center to center and are often based more on financial exigencies than on scientific or other less acceptable evidence such as anecdotal evidence.

Research on intrinsically motivated behavior (behavior motivated by personal enjoyment of performing a task, rather than by external rewards) provides an interesting insight into factors that *may* affect mediator motivation. In one noteworthy study, Pearce (1983) compared volunteers and paid employees across a variety of comparable occupations and found that volunteers reported greater job satisfaction and less intent to leave their work. This and related research on intrinsic motivation (e.g., Deci & Ryan, 1985; Staw, 1976) suggests that mediators who enjoy mediating cases might feel less motivated if they were paid for rendering the same service. The reader is reminded that in Chapter 2, Karen Duffy reported the research of

Susan Rogers and her colleagues (Rogers, Kanrich, & Steinhauser, 1989); these authors found that volunteer mediators were motivated to volunteer at the centers for altruistic reasons rather than for pragmatic reasons, and that the primary reason why mediators left service was underutilization. These results nicely fit the intrinsic motivation literature. However, it is unlikely that as public policy mandates more advanced education and fancier degrees for mediators, highly educated professionals will be content to donate their valuable time to ADR forums. We therefore need further research to guide policy decisions, not just about credentialing, but also about payment to and motivation of mediators.

With regard to the matching of mediators to disputants, Peter Carnevale, Linda Putnam, Donald Conlon, and Kathleen O'Connor (Chapter 8), while describing what mediators do that makes them more or less effective, also touch upon the issue of the demographic characteristics of mediators and the influence of those characteristics on the course of mediation. Carnevale and his colleagues found differences in the mediation styles of male and female mediators, but these had no subsequent differences in effectiveness. However, other mediator characteristics (e.g., ethnic identity, cultural background, age, etc.) may have an impact on the effectiveness of the mediator and therefore on the course of mediation. For example, Folberg and Taylor (1984) strongly suggest that socioculturally derived attitudes and perceptions influence mediation both in small ways (such as the punctuality of disputants for hearings) and in much more significant ways (such as the tendency to comply with written or oral agreements and contracts).

Many mediation centers attempt to match demographic characteristics of mediators to those of disputants; mediators are often matched to parties in terms of age, gender, ethnic background, race, and so on. We even know of one juvenile mediation program that uses both a juvenile and an adult mediator when the parties are a juvenile and the juvenile's parent(s). This seems intuitively to be a good idea, but there is little evidence in the mediation literature that matching indeed works. Given that some centers are small and retain only a handful of mediators or mediators who as a group are basically homogeneous, we should all be asking whether we are making a fuss about nothing. Again, the solution to this dilemma is to conduct more research. Only when researchers listen to practitioners, and vice versa, will this question be answered.

External Issues

Credentialing

We look now at some other issues that, while important to practitioners, are often influenced as much by outsiders as by insiders to the mediation centers. One such issue raised earlier in the book is credentialing. As the issue of credentialing mediators continues to be debated, it is important for practitioners to be aware of the complexity of the issue and to take an active role in setting guidelines for ensuring quality control within the field. We feel that research can play a vital role here, too. We already have some research on mediator effectiveness (see Part II of this book), but more is needed. This research is important, in that beyond the credentialing issue is the issue of mediator effectiveness. The fact that someone is a certified mediator does not mean that he or she is necessarily competent or effective. Like Albie Davis (see Chapter 13), we too are concerned about credentialing mediators, and maintaining quality control through continuing education, recertification, and so on. Of course, as ever, we feel that research can play a valuable role.

Ethical Dilemmas

Another issue of growing concern, and one seemingly controlled by outsiders as well as insiders to the mediation process, involves the ethical dilemmas a mediator may face. Since the role of a mediator is typically much different from that of a lawyer or judge, the proper code of conduct for a mediator is sometimes not clear. For example, what responsibility does a mediator have to the disputants if he or she is subpoenaed in connection with a dispute that later ends up in court? Also, what kinds of information disclosed by a party during a private caucus is a mediator obligated to reveal? Although some states have laws that provide guidance in resolving such questions, there remain many gray areas where the proper course of action may, in effect, be left up to the mediator or program director.

Several interesting documents exist on ethical and other standards for mediation services. One comprehensive document is a comparative analysis of mediation standards, performed by the Crime and Justice Foundation for the Office of the Chief Administrative Justice of Massachusetts (Adrian & Brophy, 1989). In this document, in which 18 separate sets of guidelines were studied, there were more than 500 individual standards embracing more than 60 subject areas. The examiners concluded that guidelines differed in their focus according to the originators of the standards. Legislatures and courts addressed pragmatic issues, for example, whereas professional associations focused on professional conduct. Moreover, the standards varied greatly in organization and subject areas, and identical issues were often addressed differently. The only issue covered in all guidelines was that of confidentiality. This mishmash of guidelines is disconcerting to us and probably to most professionals in the field as well. Again, only through insightful research and cooperation among professionals in the field will we know which standards are best and are workable and which should be discarded.

Increasing General Awareness of Mediation

Yet another relevant issue that practitioners must be aware of is the continuing need to educate the public, judges, and others about the process of mediation, to ensure that mediation does not become a "dumping ground" for cases unwanted by an overburdened judicial system or other human service agencies. The "multi-door" concept discussed by Melinda Ostermeyer (Chapter 6) and Larry Ray (Chapter 12) is a particularly attractive approach, in that it allows the parties to have some input into the type of dispute resolution method in which they participate. Research in social psychology, beginning with Brehm (1966), has repeatedly found that people are more likely to accept an alternative when they are given some degree of choice in its selection. In the multi-door approach, mediation also becomes one of many alternatives (instead of a mandatory requirement) and is used when it seems most appropriate to the characteristics of a given dispute. This recognizes the fact that mediation works better for some types of conflicts than for others (Lempert & Sanders, 1986; McFadgen, 1972). Part of the philosophy of mediation is empowerment of the participants. Therefore, mediators should buy into the multi-door approach, which sometimes empowers the parties to opt for other ADR techniques or for court. These other options, though, will compete for cases with the mediation centers.

In terms of increasing public awareness of mediation, Ellen Cohn and Mae Lynn Neyhart (Chapter 11) have described many of the factors that may serve as obstacles to widespread public awareness. Clearly, practitioners and program coordinators need to be aware of issues related to marketing their services (see Hicks, Rosenthal, & Standish, Chapter 5) and doing a needs assessment (see Folger, Chapter 4) to make sure that a mediation program is needed in the first place. Program managers also need to be able to demonstrate the effectiveness of their programs (an issue discussed below and by Wong, Blakely, & Worsham, Chapter 3) in order to obtain continued support and external funding. Practitioners and researchers need to work conjointly to lobby legislators and other public policy formulators for continued and increased funding, both for the mediation programs and for the research related to the programs and the process of mediation. By presenting a united, well-reasoned, and well-documented front to lawmakers and funders, mediation can attain the regard and use we feel it so deserves.

Although public policy formulators are usually neither practitioners nor researchers, most are trained in law, an area psychologically adjacent and akin to mediation; therefore, mediation experts may have an easier time of attracting legislators' attention than other lobbyists may. And lest any mediation professionals, researchers or practitioners, become discouraged, there is evidence that public policy makers do utilize social science research results to guide their policy and funding decisions (Beyer & Trice, 1982; Caplan, Morrison, & Stambaugh, 1975). Again, we could not possibly agree more with others (e.g., Miller, 1986) who state that legislation can go a long way in advancing the practice and the science of community mediation.

Expanding Mediation Services to Other Forums

One final practitioner issue is the expansion of mediation services to other forums. In Part IV of this book, we have examined settings into which mediation services have expanded in the past, such as family, school, consumer, and environmental and other political disputes, as well as victim–offender reconciliation. In the future, we see mediation services being extended to and accepted in other places. Where? For one, there is currently an interest in offering mediation services on college campuses. A recent conference (Warters, 1990) held on the campus of Syracuse University was designed specifically to demonstrate to institutions of higher education how to establish, promote, maintain, and use a mediation program on a college campus. An incomplete list of colleges and universities currently providing some type of dispute resolution service was developed at this conference and came to 24 campuses, some of which are highly prestigious institutions. Campus mediation programs offer the promise of alternative means to settle roommate, disciplinary, academic, interpersonal, and other disputes that arise. Such campus centers also offer the exciting possibility of built-in research laboratories for scientists interested in conflict resolution.

We also feel that as society becomes more complex, technological, and crowded, there will be an increased call for alternative means for the settlement of public and/or public policy disputes. Susan Carpenter mentions in Chapter 19 the use of mediation for a highway expansion dispute and for a dispute between groups interested in historic preservation versus economic expansion of a city. We see also the possibility of the use of neutral third parties in disputes involving the siting of housing projects, factories, landfills, and so on, as well as in many other disputes where the public will insist on being involved. We also feel that this market may develop so fast that it will quickly exceed the present capacity of mediation, given the scant number of mediators currently trained to manage such large-scale conflicts.

As the world economy and politics change (and who has not witnessed the rapid, recent changes in Eastern Europe or the continual discontent and upheaval in the Middle East?), there will be a call for mediators well versed in "shuttle diplomacy"—individuals who know and can manage the customs, culture, politics, and history of diverse but conflicting countries. One of us returned from a trip to the Soviet Union in August of 1990, where after polite, obligatory introductions followed the question, "What do you think about the reunification of Germany?" It became quickly apparent that the Soviets' history with the Germans was more intense and personalized than Americans' histories, and that Americans and Soviets (not to mention other countries) might have different views regarding the reunification or extent thereof of the two Germanies. Likewise, in the summer of 1990, the invasion of Kuwait by Iraq was a prime opportunity to utilize some neutral intermediaries to assist in settling what at this writing appears to be turning into a global dispute. Who would ever mediate such large-scale disputes, given that there are few Henry Kissingers (Rubin, 1981) in the world? We believe that there is a need for such people, but few individuals can fill this bill.

The solution we offer, although perhaps somewhat idealistic, is to provide training to prepare for the need we predict will exist in both the public policy and international arenas. Experienced mediators in these forums will need to make themselves available to conduct the training of neophytes. As Carpenter (Chapter 19) maintains, these large-scale conflicts necessitate mediation skills beyond those learned at neighborhood dispute resolution centers.

There is one other setting in which we feel mediation will play an ever-expanding role: the area of labor relations. We are aware that most union contracts provide for *arbitration,* but as a *last* step, especially in contract and disciplinary grievances. We are cognizant of the fact that mediation is used in the labor relations arena (typically in impasses during contract negotiation), but there seems to be an assumption that most other labor management disputes are unsolvable or too difficult for mediation. We see a place for mediation at the *beginning* of more labor–management disputes—in contract and disciplinary grievances, as well as in areas where labor and management have agreed to work together (e.g., a jointly sponsored drug and alcohol awareness and rehabilitation program) but in reality are disagreeing about implementation, costs, and the like. Again, this is an exciting possibility for mediation services.

RESEARCHER ISSUES

We now examine some final research-related matters. First, we feel that while this book has highlighted much valuable research, the research that exists needs to be replicated and refined. Likewise, we also feel that much research has yet to be completed (e.g., see Kressel, Pruitt, & Associates, 1989). The preceding section on practitioner issues elaborates on some of the areas where research needs to be conducted. However, in this section we continue the discussion of what research might be conducted, as well as explore some other issues related to research.

"Does mediation work?" seems to be a reasonable question that may be asked by practitioners and researchers alike. Practitioners may answer quickly, "Well, of course," but often this response is based only on their own experiences or the observations or verbal assurances of several others. Practitioners of mediation have no doubt observed their own work, reflected on it, and discussed it with others; perhaps they have even reported a particular mediation proceeding at an in-service session, or attempted to tally and keep track of successes and failures in some fairly simple, uncontrolled fashion.

On the other hand, researchers may also answer the question in the affirmative, but with some skepticism, as they await more compelling evidence on mediation's efficacy before becoming true proselytes. In our efforts at fostering a meaningful dialogue between these two groups, we attempt to address several questions regarding effectiveness from both perspectives.

Program Evaluation

First is the question of program evaluation: Is our neighborhood justice center or local center for dispute resolution working? As discussed earlier by Wong et al. (Chapter 3), applied research techniques have much to offer practitioners and researchers alike. Frequently programs of this type, struggling simply to survive or to justify their future existence, attempt to track and report what Bloom (1972) calls "program descriptions" rather than to perform true program evaluations. Included here would be the maintenance of various descriptive statistics (e.g., averages) by project staff, such as who uses the service, caseloads, and the like. Unfortunately, popularity of some option or program is not a guarantee of its quality. To claim that a program is successful requires that relevant target behaviors be changed by the program. The hypothetical example provided in Chapter 3 by Wong et al. suggests a typical question: "Does our mediation program reduce juvenile delinquency in our town?" To answer such a question requires that we go well beyond simply a description of our program, or who uses it, toward a program evaluation aimed at providing a more definitive answer to the question. For example, since the initiation of a peer mediation program throughout the school district last year, has there been a significant reduction in acts of vandalism within the community?

According to Bloom (1972), a viable program evaluation involves four major steps. First, one must specify the objectives of the program. Second, one must define relevant parameters (e.g., who the target population is, how delinquency will be measured, etc.). Third, one must specify what techniques will be used to attain these objectives. And finally, one must decide who will collect what information or data on the above-stated objectives.

Too often, however, project staff members become overworked by huge caseloads and other vagaries in the lives of mediators or program directors to maintain some "idealized" measures drawn up by researchers at the local university. On the other hand, researchers clamor for greater objectivity in the measures, as well as more of them, to answer pertinent questions.

It is here that increased dialogue can benefit both groups. Each side needs to be sensitive to the fact that program evaluation is most effective if it is made an integral part of a service program at the outset, and not simply "thrown in" later, as is too often the case (Korchin, 1976). Thus, what is necessary from the beginning is a program director or mediator who is sensitive to the researcher and data collection issues, as well as a researcher who is sympathetic to the aims of the program and compatible with the staff members and their everyday problems in running their program. As Korchin (1976) states:

> Tension between research and service staff, mutual misunderstandings of purposes and ways of thinking, and the like have undercut many evaluation projects. While each has his area of expertise, mutual respect and basic understanding are necessary. (p. 568)

Evaluation of Outcome versus Process

In trying to answer the question of "Does our mediation program work?", a number of other issues are immediately of concern. Do we simply want to assess the outcome of the mediation, or are issues related to understanding the process critical?

In clinical psychology—specifically, in the area of psychotherapy—increasing attention is being given to this distinction (e.g., see Bergin & Strupp, 1972). First, researchers have moved from a focus on outcome ("Did it work?") to a concern with the process ("What goes on between the therapist and patient?"). Second, this apparent change has resulted in a conceptual shift, in that greater attention is now being given to the myriad of complex interactions occurring among the therapist, the patient or client, and interrelational and situational variables, as they affect the therapeutic outcome (Korchin, 1976). Perhaps something similar is true of mediation as well. In the area of mediation, McGillis (1986) has noted that assessment of the impact of any community dispute resolution program is a complex issue, because of problems inherent in the measurement of such outcomes as the "quality of justice" delivered, "case-processing efficiency and costs," and "access to justice."

For years, research in the area of psychotherapy was hampered by what Donald Kiesler (1966) called the "uniformity assumption myth," or the belief that all patients, therapists, and treatments are homogeneous or somehow alike. Thus, researchers (and perhaps the public as well) tried to answer what is now considered an unanswerable question: "Does therapy work?" From the perspective of the uniformity assumption myth, asking "Does mediation work?" is perhaps akin to asking "Does therapy work?"—or else asking "Is higher education effective?" without specifying a particular university or the particular participants (both faculty and students) involved (e.g., see Hyman & Breger, 1965; McGillis, 1986).

Thus in the practice and evaluation of mediation, as in the practice and evaluation of psychotherapy, there has been a movement toward greater awareness and recognition of the complex interactions possible between the participants (e.g., mediator and disputants), as well as the style and/or tactics used by the mediator, type of case heard, and so on (e.g., see Kressel et al., 1989). Today, dialogue between the researcher and practitioner has led to the formulation of a much more sophisticated but accurate question: "What type of mediator, for what type of disputants, using what kinds of tactics, for what type of case, leads to what outcome?"

For example, recent research by Peter Carnevale and his colleagues (see Chapter 8) using this kind of contingency analysis has shed some valuable light on the complexities of mediation that may be involved in producing successful or unsuccessful outcomes. Their results clearly indicate that success in mediation may be much more complex than simply assessing "agreement." This result has profound implications for both practitioners and researchers in the field of mediation (see Lim & Carnevale, 1990).

Interaction between Researchers and Practitioners

Practitioners in a variety of fields, including perhaps mediation, have long viewed research as being irrelevant or not very useful to professional practice (e.g., Luborsky, 1972; Strupp, 1989). There is increasing evidence, however, to indicate that productive dialogue and continued interaction between practitioners and researchers can lead to empirically established findings with practical value for the practitioners (e.g., see Welton, Chapter 7; Carnevale et al., Chapter 8; McGillicuddy, Pruitt, Welton, Zubek, & Peirce, Chapter 9; and Olczak, Chapter 10).

Polarization or a lack of interaction between these two sides can only be destructive to both. The reasonable practice of mediation requires mediators to keep abreast of the latest usable research findings, whereas doing relevant research often demands that researchers "fine-tune" their skills and even the questions asked by participating in the process. Research by Dean Pruitt and his colleagues (see Chapter 9) perhaps has been an example of this ongoing dialogue, in that much of it has been conceptualized and carried out in the field by investigators who also periodically serve as mediators. We believe that much more of this type of collaboration or symbiosis is needed in the future. Interaction of this type also has far-reaching implications for the future practice and regulation of mediation, including degree of professionalization, training, licensure, continuing education, competency-based evaluation, and so forth (see Davis, Chapter 13).

If the practice of mediation meets the requirements often thought to delineate or define a "profession," then issues of education and training become paramount. Most professions view education and training as a lifelong process. Physicians are required to keep abreast of the latest developments in their field, as are attorneys. Mediators then must also continually read journals or other significant and relevant publications to remain on the cutting edge of their field. A failure to keep abreast of the latest developments in the field that researchers have found to be effective will lead to an inferior brand of practice, particularly if the complexities of mediation are amenable to scientific study—a position we obviously support.

Finally, practitioners and researchers can benefit from continued interaction by attending any one of a number of regional, national, or international meetings on mediation and other ADR forums. Here, participants not only share ideas and exchange information informally, but interact in various symposia, workshops, seminars, and demonstrations. These interactions then continue to fuel the process, leading both to improved or continued high-level practice and to better and more meaningful research. In fact, it was a joint conference of New York mediators and researchers that inspired this book!

RETROSPECTS AND PROSPECTS

We feel we have demonstrated the need for continual dialogue between practitioners and researchers, especially since the research in mediation needs to catch up with the practice, as Kressel et al. (1989) have concluded. Collaboration is the best means to ensure both high-quality service and research designed to serve the community. Collaboration is also the key to presenting a united front to outsiders such as public policy makers and funders. As the economy shifts and more attention is focused on the justice system, we predict that these outsiders will become more important than ever in determining the direction of the mediation field.

Another benefit of collaboration between researchers and practitioners in the area of mediation is that it produces a system of checks and balances. For example, researchers can scrutinize the practices in the field to ensure that they are scientifically sound and efficacious. Similarly, practitioners can monitor research to ensure that the research not only is applicable but improves practice. Too often in other fields, such as the social sciences, "the oft-proclaimed 'publish or perish' syndrome in the academic-research establishment" (Phares, 1988, p. 31) drives the research. In defense of researchers in the mediation field, we believe that most research already completed is meant to advance knowledge in the field rather than simply to advance an individual's career. We are confident that this trend of advancing the discipline will continue, because many researchers are becoming practitioners—a strategy we applaud.

We also understand that collaboration within a discipline or between disciplines can be troublesome. Because of the collaboration that has already occurred in the mediation field, the intellectual underpinnings of and contributions to mediation have been extremely diverse. For example, the authors of this book represent the areas of law, government, social psychology, management science, public policy, counseling, and education. While we encourage pluralism, we also encourage the sharing of information *across* disciplines to prevent fragmentation in the research and stagnation in the field.

Another consequence of collaboration can be conflict among collaborators. We have observed recent conflicts both *within* disciplines (psychology, as represented by the American Psychological Association [APA]) and *between* disciplines (clinical psychology vs. psychiatry). In terms of conflict within a discipline, the APA was established for *all* psychologists, many of whom are practitioners (e.g., counseling psychologists) or academics/researchers (e.g., physiological psychologists); however, a noticeable rift has recently developed in APA between these two groups. The disputes range from the timing of the national convention ("too close to the beginning of the school year," say the academics) to more basic questions regarding the primary role of the national organization or the definition or direction of contemporary psychology. As for conflict between disciplines, there exists an ongoing controversy between the disciplines of clinical psychology and psychiatry. For instance, at issue are the dispensing of medications (long the exclusive turf of psychiatrists only), hospital admission privileges, provision of expert testimony at disability hearings and criminal trials, and inclusion in national health insurance.

"Growing pains" in any field are to be expected, and they have indeed occurred in the field of mediation. During the next decade, many new challenges face mediation practitioners and researchers. By the year 2000, it will be interesting to see how the following questions may be answered:

- Will the phenomenal growth of mediation continue (perhaps as the courts become overburdened by drug cases), or, as McGillis (1986) conjectures, will it start to wane?
- How will the issue of credentialing be resolved? That is, will mediation become a profession with rigorous licensing and certification standards, or will it remain a trainable, learning-based skill, open to almost anyone with the necessary motivation and interpersonal skills?
- Will the high user satisfaction rates found in today's research actually translate tomorrow into a better quality of justice?
- Will mediation practices across the nation become more standardized as research reveals which practices yield better outcomes?
- Will programs see more walk-in clients than court referrals as word spreads about mediation? If so, will such volitional participation enhance the benefits of mediation beyond those we already know?
- Into which markets will mediation expand, and for which of these areas will it prove most useful?

• How will justice system innovations, such as the multi-door concept, affect mediation's use and acceptability?

Despite these and other unanswered questions, we hold great hope that professionals interested in conflict resolution will not fall into conflict themselves, but rather will cooperate harmoniously to advance the goals of their profession.

REFERENCES

Adrian, A. L., & Brophy, C. (1989). *Comparative analysis of mediation standards.* Boston: Crime and Justice Foundation.

Bergin, A. E., & Strupp, H. H. (Eds.). (1972). *Changing frontiers in the science of psychotherapy.* Chicago: Aldine-Atherton.

Beyer, J. M., & Trice, H. M. (1982). The utilization process: A conceptual framework and synthesis of empirical findings. *Administrative Science Quarterly, 27,* 591–622.

Bloom, B. L. (1972). Mental health program evaluation. In S. E. Golann & C. Eisdorfer (Eds.), *Handbook of community mental health.* New York: Appleton-Century-Crofts.

Brehm, J. W. (1966). *A theory of psychological reactance.* New York: Academic Press.

Caplan, N., Morrison, A., & Stambaugh, R. J. (1975). *The use of social science knowledge in policy decisions at the national level: A report to respondents.* Ann Arbor: Institute for Social Science Research, University of Michigan.

Deci, E. L., & Ryan, R. M. (1985). *Intrinsic motivation and self-determination in human behavior.* New York: Plenum.

Folberg, J., & Taylor, A. (1984). *Mediation: A comprehensive guide to resolving conflicts without litigation.* San Francisco: Jossey-Bass.

Hyman, R., & Breger, L. (1965). Discussion of H. J. Eysenck, "The effects of psychotherapy." *International Journal of Psychiatry, 1,* 317–322.

Kiesler, D. J. (1966). Some myths of psychotherapy research and the search for a paradigm. *Psychological Bulletin, 65,* 110–136.

Korchin, S. J. (1976). *Modern clinical psychology.* New York: Basic Books.

Kressel, K., Pruitt, D. G., & Associates. (Eds.). (1989). *Mediation research: The process and effectiveness of third party interventions.* San Francisco: Jossey-Bass.

Lempert, R., & Sanders, J. (1986). *An invitation to law and social science.* New York: Longman Press.

Lim, R., G., & Carnevale, P. J. (1990). Contingencies in the mediation of disputes. *Journal of Personality and Social Psychology, 58,* 259–272.

Luborsky, L. (1972). Research cannot yet influence clinical practice. In A. E. Bergin & H. H. Strupp (Eds.), *Changing frontiers in the science of psychotherapy.* Chicago: Aldine-Atherton.

McFadgen, T. (1972). *Dispute resolution in the small claims context: Adjudication, arbitration, or conciliation?* Unpublished master's thesis, Harvard University Law School.

McGillis, D. (1986). *Community dispute resolution programs and public policy.* Washington, DC: National Institute of Justice.

Miller, R. A. (1986). Crossing the legislative barrier: State legislation and the implementation of alternative methods of dispute resolution. In J. E. Palenski & H. M. Launer (Eds.), *Mediation: Contexts and challenges.* Springfield, IL: Charles C Thomas.

Pearce, J. L. (1983). Job attitude and motivation differences between volunteers and employees from comparable organizations. *Journal of Applied Psychology, 68,* 646–652.

Phares, E. J. (1988). *Introduction to personality.* Glenview, IL: Scott, Foresman.

Rogers, S. J., Kanrich, S., & Steinhauser, I. (1989). *Understanding our criminal justice volunteers: A Study of community mediators in New York State.* New York: Brooklyn Mediation Center.

Rubin, J. Z. (1981). *Dynamics of third party intervention: Kissinger and the Middle East.* New York: Praeger.

Staw, B. M. (1976). *Intrinsic and extrinsic motivation.* Morristown, NJ: General Learning Press.

Strupp, H. H. (1989). Psychotherapy: Can the practitioner learn from the researcher? *American Psychologist, 44,* 717–724.

Warters, W. (1990). *First national conference on campus mediation programs.* Syracuse, NY: Campus Mediation Center, Syracuse University.

Index